# About This Book

First off, I'd like to congratulate you on embarking on this journey of educational enlightenment. To come to the realization that you want to be among the best in your field truly carries with it a daunting task. Fortunately, it comes with great reward. You obviously have made the decision to prepare for a difficult critical care certification exam, but once you pass you will have validated yourself as an entry level practitioner for a multitude of critical care roles. I'm excited for your desire and potential.

This book is designed around a progression of content delivery. The first section and largest is the resource and reference material. Here, I explain and test you on all the concepts used in critical care transport. The test questions are specific to the certification exams you will be studying for, but the material is all encompassing. The reason for this is that I'd like you to be ready for both the certification exam you are preparing for as well as the proverbial "medical jungle" you are about to dive into.

The second section is a series of case studies with questions, explanations, focus points, and topics within the text to review for further study. The case study section helps you apply the knowledge you've learned and/ or reviewed. Lastly, in section 3, I have provided QuickLook Sheets for you to study the last few days before an exam. These QuickLook Sheets contain small memory joggers to help with cognitive recall the day of, or day before, an exam to ensure there are no weak spots in your knowledge base. Use these sections in tandem: learn the content (section 1), apply and practice the content (section 2), hit some valuable last-minute reviews (section 3), and then pass the exam.

I dubbed this study progression the Triple Threat because of the three sections of progressive learning and understanding. You can't just study the QuickLook Sheets and be able to recall fine details of a topic unless you are already intimate with the resource material. However, by studying them all in tandem, you will be well-prepared come test day. My hope is that this becomes an industry standard-setting resource, but ideally, I just want you to pass. However, I do not plan to stop there. We want our students to pass difficult certification exams with ease, and to stay sharp as they progress through their career. We will offer a very affordable subscription service that will bring case studies and critical care puzzles and challenges for you to continue to apply your knowledge, broadening you medical knowledge and skill over time.

Are you ready for this?! I am, and I promise to give you my all to help you pass your exam(s).

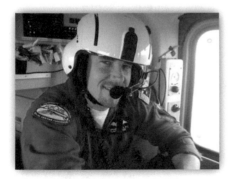

# How to Use This Book

This book is divided into 3 sections and is intended for you to use as a study guide or as a desk reference.

Section 1 is an in-depth review of the material. This section is broken into 14 different chapters. Each chapter will have three or more parts covering pertinent critical care topics. At the end of each chapter, there are sample exam questions with answer rationales.

Section 2 is a selection of 20 case studies that you should use to practice what you learned in section 1. These have been peer reviewed from experts in the field to ensure you are engaging in a quality educational experience.

Section 3 is only a few pages long, and is broken into 14 components, one from each chapter. In each chapter component will be short fact blurbs that are designed to jog your memory for a particular topic or concept. The idea is to provide you a review of the entire chapter in less than a page.

These three sections, when taken and exercised in tandem, funnel a student's study effort from initial review, to focused practice, and finally provides a bird's eye view of the entire scope of the material. In all my educational endeavors, I have yet to find a book like my Triple Threat study system I created to study for the FP-C in 2004.

Additionally, throughout this text are QR codes. These are square, geometrical pictures which are like barcodes in that they direct you to information. In the case of this text, they guide you to an audio or video file. To listen, you'll need a QR code reader– download one for free on your smart phone. There will be multiple locations throughout the text where I will interact with you by explaining concepts or demonstrating a skill or calculation.

BOTTOM LINE: study, practice, review and then go crush your exam. It seems simple, right? Well, it is. If you put in the time to understand and practice these concepts, you will be successful. So, let's punch the clock and get to work!

# Acknowledgements

To say that I have accomplished anything on my own would be a farce. Many thanks to the following professionals that influenced me as I progressed through my career.

**Clyde Deschamp**: Clyde, you were my first educator in this field. I was lucky to have had you because of the professional skill and integrity you exercise as an educational leader. IT would have been very cool to have flown with you at some point, and I am grateful you are at my side through this endeavor. Thanks for always being welcoming and encouraging.

**Kevin King**: You were my first mentor in this exciting field. I appreciate your continued hunger for EMS knowledge and emergency medicine. You were always eager for the next call that would really challenge you, and I was highly influenced by this behavior and mindset. You were the first amongst a family of clinicians who convinced me that "good" wasn't enough because there was always something you could do or study that made you a little bit better. Thank you for your mentorship and friendship.

**Donna Norris**: I remember you telling me I was hired at AirCare due to of a "lack of options", despite this mystery, you gave me a chance. You wrote the book on how to lead and how to care for your employees at the same time. Still to this day, I work hard to not let you down.

**Mark Randall**: You always had a capacity to be yourself (a good ol' southern boy) and a medical genius all at the same time. You were one of the few who influenced me to constantly sharpen my skills and knowledge base. From you I learned that reaching my best wasn't attainable; rather it is a virtue that would take a career to achieve.

**Bill Bailey**: I still refer to you in stories as my partner. I undoubtedly will have great partners in the future, but none like you. You were my confidant and my friend. You challenged and trusted me at the same time and made me feel that my contribution truly mattered. You are flat out just a good person with a big heart. That is something we need more of in the world. Thank you for always being there for me.

**Dan Turner**: if I had to describe a word that conveyed and embodied what I learned from you, that word would be professionalism. It was important to you that not only were you professional, but other people perceived it. You taught me the importance of stopping, letting the family touch and talk to the patient before departure, and to make sure they knew what was going on before we left. It is a practice that I, still to the day, am occasionally complimented on, and it makes me proud to continue this practice. Thanks for always making me better.

**Leaugeay Barnes**: You taught me how to run a program. I use skills that I learned from you in my daily work life and can attribute that to your influence. I always appreciated how you always strived for the next rung on the achievement ladder. You're always looking for the next big project, and I always try to follow in your footsteps. You were my friend through a very tough time in my life, and provided me with tough love, and guidance. Thank you for that.

**Harvey Conner**: You, sir, always hold scholastic lamp high for everyone to see and to guide the way. You have positively impacted so many clinicians in Oklahoma and the world. I have made it my mission to do the same.

**Brent Stafford**: Thank you for being a friend of mine and mentor during a very difficult transition in my life. I can always have a laugh with you. I appreciate how you always knew how to take a complicated situation, simplify it, and then serve it with a slice of poignant advice. I wish there were more people like that in the world. Thanks for always being that guy for me.

**Justin Hunter**: Sit down, because this is the last time I will be this nice to you. You always impressed me with your ideas to make the EMS world, along with the communities it serves, a better place. You're not only an idea guy, but you also follow through on the tiniest of details for every plan you conceive, and you never miss a single detail. Thanks for influencing me to be more like that. Let's hang out sometime soon.

**Cub Bercier**: I was terrified when I was considering leaving Mississippi and AirCare to move to Oklahoma to train with team USA. I randomly called an Oklahoma based air medical base and you were the one who answered. You kindly listened to my concerns and gave me sound and solid advice. Years later, when I met you in person you extended that same kindness along with an incredible grasp of emergency medicine. Thank you for being a mentor of mine while in Oklahoma as well as for my new life in Denver. You are absolutely the man.

**Kevin Ring**: Kevin, thank you defining what cool really is in the EMS world, and for introducing me to Hendricks Gin. You're "take shit from no one attitude" paired with your uncanny ability to detect bullshit is why I'm a big fan of yours. We need that in this field.

**Dr. Patrick Cody**: Doc, thanks for the consistent feedback during this project. You married being positive with being direct; a feat I am sure is difficult to accomplish. Without you, this project would not have been accurate and thorough. I appreciate all the emails, printing and editing files late at night when the ER was quiet, and again– the solid advice you gave me throughout this endeavor. It has been an honor to learn from you.

**Dr. Randall Herrin**: Ok, I have decided that being sappy just doesn't match how our friendship functions. I will thank you for all the assistance and encouragement you have given me during all the late night beer summits, early morning brunches with the girls, excursions to NOLA, NYE debauchery, shifts at the ER, and last, but certainly not least, nights at a great bar with an ever better scotch. Basically, our entire friendship revolves around us challenging the world and alcohol– and I completely dig it. Looking forward to a drinking/ sushi hang out session soon. Thanks for your friendship, advice, and encouragement.

**Enrique Murguia**: Enrique, I did not know you when I first started this project. It is important that I mention that you have influenced me significantly in multiple decisions throughout my time at Mediflight. Honestly, you are the catalyst to where I am today. You have always offered solid and poignant advice, and you knew when to give me a little nudge when I needed it. Thank you for positively influencing me in so many ways.

**David Olvera**: My man. Thanks for always helping me stay afloat, and to remind me when I had missed something. You helped me usher in a new era of my life– both professionally and personally. Thanks for being there so often. We are going to crush the critical care transport research world.

**Allen Wolfe**: Thanks for always pushing me to be better than I was yesterday. I'm influenced by your fantastic attitude with respect to your field and your passion for taking care of others paired with an unbelievable grasp of critical care. Well, that and all the sass you spread around. I enjoyed working in an environment where I am constantly challenged, yet there is so much laughter. Thanks for believing in me.

**Mom and Dad**: While I will never understand the decisions you had to make in the fall of 1977, I can truly say that I never felt disabled. Thank you for making it important to teach me how to interact with the world with what I was given. Thank you for omitting the word failure out of the English language while raising me. It's that mindset and your love that helped fuel by desire to want to make the world a better place, and I love doing it by taking care of other people as well as showing others how to take care of sick and injured people. I love you, both. Thank you.

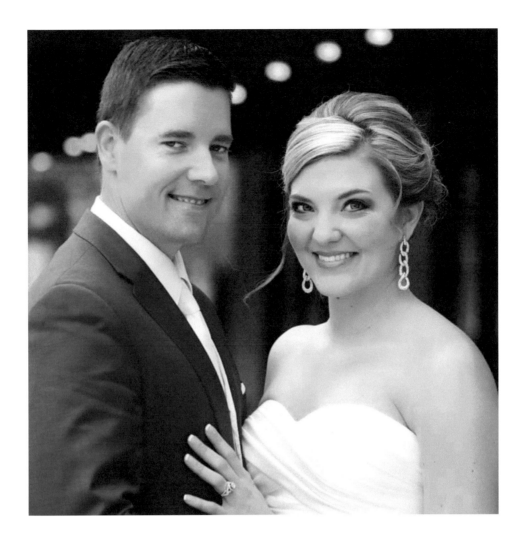

**To My Marge:**

You've sacrificed hours and hours of time allowing me to work on this project.  I hope with everything in my heart that I was able to show you thanks enough during that time.  I plan on spending a lifetime showing you just how special you are to me.  For anything that I accomplish, please know that it would not have been possible without your love, support, and your friendship.  My world is a paradise, and it is because you are in it.

I want to say thank you for always supporting my ideas and desires, because you truly helped me accomplish these goals. And as I said the day we were married in a toast to our closest friends and family playing off my USA Volleyball involvement,

"I came to Oklahoma looking for a gold medal. I found her. Marge, you are my gold medal. You are my World Record. Winning your love was, is, and will forever remain my greatest accomplishment."


Lovingly yours,

Charlie

# Editing and Reviewing Team

**Patrick Cody, DO**

*Emergency Physician, Norman Regional Hospital*

*Medical Director, EMSStat*

*Norman, OK*


**Clyde Deschamp, PhD, NRP, FP-C, CFRN**

*Flight Nurse, AirCare*

*University of Mississippi Health Care*

*Jackson, MS*


**Josh James, NRP, FP-C**

*Flight Paramedic, Memorial Herman Lifeflight*

*Houston, TX*


**Mark Galtelli, NRP, FPC**

*Flight Paramedic,*

*Critical Care Educator, Holmes Community College*

*Madison, MS*


**Parker Martin, PA-C, NRP, FPC**

*Physician Assistant, Flight Paramedic*

*Oklahoma City, OK*


**Sam Marshall, NRP, FP-C**

*Flight Paramedic, AirCare*

*University of Mississippi Health Care*

*Jackson, MS*


**Iain Holmes, RN, MSN, EMT**

*Flight Nurse, Lifenet of New York*

*Saratoga Springs, NY*

**Alex Black, MD**

*Emergency Physician, Parkland Medical Center*

*Dallas, TX*


**Justin Hunter MS, NRP, FP-C**

*Program Director, Oklahoma State Univ.– OKC*

*Paramedic, EMSStat*

*Oklahoma City, OK*


**Kevin King, RN, NRP, FP-C, CFRN**

*Flight Nurse, AirCare*

*University of Mississippi Health Care*

*Jackson, MS*


**Randall Herrin, MD**

*Chief of Emergency Medicine, Oklahoma University*

*Edmond, OK*


**Mark Randall, RN, NRP, CFRN**

*Flight Nurse, AirCare*

*University of Mississippi Health Care*

*Jackson, MS*


**Kyle Hurley, MS, NRP**

*Paramedic, EMSStat*

*Norman, OK*


**Brent Stafford, BS, NRP**

*Faculty Instructor, Oklahoma City Community College*

*Oklahoma City, OK*

# Table of Contents

# SECTION 3: DUMP SHEETS & MORE     392

# APPENDICIES A-E     429

# SECTION 1

## RESOURCE MATERIAL

# CHAPTER 1: AIRWAY MANAGMENT

## PART 1: AIRWAY MANAGEMENT BASICS

### INSPIRATION VS. EXPIRATION

1. Inspiration
   a. Normally nervous stimulation of the diaphragm (phrenic nerve) and intercostal muscles causes the diaphragm to drop down and the chest wall to increase.
   b. This results greater volume within the chest cavity simultaneously creating an increased negative pressure- and air rushes into the chest.
   c. This requires energy, and thus occurs quicker than expiration.

2. Expiration
   a. Once the respiratory centers of the brain deem the breath complete, the nervous stimulation from the diaphragm and intercostal muscles are removed and those muscles begin to slowly retract back to their normal size.
   b. This causes the chest cavity volume to decrease and simultaneously increase the pressure- which pushes out the air in the chest.
   c. This does not require energy, and therefore happens twice as slow as inspiration (normally).

### GAS EXCHANGE

1. External Respiration:
   As air is drawn down into our lungs, it terminally reaches the alveoli, one of the thinnest membranes in the body. This membrane (alveolar capillary membrane) is designed this way to allow oxygen to be pulled though it and onto the red blood cell in the alveolar capillaries. Simultaneously, $CO_2$ is pushed from the red blood cell and across the alveolar capillary into the lung. This is external respiration, or external gas exchange.

2. Internal Respiration
   The circulatory system propels the blood from the alveolar capillary membrane to the distal tissues. Here $O_2$ is pulled off the red blood cell and toward the tissue bed and ultimately towards the cells of that tissue. Again, simultaneously, $CO_2$ is pushed from the tissues and pulled towards the red blood cell. This is internal respiration, or internal gas exchange.

## VENTILATION VS. OXYGENATION

1. Ventilation
   a. The action of pulling negative pressure (breathing) or pushing positive pressure (mechanical ventilation) into a patient's lungs, thus allowing $CO_2$ to be exhaled.
   b. Key Indicator: EtCO2
   c. Normal Range: 35-45 mmHg
2. Oxygenation
   a. The action of delivering oxygen to the cells of the body.
   b. Key indicator: pulse oximetry
   c. Normal Range: $\geq$ 94%

## GENERAL RESPIRATORY ABNORMALITIES

1. Respiratory Difficulty (Insufficiency)
   a. Some pathophysiology causing a reduction in oxygen delivery to the cells of the body causing poor function to pathology-specific organs and tissues.
   b. This leads to varying degrees of compensation, but typically the patients are **not yet acidotic**, or only just barely acidotic.
   c. Identify these patients by observing low O2 saturations (<92%), **normal pH**, increasing pCO2, abnormal breath sounds, tripod position, increased RR and HR, and accessory muscle use.
2. Respiratory Failure
   a. When the body can no longer compensate, then a change in vital signs occur as the respiratory system fails to meet body's metabolic needs.
   b. **COMPLETE** failure to compensate- ACIDOSIS (pH < 7.35); persistently high pCO2/ EtCO2 (> 45 mmHg).
   c. Oxygenation or ventilatory failure (see table below for respiratory failure criteria). Each of the three criteria below exhibit respiratory failure: pH and PaCO2 represent ventilation failure, and PaO2 represents oxygenation failure.

| | |
|---|---|
| **pH** | < 7.35 |
| **PaCO2** | > 60mmHg |
| **PaO2** | < 50mmHg ( Expect AMS at levels 50- 75 mmHg for normal individuals and 90-100 mmHg in patients with COPD) |

## BASIC AIRWAY MANAGEMENT

1. Positioning
    a. "Sniffing" position optimal for patient
    b. Manual maneuvers include head-tilt chin-lift, tongue-jaw lift, jaw thrust
    c. Consider elevating the head of bed (HOB) to at least 35°. This allows normal dependent lung fluid to drop to the lower lung fields, preventing such fluid to coat the entirety of the back of the patient's lungs. This leads to higher and faster oxygenation.

2. Supplemental Oxygen Administration
    a. Nasal cannula
        i. Can provide 22-44% of FiO2.
        ii. PASSIVE OXYGENATION: this is a technique where a nasal cannula is used at high flow rates (10-15 L/min, or more) which helps wash out the nitrogen out of the lung and increase the concentration of oxygen, and is strongly supported in the literature as responsible for increasing first-pass intubation success.
    b. Non-rebreather mask (provides up to 95% FiO2)
    c. Bag-mask ventilation (BVM) with reservoir (provides up to 95% FiO2)
        i. Thenar eminence technique: this is sweeping through the critical care transport world and competes with the traditional EC grip. The thenar eminence (TE) technique uses a 2 handed, thumbs up style grip allowing one clinician to focus on the seal of the BVM. The is incredible support for this grip in the current literature.
        ii. Seated Ventilation: this is a technique marring an elevated HOB with the TE technique and has shown great strength in the literature with improving first-pass intubation success.

3. Airway Adjuncts
    a. OPA
        i. Indicated: Unconscious patients
        ii. Contraindicated: Present gag reflex
    b. NPA
        i. Indicated: Unconscious patients
        ii. Relatively contraindicated: Nasal fractures and basilar skull fractures (stop if resistance is met).

## ADVANCED AIRWAY MANAGEMENT

### *Indications for Endotracheal Intubation*

1. Failure to Protect Airway

    a. Absent or diminished gag reflex (can swallow)

    b. Glasgow Coma Scale score of 8 or less (can't follow commands)

2. Failure to Oxygenate

    a. Pathology present that prevents oxygenation at the tissue level (resulting in poor pulse oximetry readings).

    b. Causes: Non-patent airway/ Poor perfusion/Low cardiac output/ carbon monoxide poisoning.

3. Failure to Ventilate

    a. Pathology or trauma present that prevents ventilation, which can be mechanical or cellular in nature (resulting in an elevating pCO2 or EtCO2).

    b. Causes: Airway obstruction/ overdose/ C3-C5 fracture/ diaphragmatic rupture/ facial hair

4. Need for prolonged ventilatory support

5. Patient and Crew Safety

    a. Remember that combative patients or those who do not follow commands can cause a significant safety risk by reaching for the pilot, crew member, the aircraft controls, or an aircraft door handle.

    b. In cases like these, the patient may need to be electively intubated to protect the crew, pilot, and patient from any consequence of an out-of-control patient in the back if the aircraft.

    c. It's always best to err on the side of caution in this field.


### *Predicting the Difficult Airway*

#### In General

1. Allow MOANS (or alternatively ROMAN), LEMON, RODS, and SHORT to guide your airway clinical decision making

2. The benefit of these acronyms (for testing) is they provide an easy way to remember all different kinds of difficult situations. **MEMORIZE THEM.**

3. For practical use, they will help you prepare for the worst-case scenarios. It's always better to be prepared and it be an easy intubation, than to underestimate the airway and kill the patient. Write that down...

**Assess for difficult <u>BVM VENTILATION</u>:**

1. (**M**)ask– hair and odd anatomy may prevent a good mask seal → potential for 'failure to ventilate' (FTV) scenario.

2. (**O**)besity/ Obstruction– larger BMI and abnormal masses in airway indicate the potential for FTV scenario.

3. (**A**)ge– Patients older than 55 indicate a potential FTV scenario

4. (**N**)o Teeth– the BVM requires the teeth in place as a solid base to press against to create a good seal

5. (**S**)tiff Lungs– poor compliance (sick, stiff lungs) also potentially creates a FTV scenario

6. An alternative **ROMAN** is a similar acronym where the 'R' stands for radiation/restriction. The 'R' is essentially explaining the stiff lungs element from MOANS, where the lungs are poorly compliant, such as with radiation sickness (radiation) and ARDS (restrictive).

**Assess for a difficult <u>INTUBATION</u>:**

1. (**L**)ook– inspect external anatomy

2. (**E**)valuate- the 3-3-2 Rule: 3 fingers into mouth/ 3 fingers from bottom of chin to the larynx/ 2 fingers from bottom of jaw to cricothyroid membrane

3. (**M**)allampati- Grade I (good) to grade IV (bad)

4. (**O**)bstruction– evaluate for angioedema, foreign body, abnormal masses or structures in airway

5. (**N**)eck Mobility– poor neck mobility (elderly, trauma patients, cervical fusions) has potential to make intubation difficult

**Assess for difficult <u>RESCUE</u> device placement:**

1. (**R**)estricted Oral Opening– supraglottic and other rescue devices need adequate oral opening– less than 2 fingers is potentially a FTV scenario

2. (**O**)bstruction– as already mentioned, larger BMI and abnormal masses in airway indicate the potential for FTV scenario

3. (**D**)isrupted/ Distorted– odd external anatomy indicates the potential for FTV scenario

4. (**S**)tiff Lungs– poor compliance (sick, stiff lungs) also potentially creates an FTV scenario.

**Assess for difficulty in performing a <u>CRICOTHYROTOMY</u>.**

1. All the following indicate the potential danger in the performance of surgical cricothyrotomy:

2. (**S**)urgery/Disrupted Airway- abnormal external anatomy = abnormal external anatomy

3. (**M**)ass- Can't assess landmarks/ bleeding risk from hematomas, abscesses, or other mass.

4. (**A**)natomy Problems– Obesity, poor landmarks, etc

5. (**R**)adiation– scarring/ tissue deformity from radiation

6. (**T**)umor

## *Various Intubation Attempts*

1. Direct Laryngoscopy (DL)

    a. MacIntosh blade (curved)

    b. Miller blade (straight)

2. Video Laryngoscopy (VL)

    a. There exist a wide range of products utilizing a camera at the distal tip of the endotracheal blade, and there are 2 main types: traditionally-angled devices and hyper-angulated devices. Most companies offer BOTH traditionally-angled and hyper-angled video laryngoscopes, so it is important to understand the differences in them.

        i. Standard Macintosh Blade

            a) The standard blade gives about 15° of view along the optical axis of the blade.

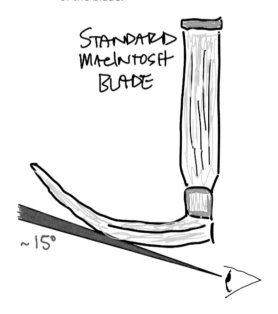

b) Here in lies the difficulty of intubation. As clinicians, we much be able to retract away tongue, neck tissue, and mandible anteriorly to view the glottic opening. Sometimes strength or leverage can be problematic.

ii. Hyer-angled Video Laryngoscope Devices

    a) Companies have devised devices that provide an expanded blade angle with the addition of a camera to provide a larger viewing angle.

    b) Glideslope was one of the first of these, although now Glideslope produces both hyper-angled blades as well as those with more standard geometry for their video laryngoscopes.

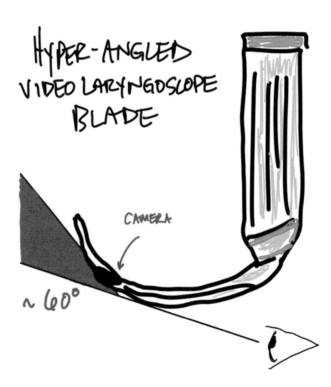

    c) These typically extend the viewing angles to ~ 75°, which includes 60° for the camera and 15° of traditional optical view.

    d) These are beneficial in the increased viewing angles, but with each use can reduce the skill of the clinician due to not using the traditional intubation approach.

iii. Standard Geometry Video Laryngoscope Devices

a) These devices have harnessed the best of both worlds, with the pocket CMAC device, and have shown strong clinical significance in improving first pass intubation success.

b) These types of devices provide a unique opportunity to the clinician, and ultimately patient by providing 2 'first looks' rather than one; it is a two bang for your buck approach.

c) An intubation 'attempt' is typically defined as the insertion of a laryngoscope into the posterior oropharynx with placement of the distal tip against the epiglottis or into the vallecula. It does not matter if the clinician attempts to intubate or not- simply the placement of the blade establishes the first 'attempt'.

d) With these standard geometry video laryngoscopes that merge the viewing angle, the clinician can place the blade and EITHER look along the optical angle (as with a standard Macintosh laryngoscope) or look at the vide on the display. If one isn't optimal, the clinician can immediately switch to the other view. Because the blade can remain stationary which switching to

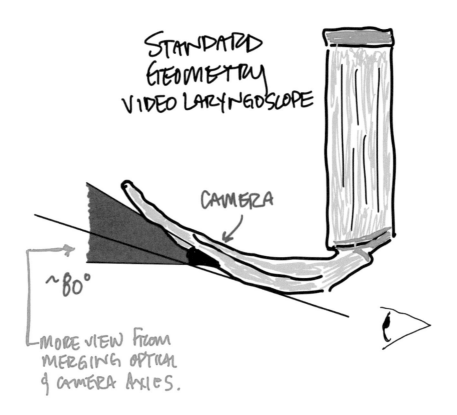

STANDARD GEOMETRY VIDEO LARYNGOSCOPE

CAMERA

~80°

MORE VIEW FROM MERGING OPTICAL & CAMERA AXIES.

optical or camera view, it all counts as 1 look. Therefore, you get 2 looks for the price of one.

    e) The clinical researchers, lead by David Olvera, has proven this maneuver to dramatically increase first-pass intubation success and therefore has saved countless lives over the last 7 years.

b. HEAVEN Criteria

    i. The HEAVEN criteria is a acronym to assist the clinician in determining which approach is statistically better considering a set of conditions.

    ii. (H)ypoxemia- if hypoxemia is the only problem, research shows DL is faster and more successful in first-pass intubation success (FPIS).

    iii. (E)xtremes of Size: a straight blade for pediatrics is statistically stronger in achieving FPIS. There is no favor of DL or VL if extremes of size is the only criterion present.

    iv. (A)natomic Disruption/Obstruction: with anatomical abnormalities are present (small mouth opening, fractured facial bones, abnormal growths or swelling), VL is favorable for FPIS- if there is not blood or vomit in the airway. Such fluids in the mouth obstruct the camera making VL a poor choice.

    v. (V)omit/Blood in the airway: as just mentioned, if ever there is blood or vomit in the airway, the research shows DL is favorable over VL in FPIS.

    vi. (E)xsanguination: if the patient has shock or is bleeding out (as long as they are not bleeding into the airway), then like hypoxemia, research shows DL is faster and more successful with respect to FPIS.

    vii. (N)eck Mobility: when the patient cannot move their neck easily (like when a c-collar is in place, or kyphosis is present), the VL shows greater success with respect to FPIS over DL and is also shown to be gentler to the patient.

3. Nasotracheal Intubation

a. Traditionally, this was the go-to advanced airway procedure for patients with cervical injury and/or trismus because it is a blind technique (insertion without visualizing the vocal cords). The RSI procedure has nearly eliminated this skill in practice.

b. The only absolute contraindication is apnea, but there are a few relative contraindications: basilar skull fracture, severe facial fracture, anticoagulation therapy, and epiglottitis. All of these relative contraindications would cause airway damage or could introduce the tip of the tube into a non-airway space (like the cranium).

    c. Generally, an ETT is inserted into a nare until the sound of air going in and out of the tube dramatically drops. The ETT is withdrawn slightly, put thumb on proximal ETT opening, and advance the tube. Directional-tip ETTs and whistling devices can aid in this procedure.

4. Digital Intubation

    a. This is another blind technique where the clinician inserts the middle fingers of their non-dominant hand into the mouth and use them to pull anterior traction on the tongue and airway. With the clinician's dominant hand, an ETT is advanced. The traction hand fingers may also help guide the ETT towards the airway.

    b. Like nasotracheal intubation, the RSI procedure has nearly eliminated this skill in practice.

5. Tomahawk Intubation

    a. This is a face-to-face approach typically utilized when there is limited access to the patient, such as being entrapped in a vehicle, buried, or in a confined space.

    b. The clinician approaches the patient from the front and wields the laryngoscope in an orientation 180° from normal, inserts the blade into the mouth and along the anatomical curvature of the tongue, and then pulls anterior traction by pulling the laryngoscope handle toward themselves. Then, the clinician should look straight down into the airway and place the ETT.

## *Confirming endotracheal tube (ETT) placement:*

1. BEST: continuous EtCO2 waveform monitoring.
2. Others: equal and bilateral lung sounds, visualization of ETT bisecting the vocal cords, ~~condensation in the ETT~~, bilateral chest wall excursion, (-) epigastric sounds.
3. You can see I scratched the 'condensation in the tube'. While it is still in the literature, but falling out of favor because our patient's perhaps needing intubation routinely consume CO2 based beverages and foods that can cause gas in the GI tract, thus reducing the sensitivity of this test.

## *Intubation Complications:*

1. Failed Airway

    a. Most agree that this constitutes 2-3 missed attempts via laryngoscopy and represents an immediate need to identify an alternative ventilation device.

    b. CAN ventilate, **CANNOT** intubate:

      i.   You have time to identify an alternative airway method (LMA, King, etc).

      ii.   AVOID doing the same exact attempt– change something in subsequent attempts (different tube, blade, technique, etc).

      iii.   **CANNOT** ventilate, **CANNOT** intubate:

         a)   This is a tough situation

         b)   Surgical cricothyrotomy right away!!!

2. Misplaced ET tube

    a. No EtCO2 Waveform/ EtCO2 measurement of zero:

      i.   w/ HYPOXIA: IMMEDIATELY remove the tube, ventilate, oxygenate, and then reintubate. Consider more medication if the patient is not well sedated and/or paralyzed.

      ii.   w/ SpO2 $\geq$ 94%: immediately visualize the glottic opening to confirm placement.

         a)   If ETT is in the trachea, consider changing the EtCO2 sensor.

         b)   If ETT is **NOT** in the trachea, extubate, ventilate, oxygenate, and then reintubate.

    b. Breath sounds not heard: **esophageal intubation** suspected. The clinician should extubate, suction, and repeat the oxygenation and intubation processes.

    c. Breath sounds heard on right side only: **right mainstem intubation** suspected. The clinician should deflate cuff, retract ETT 1-2 cm per attempt until breath sounds auscultated bilaterally. Then secure the ETT.

    d. Mid-transport Tube Dislodgement: at any point during transport, the ETT can become dislodged. Each time the patient is moved, the ETT placement and depth should be remeasured.

3. The Poor Perfusion Gremlin

    a. There are hundreds of cases where patients precipitously become acutely hypoxic, hypotensive, and shortly thereafter, bradycardic following intubation, particularly with RSI.

    b. Aggressive focus should be centered on the SHOCK INDEX, if not intuitively monitoring HR and the patient's blood pressure.

    c. A shock index (SI) is measured by dividing HR by the patient's systolic BP (SI = HR/systolic BP). A value **greater than 0.8 positively predicts** post-intubation hypotension. Therefore, prior to intubation, if the SI is > 0.8, then a fluid bolus (or multiple) should be considered as well as formulation of a plan for vasopressors should fluids not be effective. At any point hypotension and bradycardia be seen, THEY SHOULD IMMEDIATELY BE TREATED.

d. Unless the airway is an acute problem, the literature supports managing the BP prior to performing intubation, thus preventing hypotension, bradycardia, and potential death.

# PART 2: RSI AND PHARMACOLOGY

## THE BEST-PRACTICE MINDSET

It is imperative to remember that just because the procedure is called "rapid" sequence intubation, doesn't mean the procedure has to be conducted swiftly.

1. RSI does not begin as medications are being pushed but rather begins much earlier.
2. It starts when you are first dispatched and are first considering your patient and how they need to be managed.
3. Even with patients who do not require intubation during your initial impression, you should cultivate a readiness to RSI every one of your patients, should they need to be intubated acutely.
4. Planning, preparing, and always thinking multiple steps ahead will keep you alert and ready.

## THE PROCEDURE

### *Prepare*

1. Gather all needed equipment and don't just have a plan A, but also a plan B and plan C.
2. Laryngoscope/ ETTs/ back-up ETTs and blades/ BVM with mask/ suction/ supraglottic devices/ a backup person to call/ tube securing device.
3. Consider the SHOCK INDEX when preparing, since cardiac compromise can occur out of the intubation/ RSI procedure.
    a. SHOCK INDEX = [Heart Rate / Systolic BP].
    b. Normal: 0.5- 0.7
    c. Clinically significant: > 0.8
    d. In these cases of clinically significant shock index, be more aggressive with correcting the blood pressure.

## Pre-oxygenate

1. Significant studies have shown improved outcomes with effective pre-oxygenation and nitrogen washout.

   a. Since our atmosphere is mostly nitrogen, it is safe to assume that most of the air in our lungs is made up of nitrogen– if we are breathing room air (21% oxygen).

   b. When we add higher concentrations of oxygen, then we replace the nitrogen with the increasing oxygen concentration. This is called nitrogen washout. It basically turns your lungs into a reservoir mask.

2. Target ~2-3 minutes and/or an SpO2 >94%.

3. In recent years, multiple academic centers have been utilizing a high flow nasal cannula approach to increase the oxygen concentrations in the oropharynx, nasopharynx, and lungs.

   a. This is being achieved by utilizing a nasal cannula at flow rates up to 12-15 L/min.

   b. This has been shown to significantly reduce desaturations during intubations and improve first-pass intubation success.

| Medication | Sedation | Anxiolytic | Hypnosis | Amnesia |
|---|---|---|---|---|
| Versed | x | | x | x |
| Ativan | x | x | x | x |
| Barbiturates | x | x | x | |
| Propofol | x | | x | |
| Etomidate | | | x | |
| Ketamine | x | | | x |
| Fentanyl | x | x | x | |

## Pre-medications

1. It is important to have a concept of the mechanisms of the medications available for use in RSI.

   a. Analgesics– reduce the pain response and some cause patients to fall asleep, help to blunt the sympathetic response of the patient

   b. Anesthetics– this is a catch all term for the various types of medications that reduce mentation to produce a sleep– like state.

   c. Anticholinergics– prevents increased vagal tone (which would slow HR) in pediatric patients caused during intubation. Additionally, with repeated succinylcholine doses, bradycardia can occur.

d. **Lidocaine**– an antiarrhythmic which was once thought to be able to blunt ICP spikes during intubation. This has fallen out of vogue on account of little scientific support. Currently, the literature shows no benefit, but also no harm. You may still see it on exams.

2. The 4 Types of Anesthetics
   a. Most of the literature commonly utilizes the term 'sedative' to communicate its properties to put the patient to sleep.
   b. In addition to sedative, there are multiple terms that gets confusing: induction agent, anxiolytic, hypnotic, etc. Let me explain.
   c. It is important to note that specific anesthetic medications are utilized for their specific properties.
   d. The 4 anesthetic properties include: sedation, anxiolysis, hypnosis, and amnesia.
      i. **Sedation** is achieved by depressing a patient's awareness to the environment and reducing his or her responsiveness to external stimulation.
      ii. **Anxiolysis** is achieved by reducing the physiological effects of anxiety, which can be triggered by fear or concern for a situation.
      iii. **Hypnosis** is achieved by simply inducing sleep in a patient.
      iv. **Amnesia** is achieved by putting the patient into a deep enough sleep such that short term memory of a traumatic or frightful event is not even recorded.
   e. The term sedative is commonly used as a catch all term for these anesthetic medications because most all of them result in sleepiness. The table on the next page illustrates the commonly used medications in RSI and their respective properties.
   f. There isn't a single anesthetic that is best for **_all_** patients. It is important to consider what you are trying to accomplish with them. Sedatives induce sleep, but typically comes at the cost of a lower BP (benzos). Hypnotics cause a dissociative effect, and are typically safe on BP, but can affect adrenal sufficiency (etomidate, ketamine). Anxiolytics also can lower BP, and amnestics make people forget, but also can lower BP. Consider your patient and the situation.

## Paralytics

1. These medicines cause flaccid muscles, but completely allows for the sensation of pain, temperature, and touch.

2. There are 2 types: Depolarizing and non– depolarizing

3. **DEPOLARIZING NEUROMUSCULAR BLOCKERS**

   a. Succinylcholine is the only depolarizing NMB in the United States

   b. This medication is shaped molecularly like acetylcholine

   c. It leaves the nerve terminal and crosses the neuromuscular junction where it finds and enters an acetylcholine receptor; this causes a small release of potassium.

   d. The difference between succinylcholine and acetylcholine is that acetylcholine is immediately metabolized and cleared from the receptor, but succinylcholine stays in the receptor for 3-5 minutes until it is finally metabolized and kicked out of the receptor.

   e. The depolarizing action (acetylcholine or succinylcholine crosses the neuromuscular junction) causes the fasciculation's you see when this medication is administered.

   f. In patients without neuromuscular diseases there are a normal amount of acetylcholine receptors. Depolarization results in a small release of potassium.

   g. For patients WITH neuromuscular diseases (multiple sclerosis, cerebral palsy, myasthenia gravis, paraplegia, quadriplegia, patients bed bound for at least a week, etc), their muscles build millions more acetylcholine receptors to try to catch acetylcholine thus stimulating the muscle to contract. This increase in receptors causes a very dangerous situation, should succinylcholine be administered.

   h. If succinylcholine is administered to ANY patient with a neuromuscular disease, then a massive potassium release can occur from all the extra acetylcholine receptors which results in a potentially lethal hyperkalemia.

   i. Additionally, any pre- existing hyperkalemia would obviously exacerbate the potassium release caused by succinylcholine administration.

j. Bottom line: any patient with a neuromuscular disease or hyperkalemia contraindicates succinylcholine. This includes the patients we have already mentioned, in addition to burn patients 24 hours status post burn, and dialysis patients.

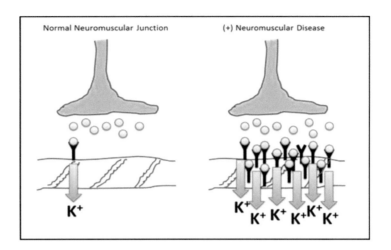

4. **NON-DEPOLARIZING NEURO MUSCULAR BLOCKERS**

   a. These medications prevent depolarization, thus do not fasciculate, do not release potassium, and last much longer than their succinylcholine.

   b. If you suspect a neuromuscular disease, a significant burn > 24 hours old, a dialysis patient, or any patient with a potassium > 5.5 mmol/L (when you'll normally see ECG changes) then you should choose a NON-DEPOLARIZING NMB.

## Place the ETT.

1. Consider using HEAVEN criteria to predict the best approach: direct or video laryngoscopy.

2. Be prepared to HALT the intubation attempt should SpO2 drop below 93%.

3. To estimate ETT size: [(Age + 16)/4].

4. To estimate proper ETT depth: [ETT size x 3].

## Confirm Placement

1. In Trachea: **(+) upright waveform on EtCO2 monitoring**; (+) witness tube pass cords; (+) condensation in ETT upon exhalation; (+) equal chest wall excursion; (-) epigastric sounds

2. In Esophagus: Opposite findings than the above.

3. X-ray– only confirms depth of tube, but not a true measure of placement.

4. The current medical literature identifies graphic EtCO2 waveform on perfusing patients as the best indicator of correct ETT placement.

5. WORST CASE SCENARIO: SpO2 100% and EtCO2 0 with a sending clinician not wanting you

to investigate the airway. Anytime EtCO2 is zero (0), you MUST quickly re-evaluate the ETT placement via laryngoscopy. If the ETT is out, then pre ready to replace the ETT.

## Secure the Tube

Be sure to use either a commercial device or other secure means to ensure the endotracheal tube (ETT) doesn't wander from the position where you secured it.

## Post– Intubation Management

1. Re– confirm positive placement and ETT depth with each patient movement.
2. Be cognizant of upcoming medication needs: analgesics, sedatives, paralytics.
3. Apply the mechanical ventilator and the appropriate strategies (see Part 4 of this chapter).
4. Be ready to aggressively treat hypotension and bradycardia.


# RSI PHARMACOLOGY

We will not cover a broad selection of RSI pharmacology here, but rather the ones you will most likely use in the field, and the ones you're most likely to see on a certification exam.

## Analgesics

### In General

1. Problem: some of these medications drop blood pressure as a result of HISTAMINE release, so it is important to know which ones to AVOID during hypotension or peri-hypotension.
2. Peri-hypotension is defined as a state where the patient is perfusing, but just barely. Any reduction in blood pressure can result in frank hypotension.
3. The release of histamine is characteristic of opiates, except for fentanyl. Fentanyl is dosed in micrograms, while the others are dosed in milligrams. Because the dosing for fentanyl is so small, it DOES NOT cause excessive histamine release while it is achieving pain control. This makes it a favorable drug for hypotensive patients.
4. A big concept to understand: an unconscious patient CAN still feel pain, so be sure to dose these patients with adequate pain medication, just don't cause hypotension with medications.

**Fentanyl**

1.  Class: Narcotic/ Analgesic

2.  Mechanism: Competitively binds with narcotic receptors and prevents the sensation of pain.

3.  Indications: pain control

4.  Contraindications: Allergy/ History of rigid chest syndrome

5.  Hemodynamics: (~CVP/ ~PCWP/~CO/~SVR).

6.  Adult Dose: 1-2 mg/kg IV. Peds Dose: 1-2 mg/kg IV.

7.  Very safe hemodynamic profile (does not drop blood pressure significantly).

8.  Can be used in the hypotensive setting when a benzodiazepine would be unsafe for perfusion.

**Morphine**

1.  Class: Narcotic/ Analgesic

2.  Mechanism: Competitively binds with narcotic receptors and prevents the sensation of pain.

3.  Indications: pain control

4.  Contraindications: Allergy/ History of rigid chest syndrome

5.  Hemodynamics: (~CVP/ ~PCWP/~CO/↓SVR).

6.  Adult Dose: 2-5 mg IV; Peds Dose: 0.1 −.02 mg/kg

7.  Can precipitously drop blood pressure.

**Ketamine**

1.  Class: Hypnotic

2.  Dose: 1-2 mg/kg IV

3.  Indications: sedation; pain control, bronchodilation

4.  Contraindications: Allergy/ increased ICP

5.  Used for both analgesia and sedation.

6.  Ketamine will help to increase BP– ideal in trauma, but not in increased ICP conditions; ketamine also will reduce bronchospasm.

7.  Hemodynamics: (~CVP/ ~PCWP/↑CO/↑SVR)

## Sedatives and Hypnotics

There are essentially 2 common classes: benzodiazepines and hypnotics.

**Benzodiazepines:**

This drug class can precipitously drop blood pressure and cause hypotension. Close attention and focus should be placed on the patient's BP and HR during the procedure. Any worsening SHOCK INDEX, especially with EtCO2 values dropping into the low 30s and upper 20s, should prompt **IMMEDIATE MANAGEMENT** of the shock state.

Versed (midazolam)

1. Dose: 2-5 mg IV
2. Indications: sedation; seizures
3. Contraindications: Allergy/ hypotension
4. Hemodynamics: ($\downarrow$CVP/ $\downarrow$PCWP/$\downarrow$CO/$\downarrow$SVR)

Ativan (lorazepam)

1. Dose: 0.05 mg/kg IV
2. Indications: sedation; seizures
3. Contraindications: Allergy/ hypotension
4. Hemodynamics: ($\downarrow$CVP/ $\downarrow$PCWP/$\downarrow$CO/$\downarrow$SVR)

**Hypnotics**

Etomidate (ethomidate)

1. This is an ultra-short acting hypnotic that has a very stable hemodynamic profile– does not lower blood pressure.
2. Dose: 0.3 mg/kg IV
3. Indications: To cause sedation for the facilitation of intubation
4. Contraindications: Allergy/ adrenal insufficiency
5. Hemodynamics: ($\sim$CVP/ $\sim$PCWP/$\sim$CO/$\sim$SVR)

**Anti-cholinergic (atropine)**

1. This is an anti– cholinergic and is used to blunt the bradycardic effect caused when the laryngoscope blade touches a pediatric posterior pharynx (vagal stimulation)
2. It combats bradycardia by simply increasing the heart rate
3. Dose: 0.01– 0.02 mg/kg IV (min. 0.1 mg ; max 0.5mg)
4. Indications: prevent vagal stimulated bradycardia
5. Contraindications: Allergy
6. Hemodynamics: ($\sim$CVP/ $\sim$PCWP/$\sim$CO/$\sim$SVR)

**Xylocaine (lidocaine)**

1. This is an anti– arrhythmic medication that was once thought to prevent ICP spikes.

2. It is no longer en vogue, but you'll need to be aware of it for testing purposes

3. Dose: 1 mg/kg IV; max dose 3 mg/kg

4. Indications: prevent elevations in ICP from intubation attempts

5. Contraindications: Allergy

6. Hemodynamics: (~CVP/ ~PCWP/~CO/~SVR)

## *Paralytics*

### Depolarizing neuromuscular blocker (NMB)

#### Anectine (succinylcholine)

1. Avoid in any neuromuscular pathophysiology– it doesn't matter why the nerve and muscle isn't talking, but that HYPERKALEMIA could occur if you administer to someone with a neuromuscular disease

2. These include myasthenia gravis, multiple sclerosis, muscular dystrophy, healthy people bedridden from surgery, sub– acute burns, etc.

3. Dose: 1-2 mg/kg IV

4. Indications: need for paralysis in RSI

5. Contraindications: History of hyperkalemia, predispositions to hyperkalemia, renal patients, organophosphate/nerve agent poisoning.

6. Hemodynamics: (~CVP/ ~PCWP/~CO/~SVR)

### Non-depolarizing neuro muscular blocker

#### Zemuron (rocuronium)

1. Dose: 0.6-1.2 mg/kg IV

2. Onset: ~ 120 seconds

3. Indications: need for paralysis in RSI

4. Contraindications: Allergy

5. Hemodynamics: (~CVP/ ~PCWP/~CO/~SVR)

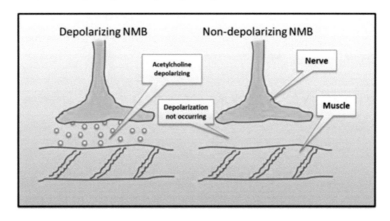

# PART 3: MANAGING INTUBATION COMPLICATIONS

## COMPLICATIONS

It is important to mention that one way to prevent complications is to be proactive and ready for them. It is imperative that you review predicting the difficult airway section (Part 1 of this chapter) and employ these skills in practice. There are two main types of complications that can arise when attempting to intubate a patient: 1) can ventilate, failure to intubate, and 2) failure to ventilate and failure to intubate.

### Can ventilate, failure to intubate

1. These are situations where an attempt to intubate has been made, however the endotracheal tube was unable to be placed.

2. These patients present with dropping oxygen saturation and an increasing heart rate (unless prolonged in which case a decreasing heart rate would manifest).

3. The saving grace is the ability to ventilate the patient, so the clinician should be prepared to utilize rescue devices (see below).

4. The oxyhemoglobin dissociation curve describes that once a patient's saturations dive below 90%, oxygen basically loses its stickiness to the red blood cell, and thus we fail to oxygenate the tissues.

### Failure to ventilate and failure to intubate

1. This is an incredibly stressful situation, in which most texts will agree, that you should not hesitate in performing a needle cricothyrotomy or a surgical cricothyrotomy.

2. At this point, every moment that goes by the patient is being deprived of cellular oxygen and thus creating acid.

3. As critical care clinicians we must act very quickly to ensure and reestablish airway, ventilation, and oxygenation.

## SECOND ATTEMPT AND RESCUE MANEUVERS

There are several alternative, or rescue airway devices and procedures that are available to the critical care clinician. It is imperative that you become familiar with these rescue devices so that when you're faced with a failed airway, you will be prepared to handle this difficult situation. No matter what your second attempt approach- **TRY SOMETHING DIFFERENT**!

### Three Curtain Method for Airway Visualization:

1. If you insert the laryngoscope blade all the way into the mouth, chances are you are in the esophagus. This is known as the first curtain.

2. If you then begin to slowly retract the blade, the epiglottis will fall from the top of your view revealing the glottic opening, aka airway (second curtain).

3. If you continue to retract the blade, the tongue will fall and occlude the oropharynx (third curtain).

4. The difficulty with intubation often centers on identifying landmarks. With this method, you have identified all 3 major structures associated with the airway: the esophagus , the glottic opening, and the oropharynx.

5. If you reinsert the blade gently  back into the airway  (all the way), then slowly retract until you again see the epiglottis fall from the top of your view. Put the tip of the blade into the vallecula (if using a Mac blade) or lift the vallecula (if using a Miller blade). This will assist you in identifying critical anatomy and place the tube once the trachea is identified.

## Swearingen's Traction Method

1. The first clinician (at the patient's head) inserts the laryngoscope into the patient's mouth while the assistant pulls upward traction mimicking a jaw thrust.

2. The assistant maintains this traction while the first clinician is able to free their right hand from the laryngoscope, and can then place the endotracheal tube.

3. Bougie

4. A bougie is a long flexible piece of plastic that is thin enough to be passed through an endotracheal tube.

5. The laryngoscope is used as normal to visualize the glottic opening, and then the Bougie is placed in between the vocal cords.

6. The endotracheal tube is then passed over the Bougie following its path into the trachea.

## Laryngeal Mask Airway (LMA)

1. This device is a noninvasive single lumen airway device that is designed to occlude the supraglottic opening and thus facilitating ventilation.

2. Once a failed intubation has occurred and the failed airway path has been initiated, a blind insertion of this device followed by inflating of the mask portion of this device should be executed.

## King LT Airway

1. This device is a supraglottic airway device that stabilize the airway at the base of the tongue.

2. This device is blindly inserted into the patient's airway and the large silicone cuff is inflated.

3. This seals off the posterior pharynx and allows air to flow from the tube opening, past the silicone to cuff, into the posterior pharynx, and then into the trachea.

4. Air is not allowed to go into the esophagus because of a distal balloon.

5. Most King airways and LMAs also offer supraglottic suctioning, which has been shown to reduce ventilator assisted pneumonia (VAP).

## Needle Cricothyrotomy

1. This procedure involves identifying the cricothyroid membrane and passing a large bore IV catheter through this membrane.

2. A size 5.5mm endotracheal tube hub should be placed inside of a 3cc syringe (plunger removed), and then attached to the end of the catheter.

3. This componentry will allow a bag valve mask to be attached to the catheter for ventilation.

4. It will not be possible to reach large, and possibly not even normal, minute ventilations with this method, however oxidation can still occur with 100% oxygen.

5. An alternative method is to use a 3.5 ETT adapter to the inside of an angiocatheter.

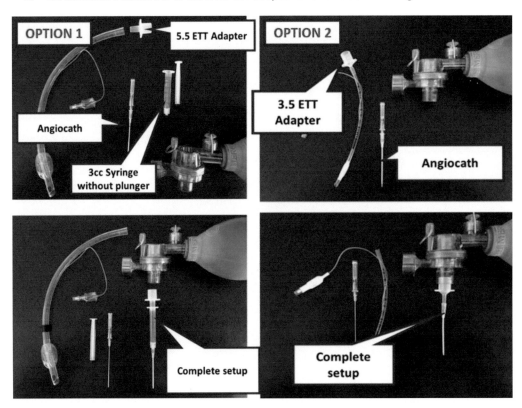

## Surgical Cricothyrotomy

1. This procedure involves it using a scalpel to incise through the cricothyroid membrane and pass an endotracheal tube through this incision.

2. Complications with this procedure can include incorrect placement into a false passage, severe bleeding, subcutaneous emphysema, and vocal cord damage.

3. There are also surgical cricothyrotomy products on the market that are designed for reduced error and simplistic use; however, the literature is inconclusive as to which of these have better outcomes, if any.

4. Whichever skill is utilized (scalpel or commercial device), the clinician must be prepared in the equipment and procedure for EVERY SINGLE PATIENT.
5. It is imperative this skill be reviewed often because it is a skill that is very high risk and very low frequency: meaning it is dangerous and you will not perform it often.

# PART 4: AIRWAY MANAGEMENT QUESTIONS

1. Your patient is showing signs of acute respiratory failure. You make the decision to intubate. The patient is 6 feet tall, weighs 190 pounds, has a full beard, and his oral opening is approximately three fingers wide. Using this information, which of the following acronym concerns you?
   a. SMART
   b. RODS
   c. LEMON
   d. MOANS

2. Which of these following patients exhibit an indication for intubation?
   a. Asthma patient on a continuous nebulizer
   b. COPD patient on CPAP at 94% SPO2
   c. Overdose patient with a pH of 7.29
   d. AMI patient breathing 22 times a minute

3. You are about to RSI your patient. Your patient is status post cardiac arrest who has had a spontaneous return of circulation. This patient has end stage kidney and liver disease and is currently hemodynamically unstable. What is the ideal RSI regime?
   a. Versed, succinylcholine, rocuronium
   b. Ketamine, succinylcholine, pancurionium
   c. Etomidate, Fentanyl, zemuron
   d. Morphine, Anectine, rocuronium

4. You are preparing to intubate your patient and considering medication selections. Your patient has the current labs and values, HR 107, BP 92/68, RR 19, SpO2 94%, CO 3, pH 7.36, pCO2 44. Which of the following medication sequences would be appropriate?
   a. Versed, etomidate, ketamine
   b. Rocuronium, ketamine, succinylcholine
   c. Succinylcholine, ketamine, versed
   d. Ketamine, succinylcholine, zemuron

5. Which of the following situations contraindicates the use of succinylcholine?
   a. 17-year-old chest trauma patient
   b. AMI patent with fibrinolytic on board
   c. Poorly ambulatory kidney failure patient
   d. Seizure patient with refractory seizures

6.  Your patient is experiencing severe bronchospasm. You have made the decision to intubate the patient. Which of the following RSI regimes would be ideal?
    a.  Versed, succinylcholine
    b.  Etomidate, zemuron
    c.  Ketamine, succinylcholine
    d.  Lorazepam, rocuronium

7.  Your patient's vital signs are BP 112/78, HR 99, O2 sats 95%, RR 21, and EtCO2 55. Which of the following is the best description of the patient's status?
    a.  Poor ventilation
    b.  Low oxygenation
    c.  Pre- hypotensive
    d.  Mild tachycardia

8.  You are caring for a seriously injured patient. During your patient assessment, you find that the patient has a decreased level of consciousness, an absent gag reflex, and a GCS of 6. Based on this information, you anticipate that this patient will require which of the following interventions?
    a.  Surgical tracheostomy
    b.  Endotracheal intubation
    c.  Supplemental oxygen
    d.  Nasal pharyngeal airway

9.  Currently, your adult patient is intubated with a 6.5 ETT, and secured with a commercial device at 22 cm at the gumline. Their vital signs are as follows: HR 121, BP is 108/74, SpO2 is 88%, and their EtCO2 is 54. Which of the following is the best immediate action?
    a.  Reduce the VE
    b.  Increase the FiO2
    c.  Back up the ETT
    d.  Increase the HOB

# PART 5: AIRWAY MANAGEMENT RATIONALES

1.  **(D)**. The beard indicates that this patient could potentially be a difficult patient to ventilate. It is important that you plan to have multiple back up plans. The point being always be prepared and never let a situation catch you off guard.

2.  **(C)**. The AMI patient is simply tachycardic and does not indicate intubation. The COPD patient does not indicate intubation either because they are maintaining their saturations. The asthmatic patient simply does not provide enough information for us to decide. The patient who does require intubation, is a patient with a pH of 7.29 who has overdosed. You could argue the reasons for intubation were 1) expected clinical course could require intubation as well as 2) failure to protect the airway.

3.  **(C)**. This is the only answer without succinylcholine (Anectine is the brand name of succinylcholine). This patient has kidney disease, so they are predisposed to high potassium which contraindicates the use of succinylcholine.

4.  **(D)**. The best sequence here should follow the sedative/ paralytic sequence and should avoid anything that could drop BP. Versed drops BP and sedatives must come first. Therefore, D is the only option.

5.  **(C)**. Succinylcholine is contraindicated in patients susceptible to hyperkalemia (like renal failure patients, patients who are bedbound, and any neuromuscular pathology). Therefore, the only patient here that is susceptible to hyperkalemia is the renal patient. They have kidney disease (therefore likely has higher potassium) and are poorly ambulatory (so they will be susceptible to hyperkalemia for this reason too).

6.  **(C)**. Bronchospasm can be attenuated by ketamine; therefore, this is the best answer in this limited information question.

7.  **(A)**. Ventilatory status is identified by evaluating EtCO2, or if using an ABG then it is evaluated by the pCO2.

8.  **(B)**. This patient is absent the mental capacity to protect their airway (decreased LOC) and has no gag reflex (that normally protects the patient from aspiration). You need to secure the airway and an NPA and suctioning will not secure the airway. A tracheostomy and ETT would do the job, so use the less invasive option: ETT, or endotracheal intubation.

9.  **(C)**. While, yes, increasing the FiO2 will normally increase the SpO2, this case requires the ETT be backed up because it is too deep, right main- stemmed, and has reduced minute ventilation (by about half) by only ventilating one lung. The only correct answer here is to back up the ETT. Remember, the appropriate depth is approximately 3 x ETT size. In this case, 6.5 x 3 = 19.5, therefore, the ETT is about 2.5 centimeters too deep- deep enough to go right mainstem.

# CHAPTER 2: RESPIRATORY MANAGMENT

## PART 1: THE RESPIRATORY ASSESSMENT

### INTRODUCTION

During the respiratory assessment, we want to determine if RESPIRATORY DIFFICULTY, or the potential progression to RESPIRATORY FAILURE, is present. If someone is breathing normally and calm, then clinically we may not be too concerned from a respiratory standpoint. However, a patient that is in respiratory, then actions are needed to correct oxygenation, ventilation or both. Ventilation describes the patient's ability to off– load carbon dioxide. Oxygenation describes the body's ability to grab environmental oxygen, force it onto a red blood cell, and deliver it to the body's distal tissues. In this chapter we will learn to assess and manage respiratory issues.

### THE INITIAL ASSESSMENT

As you approach the patient, look at their body position, work of breathing and skin condition and color.

1. Their body position tells you great information: tripod means they are short of breath/ hypoxic, laying on the ground with weak muscles mean they are extremely hypoxic.
2. Normal respiratory effort indicates they are receiving adequate oxygen, but labored respirations indicates they are hypoxic.
3. Normal skin color indicates adequate perfusion, but pale or mottled skin can indicate poor perfusion.

### ASSESS MENTAL STATUS

1. AVPU: Awake– eyes open spontaneously; Verbal- arouses to stimulation by voice; Painful– purposeful movements to painful stimuli; Unresponsive- no response to any stimuli
2. Assess GCS
   a. Eye Opening: Spontaneous (4); to speech (3); to painful stimuli (2); no opening at all (0)
   b. Verbal Effort: normal conversation (5); confused (4); inappropriate words (3); incomprehensible sounds (2); no verbal effort (1)
   c. Motor Effort: follows commands (6); localizes pains (5); withdrawals from pain (4); decorticate posturing (3); decerebrate posturing (2); no motor effort (1)

### ASSESS ABCS

1. Airway: Ensure a patent airway.
2. Breathing and Respiratory Effort: Note rate, quality (normal or labored), and rhythm (normal or abnormal respiratory patterns).
3. Circulation:
   a. Ensure the patient has a pulse and note the rate, strength (normal, bounding, or weak), and quality (regular or irregular).
   b. Obtain and assess heart rate, blood pressure, pulse oximetry, cardiac monitoring, and labs/ images if available.

# FOCUSED RESPIRATORY ASSESSMENT

## Observe Respirations

1. Rate
   a. Too fast (>30)- suggests acidosis or neuro injury
   b. Too slow (< 10)- indicates drug overdose
2. Rhythm
   a. Regular– good blood flow and temperature to the respiratory center of the brain
   b. Irregular– pathophysiology to the brain resulting in abnormal breathing patterns.
3. Depth
   a. Full– normal respiration
   b. Shallow– broken ribs, reduced airway diameter (asthma/ COPD), drug/ medication OD

## Inspection

1. Effort
   a. Normal→ calm respiratory effort
   b. Increased effort/ WOB: ↑ RR, (+) retractions, (+) tripod, (+) pursed lip breathing, (+) head bobbing
2. Excursion
   a. Full/ Normal: Appears that a full breath enters into chest
   b. Shallow/ Abnormal: Looks like only a portion of normal inspiration volume entering chest- (reduced ventilation)
3. Pattern
   a. Cheyne– Stoke: cyclical crescendo– decrescendo pattern with a short apneic period in between; seen in stroke/ tumor/ TBI/ CO poisoning/ altitude sickness
   b. Kussmauls: regular, increased rate and tidal volume; seen in metabolic acidosis/ severe hyperglycemia
   c. Biot's: irregular rate and tidal volume with varying periods of apnea; occurs with brainstem stroke/ TBI, narcotic overdoses, or damage to medulla oblongata
   d. Apneustic: each inspiration followed by a long pause, then each expiration also followed by a long pause; caused by a damaged respiratory center in the brain (upper pons)
   e. Ataxic—completely irregular breathing with irregular pauses. Caused by damage to the medulla oblongata.
4. I:E Ratio
   a. Norm I:E is 1:2
   b. Prolonged E time (exhalation time) means air trapping.
5. External Features
   a. Retractions- increased respiratory effort/ WOB
   b. Barrel Chest- obstructive disease = air trapping
   c. Chest tubes/ surgical scar/ trauma
   d. Tracheal tugging = tension pneumothorax

## Palpation

1. Pain = injury (rib fx can lead to atelectasis from not wanting to take a breath– distal alveoli begin to collapse if not inflated with each breath)
2. Masses = cancer (reduces tidal volume)
3. Subcutaneous Emphysema = injury
4. Fremitus:
   a. ↑ in consolidation
   b. ↓ over air trapping or obstructed branch

## Percussion

1. Hyperresonant: Air in chest (pneumo or air trapping)
2. Dull: Consolidation = pneumonia (or other fluid in the lungs)

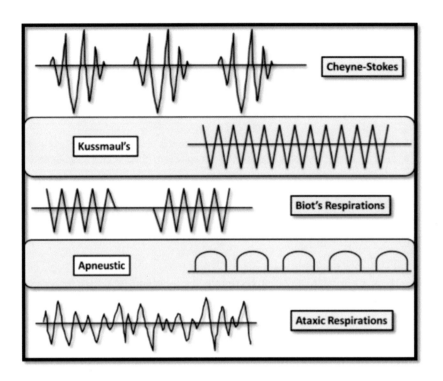

## Auscultation

1. Rales- indicates pulmonary edema/ pneumonia
2. Rhonchi- indicates pneumonia/ secretions in lungs
3. Wheezes- indicates bronchospasm
4. Friction Rub- indicates inflamed pleura from infection or pneumothorax

## X– Ray Interpretation

### Goal of Assessment

Obtain any information indicating that lung surface area is reduced or disrupted. This review will not be an in-depth review, as it is not the scope of this work.

### Tissue Appearance

1. Air- Presents as BLACK
2. Bone- Presents as GREY
3. Fluid (blood/ mucous/ infiltrates/ edema)- Presents as WHITE

### Assessment

1. Remember, this is a two-dimensional view of 3D structures.
2. Whatever assessment technique you use, use the exact same method EVERYTIME you assess an X-ray. Keep it systematic.
3. Bones:
   a. Should all be symmetrical
   b. Should all be intact (if not– consider fracture or dislocation
   c. Spine should be midline and directly behind the sternum– if not the patient is rotated, and therefore it isn't a good film (X-ray)
4. Soft tissue:
   a. Lung markings go all the way out to the chest wall– if not, pneumothorax may be present
   b. Lung markings throughout lung field– if NONE, consider pneumothorax

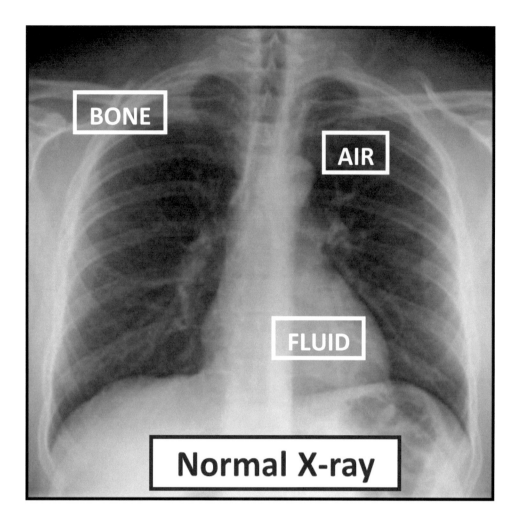

**Normal X-ray**

    c. Lung markings should be faint– bold lung markings indicate consolidation (fluid, or pneumonia)

    d. Costophrenic angles should be present and sharp– Could be:

        i.    Flat =  COPD/ Asthma (air trapping flattens the costophrenic angles of the diaphragm)

        ii.   Free air– ruptured diaphragm will reveal free air under the diaphragm

    e. Trachea– Should be midline; if not, consider pneumothorax or trauma

    f. Cardiac

        i.    Cardiac silhouette should be clear– if hazy, or unobservable, then fluid is in the way (pneumonia/ consolidation possibly)

        ii.   1/3 Rule: the heart should be 1/3 the size of the chest cavity; if its bigger, then cardiomegaly is present

**The Big Picture**

1. We do not need to be experts at x– ray interpretation. Use the above x-ray to compare with subsequent  x-rays, because this one is NORMAL.
2. We need to know any information that would worsen ventilation or oxygenation, so that we can best be prepared for any patient decline.
3. Anything that prevents air from being drawn into the lung (fluid, collapsed lung, obstruction, etc) will prevent adequate ventilation.

**Consider this X-ray.**

1. This patient has just been extubated and is about to be re-intubated. The endotracheal tube was thought to be too deep and of an inappropriate size.
2. Notice the patient's left side (ride side of the picture is the patient's left side) has a lot whiter in the lung fields– this indicates atelectasis.

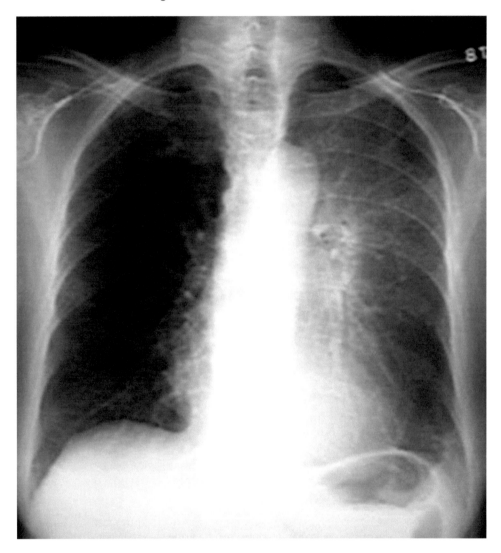

**Note the next X-ray.**

1. This is from a patient who has been ill for the last few days. Three of her family members have been sick in her household too.
2. She presents with fever and a productive cough.
3. Notice the CONSOLIDATION in the patient's right lower lung lobe? That is isolated pneumonia in that lobe.

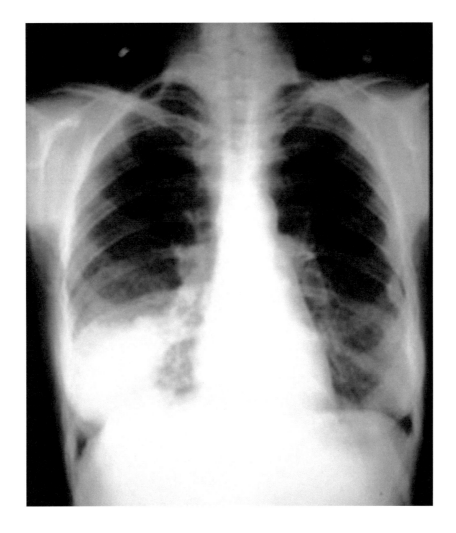

**Consider the next X-ray:**

1. The following X– ray is from a patient who was involved in a motor vehicle collision and is currently having trouble breathing. They are displaying significant air hunger and their pulse oximetry is currently 88%. The patient has clear breath sounds, but is slightly decreased on the left side.

2. Consider what would cause these findings and begin to formulate an idea of what's happening (build your differential diagnosis).

3. In this case, there is a partially collapsed lung on the patients left side (aka PNEUMOTHORAX). This patient would warrant a needle decompression or a chest tube because if this enlarges, then it can lead to TENSION PNEUMOTHORAX

4. Look to the next X-ray for a worsening of this condition. Notice the expanding left intrathoracic space from an increasing tension pneumothorax. This X-ray indicates a needle decompression or chest tube immediately before the tension significantly affects cardiac output, leading to hypoperfusion.

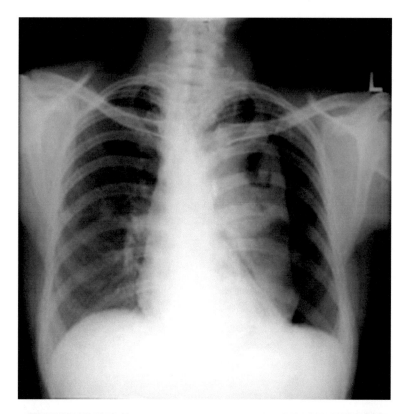

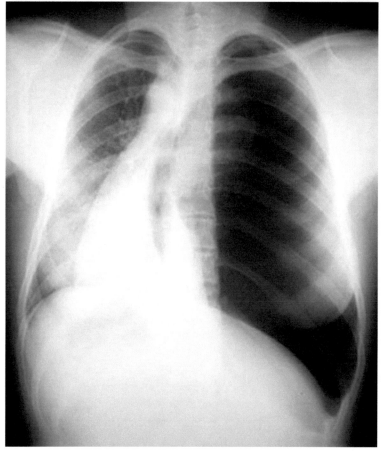

# PART 2: CONTINUED RESPIRATORY MONITORING

## INTRODUCTION

It is important to continuously monitor your respiratory patient throughout your transport. You should be looking for any and all information that will assist you in early identification of a patient that is decompensating. There are three ongoing monitoring assessments that can help identify a patient's respiratory status:

1. SpO2 monitoring (Oxygenation)
2. EtCo2 monitoring (Ventilation)
3. ABG assessment (BOTH- and most accurate).

## VENTILATION (MEASURED BY CO2)

1. Each of our cells must use oxygen (which is why we breathe O2) and glucose (which is why we eat) to create energy so that we can run all our cells, tissues, and organs.
2. When oxygen is present in this energy making process water, heat, and, carbon dioxide (CO2) are by– products.
3. As oxygen and sugar are metabolized in our body from moment to moment, there is a constant CO2 pressure in the blood that is measurable: normal is 35– 45 mmHg.
4. If we don't breathe within 12-20 times per minute with normal tidal volumes, then we either build up CO2 (from breathing too slow), or we will expel too much (from breathing too fast). Again, this occurs because our body will constantly off loads CO2 at the same rate, and if we are breathing normally, then we can adequately discard the CO2. If we breathe too slow, we build up CO2. If we breathe too fast, then we lose too much CO2. Its all a balancing.

### OXYHEMOGLOBIN DISSOCIATION CURVE

1. There is a SPECIFIC reason for this balance– you ever heard of the oxyhemoglobin disassociation curve? Well, CO2 is a HUGE factor in keeping this curve in its normal place.
2. Researchers have measured the "stickiness" of oxygen to the red blood cell, and they use a graph to describe it (psst– that's the dreaded oxyhemoglobin disassociation curve, let's call it ODC for short).
3. You do not need to know much about the ODC, other than it describes the stickiness (or affinity, to use a bigger word) of oxygen to the RBC (specifically hemoglobin).
4. When you visit a friend in another city, you most likely go to the airport, get on an airplane, fly to where your friend lives, and then get off the plane to head to their home. This is exactly what normally happens to oxygen. Normally, oxygen is bound to hemoglobin by being picked up in the lungs by an RBC (the airport in this analogy), transported in the blood to the tissues (flying to your friend's city), and then, the oxygen wants to jump off the RBC to move into the tissues (just like you do when you land). Would you ever get to the airport and not get on the plane systematically?

Would you ever fly somewhere and not get off the plane? The answer is NO, and oxygen is the same way. It is programmed to get onto the RBC and get off at the tissues.

5. There are situations where oxygen doesn't stick to the RBC very well, and there are conditions where this normal balance of stickiness is influenced to be either stickier or less sticky.

6. Conditions causing oxygen to be LESS sticky (or show less affinity) to hemoglobin on the RBC:
   a. High acid (acidosis)
   b. High CO2
   c. High temperature
   d. High 2,3-DPG (a chemical created by RBCs in low oxygen environments)

7. Conditions causing oxygen to be MORE sticky (or show greater affinity) to hemoglobin on the RBC:
   a. Low acid (aLkalosis)
   b. Low CO2
   c. Low temperature
   d. Low 2,3-DPG
   e. Lots of carbon monoxide

## PUTTING IT TOGETHER

1. Now, get ready to be "Miagi'd" (the gentle old man who taught a kid karate by making him perform chores– you'll thank me later).

2. If you turn a fan on in a room, what happens to the temperature? It gets cooler, correct? Absolutely, it does. Now, where would the temperature be cooler- in your muscles that create heat and energy? Or in your lungs with air coming in and out (like a fan)? The lungs are cooler than other tissues (muscles are warmer).

3. Notice in the above paragraph (bullet f) that "Low temperature" is a cause of MORE sticky? Therefore, greater affinity of oxygen for hemoglobin occurs when the temperature is cooler.

4. Guess what? This isn't just the case in temperature– it's the case for MOST ALL of the "More Sticky" conditions. Most of the "LOW" conditions are related. Can you think of an organ that starts with an 'L'? No, not liver– try again. LUNG! These low conditions are "lung" like, meaning most of these conditions physiologically occur in the lung: cooler temps, not a lot of metabolism (so lower CO2 and less acid), etc.

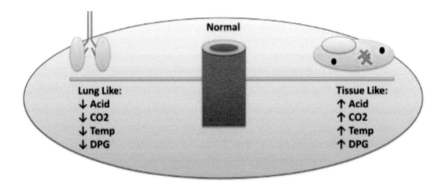

5. The "High" conditions are those found in the distal tissues (like muscles): higher temps (energy production releases heat), higher acid (less oxygen at tissues), higher CO2 (more energy produced in distal tissues), etc.

6. The bottom line: the 'LOWs' are LUNG– like, and the 'HIGHs' are TISSUE– like. This concept allows for better recall than just trying to memorize a list of highs and lows.

7. Lastly, lets tie this all together. When people discuss the oxyhemoglobin dissociation curve, they usually refer to it being shifted to the left or to the right. Guess what? You already know this: Any condition that is placed on a patient that simulates the lung conditions (cooler, less acids, etc.), then the ODC is said to have a left shift. Any condition that mimics the conditions in the tissues is said to shift the OCD to the right.

8. Therefore, with respect to ventilation, which began this tangent, we almost always want to keep the EtCO2 between 35– 45 mmHg. If we do not, then, the RBC will be either too sticky or not sticky enough for O2. Keep EtCO2 in the normal range!

9. EtCO2 and pH Relationship: There may be a situation where both pH and pCO2 are low. In this case, it is important to consider the physiologic observation that an $\uparrow$ pCO2 or EtCO2 relates to a $^-$ of pH by 0.08. Therefore, if there is a low pH and a low EtCO2, reducing minute ventilation would worsen the pH leading to worsening acidosis.

## CORRECTING CO₂

**Correct a HIGH CO2 by:**
1. Increasing tidal volume
2. Increasing respiratory rate
3. Increasing pressure control (if ventilating the patient using pressure ventilation)

**Correct a LOW CO2 by:**
1. Decreasing tidal volume
2. Decreasing respiratory rate
3. Decreasing pressure control (if ventilating the patient using pressure ventilation)

In summary, we need to be aggressive in maintaining good ventilation, which is indicated by an EtCO2/ pCO2 of 35-45 mmHg. Any deviation will cause a left or right shift in the oxyhemoglobin disassociation curve, and will result in too sticky of a RBC or a RBC that is not sticky enough relative to oxygen. RBCs that are too sticky hold on to oxygen instead of allowing the oxygen to offload to the cells (left shift). RBCs that are not sticky enough never grab oxygen in the lung (right shift). Therefore, we strive to keep EtCO2/ pCO2 in between 35-45 mmHg.

# OXYGENATION (MEASURED BY SPO2)

1. Oxygenation describes the delivery of oxygen to the distal tissues for use in metabolism, which is where we derive energy from sugar and oxygen (as mentioned earlier).

2. Basically, we need to bring in oxygenated air into our lungs, then the oxygen needs to cross the alveolar capillary membrane onto a RBC, then the RBC needs to be pumped by the heart around to the tissues, then the oxygen needs to jump off the RBC and into the tissue bed, and finally the oxygen needs to find its way into a cell and into a mitochondria so it can participate in metabolism.

3. Anywhere that oxygen is not allowed to proceed along this path will result in hypoxia, and if uncorrected, will result in acidosis and death.

4. CORRELATION: recall the types of hypoxia describe where oxygen derangements can occur: hypoxic hypoxia, hypemic hypoxia, stagnant hypoxia, and histotoxic hypoxia– the path of oxygen from the air to the tissues.

## The Difference Between SpO2 and PaO2.

**PaO2**
1. PaO2 is the direct measurement of the tension (presence) of oxygen within the blood itself and is obtained from an ABG.
2. It is measured in mmHg.

3. NORMAL: 60-100 mmHg
4. Note: with aggressive BVM ventilation and/ or high FiO2, the PaO2 can get as high as 300-400 mmHg. This is dangerous over time as oxygen in this amounts cause oxygen free radicals to be formed– these O2 molecules destroy normal tissue.

**SpO2**
5. SpO2 is the measurement of the number saturated (taken or filled) spots for oxygen on an RBC compared to the available spots for oxygen on the RBC.
6. It is reported as a percent.
7. NORMAL:  95% or greater

*You can estimate an expected PaO2 from your observed SpO2.*

| Monitored SpO2 | Expected PaO2 |
|---|---|
| 90% | 60mmHg |
| 80% | 50mmHg |
| 70% | 40mmHg |

*CORRECTING SpO$_2$*

**Correct a LOW SpO2 by:**
1. Increasing FiO2
2. Increasing PEEP
3. Reverse I:E Ratio

## THE ARTERIAL BLOOD GAS (ABG) ANALYSIS
1. Like all of the other skills in this text, a systematic approach is needed each time you execute an ABG interpretation.
2. Understanding an ABG can help you make an early intubation decision, as well provide you with information to help you make changes that result in a better oxygenated patient.

*The Players (aka the parameters):*

**pH**
1. The pH represents the concentration of hydrogen ions that are present in the blood. The more hydrogen ions there are translates into the blood being more acidic.
2. However, the pH scale is logarithmic, meaning it is upside down. This means that the LOWER the pH value then the MORE acidic the blood is.
3. NORMAL: 7.35– 7.45
4. Acidic: 7.35 and BELOW
5. Alkalotic: 7.45 and HIGHER

**pCO2**
1. The pCO2 is the tension (or presence) of CO2 in the blood. It is very close to EtCO2.
2. CO2 is known as the "respiratory" component in ABG interpretation. As the pH in our blood gets out of normal range, our respiratory system will kick in first to help to correct it. It can change the pH within MINUTES of changing the respiratory variables (RR and TV).
3. NORMAL: 35– 45 mmHg

**HCO3**
1. The HCO3, or bicarb, is the amount of buffer (a chemical that neutralizes the acid) in our blood.
2. Bicarb is known as the "metabolic" component in ABG interpretation. As the pH in our blood gets out of normal range, our renal system will kick in to assist the respiratory system. It effects change within HOURS to DAYS.
3. NORMAL: 22-26  mmol/L   (or mEq/L)

**Base Excess (BE):**
1. Base excess basically describes all the base added up and compared to the acid present. It is reported in a positive or negative number. Positive numbers mean there is a lot of base in excess, and negative numbers mean there is a deficit of base (not much) in the blood.
2. Normal: 2 to –2 mEq/L
3. Oxygen PaO2)
4. NORMAL:  60– 100 mmHg

The major players are the pH, the pCO2, and the HCO3. These are the ones that will tell us the most about what's going on with our patient.

## The Parts of the ABG Interpretation

Generally, we need to identify 3 parts of any ABG. Approaching the ABG in this way simplifies the skill. The easier a skill can be, the more likely you'll be about to use it in the field, and the more accurate you will be as well.

**First Part: Acidity**
1. The first thing to look at is the pH.
2. If the pH is acidic (< 7.35), then we have identified there is ACIDOSIS present.
3. If the pH is alkalotic (> 7.45), then ALKALOSIS is present.

**Second Part: The Culprit**
1. The second thing to look at is the culprit– which component (respiratory or metabolic) is at fault for the acidosis or alkalosis. A low HCO3 and high CO2 is acidic, while a low CO2 and high HCO3 is alkalotic.
2. If you determine that the CO2 matches the pH, then the RESPIRATORY component is the culprit, so then you'd put 'respiratory' in front of either acidosis or alkalosis in nomenclature.
3. If you determine that the HCO3 matches the pH, then the METABOLIC component is the culprit, so then you'd put 'metabolic' in front of either acidosis or alkalosis in nomenclature.

**Third Part: Compensation**
1. The third part tells us if any compensation is occurring (meaning are the respiratory/ metabolic components are attempting to normalize the pH).
2. To understand this, consider a patient without any illness.
3. Their pH begins within the normal range.

4.  Let's say they OD on narcotics and almost quit breathing. Not breathing means less oxygen in the tissues (leading to acidosis) and the low respiratory rate prevents getting rid of CO2 (worsening the acidosis). Their pH now begins to drop (so they are becoming ACIDIC).

5.  Since the breathing caused the acidosis, then the culprit is the RESPIRATORY component.

6.  As this condition first begins, only the respiratory component is acting on the pH– and there is no compensation, and it is termed ACUTE.

7.  If this condition were allowed to continue, eventually the renal system would jump in and start helping– this would be termed PARTIALLY COMPENSATION. In this case, the respiratory component would match the pH, but the metabolic component would not match.

8.  Now, if the condition were allowed to continue getting worse, then the renal system would work hard enough to correct the problem that it actually pushes the pH barely into the normal range. In this case, you'd see a barely normal pH, the respiratory component that was acidotic and the metabolic component was alkalotic. FULLY COMPENSATED.

9.  As it continues to worsen, the metabolic component would fail, and both CO2 and HCO3 would become acidic. This is MIXED.

10. Compensation is a continuum from normal to really bad. Ultimately, you will need to match the components to the pH and identify the level of compensation.

## The MeduPros Method

### STEP #1: Assign each parameter as acidic- like, alkalotic- like, or normal.

1.  Imagine this patient: pH 7.2/ pCO2 66/ HCO3 23

2.  If the components are outside of normal ranges, they can behave like acids and bases.

    a.  CO2 higher than 45 mmHg = ACIDOTIC
    b.  HCO3 higher than 26 mmol/L = ALKALOTIC
    c.  CO2 lower than 35 mmHg = ALKALOTIC
    d.  HCO3 lower than 22 mmol/L = ACIDOTIC

3.  Use this to assign a status to the pH and each component: normal, acidotic, or alkalotic.

4.  The pH is 7.2, so it is assigned as ACIDIC. The HCO3 is 23 mmol/L, so it is assigned as NORMAL. The CO2 is 66 mmHg, so it is assigned as ACIDIC.

### Step #2: Identify which component is the culprit of the pH problem. Circle those that match and put the names together

1.  In this case, the pH is acidic, so ACIDOSIS is present.

2.  Which component caused it? CO2 (the respiratory component) caused it because it matches the pH problem.

3.  Circle and put the names together. As you can see below, since both the pH and the CO2 match (acidic) it is respiratory acidosis.

### STEP #3: Assess for acuteness or compensation

1.  Abnormal pH with 1 normal component and 1 abnormal component = ACUTE

2.  Abnormal pH with both components abnormal (where one matches the pH, and one doesn't)= PARTIALLY COMPENSATED

3.  NORMAL pH with both components abnormal = FULLY COMPENSATED

    a.  In these cases, normal pH will be narrowed to 7.4 for the purpose of interpretation.
    b.  is considered alkalotic- like
    c.  7.39 is considered acidotic- like

4.  ALL match (pH, CO2, and HCO3) = MIXED

5.  3 "No" Rule: if all three (3) values answer 'No' to the question, "are these values normal," then you have a partially compensated condition.

6.  This is an achievable skill with practice.

7. EXAMPLES:
   a. Example 1: pH 7.35/ pCO2 66/ HCO3 30 (Fully compensated respiratory acidosis)
   b. Example 2: pH 7.12/ pCO2 67/ HCO3 12 (Mixed Acidosis)
   c. Example 3: pH 7.52/ pCO2 34/ HCO3 30 (Partially-compensated metabolic Alkalosis)

# PART 3: RESPIRATORY CONDITONS

## INTRODUCTION

You will be exposed, repeatedly, to moderately complex respiratory conditions, and at times, you will be forced to contend with a highly complex medical situation. Fix what you can fix and treat what you can treat. Use medical control if needed.

Consider using a system I use to study where I know the 3 domains of a medical condition: Pathophysiology, Assessment (S/S), and Management, or PAM for short. If you know the pathophysiology of a condition, you should be able to describe the signs and symptoms, as well as how to manage the condition. Similarly, if you are provided with a series of treatments, you should be able to backtrack (usually with a little history) what the pathophysiology is and therefore how to identify it. Finally, if someone gives you a set of signs and symptoms, then you should be able to identify the condition and the management. So, you see, from any of these domains are known, then you should be able to figure out the other two. Therefore, we will study the content in this way.

To recall the important pathophysiologies- those that could immediately kill the patient, or that will do so within hours, I use the pneumonic **A CAP APP**. There are a few other conditions mentioned after these in the pages below, but this is what I memorize to be able to identify and manage the primary conditions.

**A** is for ARDS.

**C** is for COPD (emphysema and chronic bronchitis)

**A** is for asthma/ status asthmaticus.

**P** is for pulmonary embolism.

**A** is for allergy/angioedema/ anaphylaxis.

**P** is for pneumonia.

**P** is for pneumothorax.

## PRIMARY CONDITIONS

### Acute Respiratory Distress Syndrome (ARDS)

1. Patho: Lung injury from disease or illness--> prolonged inflammatory response in lungs--> decrease in lung compliance (wooden box lung)--> higher pressure in lungs--> reduced blood flow into lungs--> multiple  types of hypoxia
2. S/S: Hx lung injury/ illness, progressive hypoxia, bilateral infiltrates (x-ray), PCWP < 18 mmHg and no left atrial HTN, PaO2/ FiO2 of < 100mmHg
3. MGT: keep SpO2 >90%; minimize FiO2 to maintain this SpO2; maximize PEEP, PC ventilation, reverse I:E

### COPD: Emphysema

1. Patho: airway collapse distal to terminal bronchioles (mainly alveolar)--> loss of alveolar surface area--> poor gas exchange (increase in CO2)--> hyperinflation and air trapping
2. S/S: dyspnea, wheezing, pursed lip breathing, barrel chest; poor air movement upon auscultation; a cough (with or without sputum)
3. MGT: keep SpO2 >90%; bronchodilators; corticosteroids; consider antibiotics, CPAP, and intubation

### COPD: Chronic Bronchitis

1. Patho: airway plugging with collapse of bronchioles--> no alveolar loss, but inflammation--> influx of inflammatory cells--> narrowing of small airways due to fibrosis, inflammation, mucus--> poor air movement and hypoxia
2. S/S: REFRACTORY: dyspnea, wheezing, pursed lip breathing, barrel chest; poor air movement upon auscultation; a cough (with or without sputum)
3. MGT: keep SpO2 >90%; bronchodilators; corticosteroids; consider antibiotics, CPAP, and intubation

### Asthma

1. Patho: hypersensitivity--> bronchial inflammation--> bronchospasm--> wheezing and dyspnea--> hypoxia
2. S/S: dyspnea, wheezing, cough, absent wheezing in worst cases (no air movement), 1-2-word dyspnea
3. MGT: Keep SpO2 >90%; bronchodilators; corticosteroids (PO if a mild case, IV if severe); H1 blocker (diphenhydramine), consider epinephrine, mag sulfate, terbutaline, heliox in severe cases

### Status Asthmaticus

1. Patho: hypersensitivity--> bronchial inflammation--> REFRACTORY bronchospasm--> wheezing and dyspnea despite home or initial treatments--> hypoxia
2. S/S: REFRACTORY: dyspnea, wheezing, cough, absent wheezing in worst cases (no air movement), 1-2 word dyspnea
3. MGT: SpO2 >90%; bronchodilators; corticosteroids (PO if mild case, IV if severe); WILL PROBABLY NEED AT LEAST ONE OF THESE: intubation, epinephrine, mag sulfate, terbutaline, heliox in severe cases. Intubate patients with CO2 > 55 mmHg.

### Pulmonary Embolism

1. Patho: an embolus (any source) travels into through heart and lodges in a pulmonary artery--> lung parenchyma infarction--> vent/ perfusion mismatch
2. S/S: rapid onset; (+) D-dimer; dyspnea; pleuritic chest pain; Hx of DVT
3. MGT: Anticoagulation; IV fluids/ pressors (if low BP); fibrinolysis (if not contraindicated)

## Allergy/ Angioedema

1. Patho: hypersensitivity due to histamine release from over active immune system--> uticaria, itching, wheezing (bronchospasm) and hypotension
2. S/S: dyspnea, wheezing, cough, absent wheezing in worst cases (no air movement), 1-2-word dyspnea
3. MGT: Keep SpO2 >90%; antihistamines: H1 blocker (diphenhydramine), H2 blocker (Famotidine or Ranitidine); bronchodilators; corticosteroids (PO if a mild case, IV if severe); consider epinephrine, mag sulfate, terbutaline, heliox in severe cases

## Pneumonia

1. Patho: infection of lung parenchyma--> inflammation, exudates, and consolidation
2. S/S: fever, adventitious breath sounds; productive cough; X-ray- infiltrates/ effusion; hypoxemic ABG; elevated WBCs
3. MGT: maximize oxygenation; isolation prn; broad spectrum antibiotic with also a high-power narrow target antibiotic; admit  to hospital if pt is hypoxemic or seemingly toxic

## Aspiration Pneumonia

1. Patho: AMS (from any mechanism)--> inhaled vomitus/food--> acute inflammation--> lung exudates--> hypoxia
2. S/S: fever, adventitious breath sounds; productive cough; X-ray- infiltrates/ effusion; elevated WBCs
3. MGT: prevent further aspiration; maximize oxygenation; isolation prn; broad spectrum antibiotic with also a high power narrow target antibiotic; admit if pt is hypoxemic or seemingly toxic

## Pneumothorax

1. Patho: free air in intrapleural space--> reduced lung volume--> hypoxia (size dependent)
2. S/S: acute dyspnea; unequal chest expansion; decreased fremitus; hyper resonant; decreased breath sounds; X-ray- reduced lateral lung margins
3. MGT: maximize oxygenation; consider needle decompression with 15-30% deflated lung (X-ray required to know this); consider chest tube if >30% lung deflated. Immediate needle decompression (tension pneumothorax only)

# OTHER CONDITIONS

## Pulmonary Hypertension

1. Patho: Damage to the small blood vessels in the lungs from COPD-->difficult to pump blood through the lungs--> increased blood pressure in the lungs--> SOB/ fatigue/ pulmonary edema
2. S/S: fatigue, chest discomfort, tachypnea, dyspnea with exercise; peripheral edema, JVD; Large right heart border on chest X-ray
3. MGT: maximize O2, Ca blocker, digoxin, diuretics, consider: prostacyclin analogue, Nitrous Oxide, PDE5 inhibitors

## Acidosis (General)

1. We have spent considerable time discussing how to identify if we are oxygenating our patients adequately.  However, what if we arrive and they already are acidotic?
2. Anytime we assess that oxygen is not adequately being taken from the atmosphere and transported to our patient's tissues, then, aggressive basic and advanced skills should be employed to correct the acidosis caused by inadequate oxygen supply and delivery.
3. If you cannot clearly identify and diagnose the current clinical problems, we can always fall back on basics and assess, prevent, and treat acidosis.

4. Preventing Acidosis:
    a. Ensure Oxygenation: ↑ FiO2, ↑ PEEP, Reduce/ invert the I:E ratio
    b. Ensure Ventilation:
        i. Normalize the EtCO2 (make changes to the RR and either TV or PC)
        ii. By preventing an abnormally high EtCO2, you reduce the amount of acid floating through the bloodstream, thus prevent or reduce acidosis.
        iii. The bicarbonate buffer system is the chemical pathway that helps to regulate the blood by changing CO2 into acid, or acid back into CO2. This reaction goes both directions depending on how much CO2 or how much acid is in the system. If there is lots of acid in our body, then the bicarbonate buffer system will break that acid into CO2 so that we can exhale it, reducing acidosis. If there is too little amount of acid, then our body will hold onto CO2 (by reducing breathing efforts) and convert it into acid.
        iv. With a patient on the ventilator, we can help this bicarbonate buffer system out by keeping the patient's EtCO2 in between 35- 45 mmHg.
    c. Ensure Blood Pressure: by maintaining an adequate blood pressure, you are ensuring the red blood cell can make it to the distal tissues so it can offload oxygen for cellular use.
5. Assessing for Acidosis:
    a. History and physical exam consistent with conditions or situations that could lead to pour oxygenation/ perfusion which when can subsequently lead to acidosis.
    b. Low SpO2: indicates no oxygen in the red blood cell at the level of the tissues
    c. No radial pulse: indicates that blood pressure is not adequate to get the red blood cell to the distal tissues
    d. High EtCO2:
        i. Indicates a buildup of  CO2, most likely from the body try to get rid of acid via the bicarbonate buffer system. This could also be caused by a decrease in respiratory effort.
        ii. Changes in EtCO2 of 10 mmHg equates to a change in pH of 0.08 (or about 0.1). It is uncommon to have to calculate this on the certification exams, but I would still commit it to memory.
    e. High Lactate: Lactate elevates when anaerobic metabolism occurs for too long of a period.
    f. Low pH (acidosis): this is a direct measure of the acid content in the blood. They confirmed low pH (less than 7.35) required immediate and aggressive treatment to correct the acidosis. Acidosis that is allowed to continue too long can kill patients.
    g. Acidosis-induced hyperkalemia:
        i. As your pH drops to dangerously low levels, your body will take those hydrogen ions (acids) and exchange them for potassium. This results in a falsely high potassium.
        ii. Every change in pH of 0.1, the potassium changes 0.6 in the opposite direction. Therefore, if pH is 7.4 and changes to 7.3 (a reduction), the in the potassium will increase. If it started out at 4.4 mmol/L, then it would be 5.0 mmol/L after the change in pH.
6. Correcting Acidosis: be aggressive with oxygenation, ventilation, stabilizing/maintaining blood pressure. Aggressive fluid resuscitation, pressers, and mechanical ventilation may be necessary.

## *Respiratory Acidosis*
1. Patho: this occurs when the respiratory effort is inadequate to remove enough carbon dioxide to maintain a normal pH. This can be caused by drug overdose or damage to the respiratory center that results in a reduced respiratory rate.
2. S/S: pH less than 7.35 and pCO2 (or EtCO2) greater than 45 mmHg.
3. MGT: increase minute ventilation (RR and/or either TV or PC) to remove excess CO2.

### Respiratory Alkalosis

1. Patho: this occurs with conditions that cause hyperventilation: TBI/ stroke/ DKA.
2. S/S: pH greater than 7.45 and pCO2 (or EtCO2) less than 35 mmHg.
3. MGT: reduce minute ventilation (RR and/or either TV or PC) to retain CO2.

### Metabolic Acidosis

1. Patho: this occurs when the renal system is inadequate in removing enough systemic acids to maintain a normal pH. This can be caused by renal failure, DKA, cellular poisons (cyanide, CO).
2. S/S: pH less than 7.35 and HCO3 less than 22 mmol/L.
3. Anion Gap Metabolic Acidosis: Quick trick to identify metabolic acidosis: Add up ([Na+] + [K+]) – ([Cl-] + [HCO3–]) . If this equation yields a value of 11 or more, then anion gap metabolic acidosis is present.
4. MGT: correct oxygenation and perfusion. Fluid resuscitation.

### Metabolic Alkalosis

1. Patho: this occurs with conditions that cause a decrease in hydrogen ions (acid) or an increase in bicarbonate (HCO3). Vomiting/ GI suctioning and reducing acid, while aldosteronism will increase HCO3.
2. S/S: pH greater than 7.45 and HCO3 greater than 26 mmHg.
3. MGT: fix cause; fluid resuscitation; fix electrolytes (see chapter 13)

# PART 4: RESPIRATORY PHARMACOLOGY

## INTRODUCTION

One of the most important concepts in pharmacology is understanding the mechanism by which the medicine works. If we see that the patient is experiencing bronchospasm, then we need to choose a drug that will open the airways. There are a few ways (or mechanisms) by which this can be done. Understanding pharmacological mechanisms will give you the tools to successfully choose medications, both in the field and on your critical care certification exams.

For each medication, class, mechanism, indications, contraindications, hemodynamics, and dosing will be discussed. In some cases, extra notes will be added if necessary. The hemodynamics portion provides central venous pressure (CVP), pulmonary capillary wedge pressure (PCWP), cardiac output (CO), and systemic vascular resistance (SVR). There are others, but I feel this is a great set of data to assess the patient's hemodynamic status. If you see an up arrow (X), then this medication will likely increase that value following administration. If there is a downward pointing arrow (X) next to one of these hemodynamic parameters, then it is likely the medication with reduce that parameter. If the parameter has this sign (~), then there is no expected effect to that parameter. SWEARINGEN'S RESOURCE AND STUDY GUIDE FOR CRITICAL CARE TRANSPORT CLINICIANS is the only textbook with these broken down. They have been betted by multiple PhDs in pharmacology.

## MEDICATIONS

### Albuterol

1. Class: Beta agonist
2. Mechanism: Stimulates the beta 2 receptor, which relaxes bronchiole smooth muscle, which causes bronchodilation.
3. Indications: Acute bronchospasm (from COPD, asthma, allergic reaction) or any other cause of bronchoconstriction.
4. Contraindications: tachycardia, hypertension, dysrhythmia
5. Hemodynamics: (~CVP/ ~PCWP/~CO/~SVR).
6. Adult/Peds Dose: 2.5 mg in 3 mL NS and nebulized
7. Infant Dose: 1.25 mg in 3 mL NS and nebulized

### Ipratropium Bromide

1. Class: Anticholinergic Bronchodilator
2. Mechanism: blocks acetylcholine with results in bronchial smooth muscle relaxation
3. Indications: Acute bronchospasm (from COPD, asthma, allergic reaction) or any other cause of bronchoconstriction.
4. Contraindications: hypersensitivity
5. Hemodynamics: (~CVP/ ~PCWP/~CO/~SVR).
6. Adult/Peds Dose: 500 mcg every 4-6 hours

### Xopenex

1. Class: Beta agonist (more specific than albuterol)
2. Mechanism: Stimulates the beta 2 receptor, which relaxes bronchiole smooth muscle which causes bronchodilation.
3. Indications: Acute bronchospasm (from COPD, asthma, allergic reaction or any other cause of bronchoconstriction.
4. Contraindications: tachycardia, hypertension, PEDS < 6 years
5. Hemodynamics: (~CVP/ ~PCWP/~CO/~SVR).
6. Adult Dose: 0.63– 1.25 mg in 3 cc NS and nebulized every 4-6 hours
7. Peds Dose: 0.31– 0.63 mg in 3 cc NS and nebulized every 4-6 hours

### Methylprednisolone (Solumedrol)

1. Class: glucocorticoid
2. Mechanism: steroid that has both immunosuppressive and anti– inflammatory properties
3. Indications: reduces the inflammatory causes of bronchospasm
4. Contraindications: hypersensitivity
5. Hemodynamics: (~CVP/ ~PCWP/~CO/~SVR).
6. Dose: 1-2 mg/kg IV

### Magnesium Sulfate

1. Class: Electrolyte, Muscle relaxant
2. Mechanism: decreases the excitability of muscles, therefore, relaxes skeletal and smooth muscle reduces BP, relaxes uterine contractions, bronchodilates, slows HR.
3. Indications: **refractory** bronchospasm, ventricular tachycardia refractory to other treatments, eclampsia, tocolysis for pregnancy
4. Contraindications: Bradycardia, hypotension, heart block
5. Hemodynamics: (↓CVP/ ↓PCWP/↓CO/↓SVR).
6. Adult Dose 1-2 g administered IV over 10-20 minutes
7. Peds Dose: 25-50 mg/kg IV

## Epinephrine

1. Class: Vasopressor, Sympathomimetic, bronchodilator
2. Mechanism: Markedly stimulates both the alpha and beta receptors; therefore, significant increases in heart rate, blood pressure, and cardiac output occur.
3. Indications: hypotension, low cardiac output, poor perfusion, pulseless ventricular tachycardia, ventricular fibrillation, pulseless electrical activity
4. Contraindications: Hypertension, tachycardia, acute coronary syndromes, hypersensitivity
5. Hemodynamics: (↑CVP/ ↑PCWP/↑CO/↑SVR).
6. Dose: 1-30 mg/min (typical therapeutic use is ~8-12)
7. Hypotension, adults:1- 4 mg/min
8. Anaphylaxis, adults: 0.1-.05 mg SQ/IM

9. Hypotension, pediatric: 0.1- 1.0 mg/min
10. Anaphylaxis, pediatric: 0.01 mg/kg SQ/IM

## Terbutaline

1. Class: Bronchodilator, smooth muscle relaxant (uterine relaxant)
2. Mechanism: Stimulates the beta 2 receptor, which relaxes bronchiole smooth muscle which causes bronchodilation.
3. Indications: Acute bronchospasm (from COPD, asthma, allergic reaction or any other cause of bronchoconstriction; to achieve tocolysis
4. Contraindications: Hypertension, tachycardia, acute coronary syndromes, hypersensitivity, concurrent digitalis therapy
5. Hemodynamics: (↑CVP/ ↑PCWP/↑CO/↑SVR)
6. Dose: 0.25 mg SQ every 15 minutes to a max of 0.5 in 4 hours.
7. Peds Dose: 0.01 mg/kg (max 0.4) every 15 minutes for total of 2 doses

## Diphenhydramine

1. Class: histamine 1 blocker
2. Mechanism: blocks histamine which reduces the effects of histamine release (angioedema, hypotension, etc.).
3. Indications: allergic reactions, anaphylactic reactions
4. Contraindications: none
5. Hemodynamics: (~CVP/ ~PCWP/~CO/~SVR).
6. Adult Dose: 10– 50 mg IV; avoid more than 25 mg/min administration.
7. Peds Dose: 1 mg/kg IV or IM

## Heparin

1. Class: Anticoagulant
2. Mechanism: Blocks the conversion of both prothrombin → thrombin and fibrinogen → fibrin, therefore, it prevents future clots from forming. It does not dissolve existing clots.
3. Indications: AMI, PE, A-fib, DIC
4. Contraindications: bleeding tendencies, thrombocytopenia (low platelets in the blood), intracranial hemorrhage
5. Hemodynamics: (~CVP/ ~PCWP/~CO/~SVR).
6. Dose:
7. Adults: 5000 units IV bolus; then maintenance infusion of 1000 units/hr
8. Peds: 50 units/kg IVP initially; maintenance infusion 50-100 units/kg IVP q 4 hours

### Alteplase (t-PA)

1. Class: Fibrinolytic
2. Mechanism: Causes the release of plasminogen, which is then converted into plasmin. Plasmin destroys fibrin (the clot's glue) therefore the clot breaks up, and blood flow is restored.
3. Indications: Active AMI, ischemic stroke, acute PE
4. Contraindications: bleeding tendencies, uncontrolled hypertension
5. Hemodynamics: (~CVP/ ~PCWP/~CO/~SVR).
6. Dose:
   a. Pulmonary Embolism: 100 mg over 2 hours
   b. AMI
      i. If >65 kg; 15 mg IVP over 2 minutes, followed by 50 mg IV over the next 30 minutes, followed by 35 mg IV over the next 60 minutes.
      ii. If < 65 kg; 15 mg IVP over 2 minutes, followed by 0.75 mg/kg IV over the next 30 minutes, followed by 0.5 mg/kg IV over the next 60 minutes.
   c. Ischemic Stroke: 0.9 mg/kg IV (max 90 mg) with first 10% of dose given over 1 minute

# PART 5: RESPIRATORY LAB VALUES

## INTRODUCTION

There are a handful of labs that can help assess the reason for breathing difficulty. In this section, we will look into several of these labs.

## MAIN LAB VALUES

### SpO2 monitoring

1. Reflects oxygenation
2. Norm: >94%
3. Corrective actions: ↑FiO2 and PEEP

### EtCO2 monitoring

1. Reflects ventilation
2. Norm: 35- 45 mmHg
3. Corrective actions: ↑ or ↓ RR, TV, or PC

### ABG: Arterial blood gas analysis

1. Oxygenation status
2. Adequacy of ventilation
3. Acid-base balance

## ADDIOTNAL LAB VALUES

### D- dimer

1. This lab value is a degradation product of fibrin. After a clot is formed, it begins to degrade and releases D-dimer into the bloodstream. It is used primarily to rule out DVT/ PE/ thrombosis rather than confirm it. It is more reliable with a negative result than with a positive result.
2. Normal:
    a. US: 250 [ng/L]
    b. SI: 250 [mg/L]
3. HIGH: Potential DVT/PE/thrombosis/DIC
4. LOW: VERY LITTLE CHANCE OF ANY THROMBOSIS

### Prothrombin Time (PT)

1. PT is a measure of the extrinsic pathway of coagulation and it tells us the clotting tendency of blood. Increased values tells us clotting occurs faster.
2. Normal:  11.4– 14.2 seconds
3. HIGH: DIC, massive transfusion, vitamin K deficiency, warfarin therapy

### International Normalized Ratio (INR)

1. The INR is very similar to the PT value; however, it is mathematically "normalized". It is a measure of the extrinsic pathway of coagulation and it tells us the clotting tendency of blood.  Increased values tells us clotting occurs faster.
2. Normal:  0.9– 1.2 second(s)
3. HIGH: DIC, massive transfusion, vitamin K deficiency, warfarin therapy

### Lactate

1. Produced in large amounts during anaerobic metabolism
2. Norm: 4-20 mg/dL (SI = 0.5-2 mmol/L)
3. Critical Value:
    a. >45 mg/dL this indicates that there is ischemic disease or hypoperfusion, or both
    b. (SI >4.5 mmol/L) this indicates that there is ischemic disease or hypoperfusion, or both

# PART 6: MANAGING THE MECHANICAL VENTILATED PATIENT

## INTRODUCTION

The ventilated patient provides several challenges that the critical care clinician must be able to navigate. Historically, the mechanical ventilator has proven to be a frightening piece of equipment in the critical care transport environment. With minimal study time, any clinician can learn to utilize this piece of equipment with confidence.

## MECHANICAL VENTILATION BASICS

### Types of Ventilation

**Volume Control Ventilation:**
1. this is a type of ventilation where air is forced into a patient's lungs until a particular volume of air in the lungs is reached. At this point the ventilator stops airflow into the patient's lungs.
2. This is a common setting in adult patients with relatively healthy lungs.
3. This type of ventilation can guarantee tidal volume, but not pressure. This means that you can guarantee a particular tidal volume, but the pressure will vary from breath to breath (pressure is variable).

**Pressure Control Ventilation:**
1. this type of ventilation is characterized by air being forced into a patient's lungs until a particular pressure is reached, and then the ventilator stops airflow to the patient's lungs.
2. This is a common ventilation type in the pediatric population and patients with damaged or diseased lungs.
3. This type of ventilation guarantees a particular pressure is never exceeded, however the breath to breath volume is variable.

### Modes of Ventilation

**Controlled Mandatory Ventilation (CMV)**
1. This mode of ventilation is as basic as it gets. There is no sensing of the machine for what the patient is doing.
2. Initially, you set the rate and tidal volume (very few transport ventilators offer CMV with a pressure setting). On fully programmable ventilators, like those in the hospital that respiratory therapists use, CMV can easily be set to pressure control ventilation. Here you'd set the rate and pressure control (PC) setting. IF EtCO2 was too low, you'd back off the PC setting. Conversely, if the EtCO2 was too high, then you'd increase the PC setting.
3. The danger with this mode is the result of the patient taking in a full breath in on their own (for instance if they begin waking up) and then the ventilator delivers a full pre-set breath before exhalation. This can result in twice the volume into the lung at one time- causing barotrauma if too high of pressures are reached and volutrauma over time.

4. Please note, in the picture titled, CMV with a Paralyzed Patient, the tidal volume is set at 500 (green color) and the patient is receiving that 500 mL (red) with each breath. The pressure is remaining the same (20 cmH2O PIP- also in green).

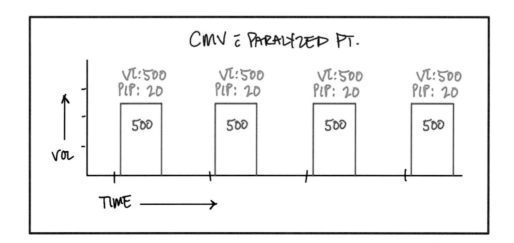

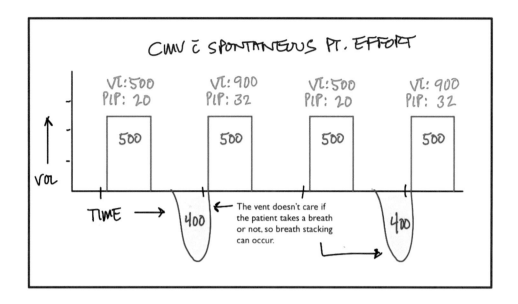

5. In these graphics, you'll see they are drafted based on volume (y-axis) and time (x-axis). On the x-axis, you'll note black hash marks, and they usually precede the machine breath (in red). The distance between each hashmark illustrates 1 breath interval (inhalation plus exhalation).

6. When the patient is paralyzed or completely apneic for another reason, they never attempt a breath. A Patient triggered breath is noted below the x-axis in blue.

7. In the second graphic, titled CMV with Spontaneous Respirations, you see downward deflections or volume- this is additive to the total volume. As you can see in the second graphic and after the first machine breath (in red), the patient takes a breath and inhales 400 mL of tidal volume before the machine is triggered (by the timing of the set respiratory rate) and then it delivers the pre-set 500 mL tidal volume. This results in a total of 900 mL of tidal volume at a single time. This happens again at the end of the graphic and is referred to as double-stacking breaths- one part of the patient's doing and the other the ventilator's part.

8. The dangers here include the potential for barotrauma and volutrauma. **Barotrauma** is due to over-pressurization as lung tissue, essentially damaged by crushing forces of the pressure (note the PIP in green when the double-stacking is occurring- it is 32 cmH2O). **Volumtrauma** is due to over-distention of the lung tissue, essentially stretching the lung tissue to microfailure resulting in injury.

9. If you are ever using CMV, be sure to keep your patients very sedated and/or pain controlled, and potentially paralyzed since any respiratory effort can result in disastrous effects on volutrauma and barotrauma.


**Assist Control (A/C)**

1. This is a mode of ventilation that is characterized by the ventilator recognizing each time the patient attempts to breathe and then delivering the preset tidal volume or preset pressure control.

2. Initially if you set the rate, and if the patient does not initiate a breath, then the ventilator will deliver breaths at this rate.

3. However, should the patient begin to initiate a breath, the ventilator will recognize it and deliver the entire tidal preset volume (if on volume ventilation) or pressure (if on pressure ventilation) that is set.

4. This means that if the patient is not adequately sedated, then the patient could be triggering a much higher minute ventilation than you set on the ventilator.

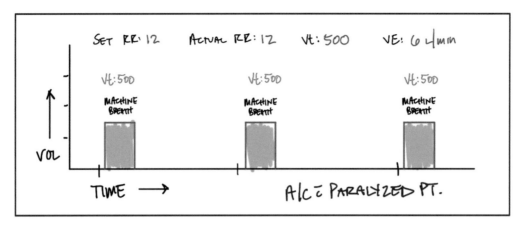

SET RR: 12    ACTUAL RR: 12    Vt: 500    VE: 6 L/min

Vt: 500          Vt: 500          Vt: 500

MACHINE          MACHINE          MACHINE
BREATH           BREATH           BREATH

VOL

TIME →                        A/C c̄ PARALYZED PT.

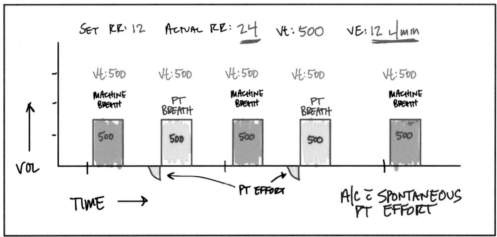

SET RR: 12    ACTUAL RR: 24    Vt: 500    VE: 12 L/min

Vt: 500    Vt: 500    Vt: 500    Vt: 500    Vt: 500

MACHINE     PT      MACHINE     PT      MACHINE
BREATH    BREATH    BREATH    BREATH    BREATH

500    500    500    500    500

VOL

TIME →              PT EFFORT        A/C c̄ SPONTANEOUS
                                        PT EFFORT

5. Example: You set the ventilator on 500 tidal volume and 12 RR, so the minute ventilation should be 6 L/min. If the patient is over breathing the vent at 20, then the real minute ventilation is 10 L/min.

6. As you can see above, if the patient is apneic for any reason, then the machine will deliver a set tidal volume or pressure control breath at the set respiratory rate.

7. Additionally, if the patient is not well sedated or paralyzed, then they will be able to trigger a breath on their own. Each time this happens in A/C, the vent recognizes this and provides a full preset tidal volume or pressure. The vent "assists" them in their effort. This can allow for over–breathing the vent and high minute volumes.

8. The take home message is this: the patient can easily over-breathe the preset ventilation rate, resulting in very high minute volumes, so be sure to sedate your patient adequately.

9. Please look at the graphic titled, A/C with a Paralyzed Patient. Recall in these graphics, you'll see they are drafted based on volume (y-axis) and time (x-axis). On the x-axis, you'll note black hash marks, and they usually precede the machine breath (in red). The distance between each hashmark illustrates 1 breath interval (inhalation plus exhalation).

10. Note there is essentially no difference in 'A/C with a Paralyzed Patient' and 'CMV with a Paralyzed Patient'. Both display machine breaths at the beginning of each interval, deliver 500 mL tidal volume, and exhibit no patient effort. We will revisit this and expand on its importance after SIMV coming up.

11. In the graphic titled, A/C with Spontaneous Patient Effort, you'll observe 2 different colors of breaths: red and blue. Red represents the machine-triggered breaths while blue represents the patient-triggered breaths.

12. Since both colored breaths are above the x-axis, they are all powered by the ventilator. Recall in CMV, the patient breath went BELOW the x-axis. In assist-control ventilation, each time the patient *ATTEMPTS* a breath, the machine (the vent) senses this patient attempt and initiates a full pre-set volume or pressure delivery (depending if you are in volume control or pressure control ventilation). The patient only inhales a few mL of air (via their diaphragm-aka negative pressure ventilation) before the vent senses this and begins a positive pressure ventilation of the pre-set volume or pressure. You can see this occurring with the small blue negative deflections, followed by almost immediate upward waveform (in red).

13. Note each breath in A/C, both in the paralyzed patient and the breathing patient, all fill to the same volume- 500 mL. This is the benefit of A/C mode- it ensures a full pre-set volume or breath WITH EACH AND EVERY BREATH. If the machine is triggered for a breath by time (RR) or by the patient's effort because they are awake, they we receive the set volume or pressure EVERY TIME. While this prevents double-stacking breaths, it can result in very large minute volumes if the patient is not paralyzed and/or sedated.

14. Note at the top of the graphic, A/C with a Paralyzed Patient, the set RR is 12, the measured RR is 12, the Vt is 500, and therefore the minute ventilation (VE) is 6 L/min (500 mL x 12 RR = 6000 mL, or 6 L/min). This is all as expected if you set a RR of 12 and a Vt of 500. Now examine the graphic, A/C with Spontaneous Patient Effort. You'll note the set RR is 12, the measured RR is NOT 12, but rather 24, the Vt is still 500, and therefore the minute ventilation (VE) is 12 L/min (500 mL x 24 RR = 12000 mL, or 12 L/min). This is due to the patient over-breathing the ventilator by 1 extra breath per 1 machine breath. It DOUBLES the minute ventilation, which illustrates the danger of A/C- without sufficient paralysis and/or sedation, the patient could wake up and begin to over-breathe the ventilator resulting in high minute volumes causing a drop in EtCO2 and an increasing pH (alkalosis).

15. If you are ever using A/C, be sure to keep your patients very sedated and/or pain controlled, and potentially paralyzed since any respiratory effort can result in disastrous effects on minute ventilation and pH.

**Synchronous Intermittent Mandatory Ventilation (SIMV)**

1. Initially, this mode is like A/C in that it senses the patient's efforts and assists their breathing effort.

2. The difference is that SIMV ensures the FIRST breath in a breath interval is a full breath, achieved by delivering the pre-set volume or pressure. Subsequent breath attempts in that same breath interval can continue physiologically- meaning the patient can breathe on their own (negative pressure ventilation) using their own diaphragm. This prevents the full ventilation with each breath attempt, and thus minimizes the excess minute ventilation caused by over breathing. Additionally, allowing the patient to take breaths on their own helps to wean them off the vent, and this is achieved by reducing the RR as the patient begins to breathe more often and with greater strength.

3. Just like in assist control, you preset the rate and if the patient does not attempt to breathe, then the ventilator will deliver breaths at that preset rate.

4. If the patient attempts to take a breath, and this attempt occurs near the beginning of a breath interval, the ventilator will detect this effort and provide the full preset volume or pressure. Recall that this is exactly what happens in assist control mode.

5. If the patient takes a breath after the beginning of a breath interval, then the ventilator will allow the patient to take a breath using their own power. The volume that is drawn into the lungs during these patient– powered breaths are dependent upon the patient's own respiratory strength.

6. What makes this mode different and unique is that it allows the patient to take breaths on their own in-between the mandatory breaths.

7. Notice how the above SIMV schematic looks exactly like assist control when there is no patient effort? What differentiates all these modes is what happens when the PATIENT takes a breath on their own while on the mechanical ventilator.

8. In this mode, each time the patient takes a breath on their own, it is either processed as an A/C (if close to the beginning of the breath interval) or as a patient– powered breath (if the attempt is NOT close to the beginning of the breath interval). This allows for a unique situation where you can allow the patient to use their own respiratory muscles to take a breath. Also, you can enhance that breath by providing a 'turbo boost' during the patient– powered attempt. This 'turbo boost'.

9. manifests in the form of positive airway pressure. This turbo boost is called pressure support. We will talk more about it in the upcoming pages.

10. Only in SIMV can you apply this pressure support (PS).

11. Additionally, when SIMV with PS is selected, you can choose a PS of 10, a PS of zero, any interval in between and even beyond a PS of 10. Note, that since A/C does not allow the patient to take their own patient– powered breath, then **PS can never be applied to A/C mode.** For PS to be added as a turbo boost, the mode must allow the patient to breathe on their own. Therefore, you will see machine breaths and patient– only breaths.

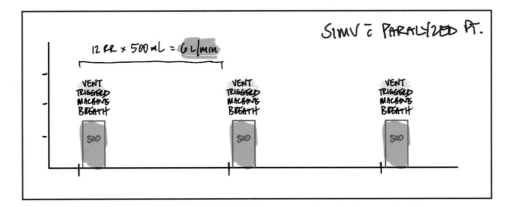

12. Please look at the graphic titled, SIMV with a Paralyzed Patient. Recall in these graphics, you'll see they are drafted based on volume (y-axis) and time (x-axis). On the x-axis, you'll note black hash marks, and they usually precede the machine breath (in red). The distance between each hashmark illustrates 1 breath interval (inhalation plus exhalation).

13. Note there is essentially no difference in 'A/C with a Paralyzed Patient' and 'CMV with a Paralyzed Patient' in addition to 'A/C with a Paralyzed Patient.' ALL display machine breaths at the beginning of each interval, deliver 500 mL tidal volume, and exhibit no patient effort. Ultimately, with the paralyzed patient, or one apneic for any other reason, will never try to take a breath and therefore will experience the ventilator just as they would if they were on CMV- a rate and volume (or pressure) is set. The ventilator will deliver that breath as often as the set rate dictates- PERIOD. This means that A/C and SIMV's true differences are what happens when the patient *ATTEMPTS* to take a breath. If they never attempt it (because paralyzed or apneic) *__then the mode doesn't matter at all__*. At least it doesn't matter until the paralysis and/or sedation wears off.

14. Now we need to discuss the 'add-on' that is available with SIMV mode: pressure support. There is no difference between pressure support (PS) and pressure control (PC) other than *WHEN* it is applied. Both delivers air into the lung until a certain pressure is measured or reached- then the airflow is terminated. When we are controlling each breath, as is the case when the patient is intubated, we can choose to set a pressure or volume to be pushed into the lung. When pressure is chosen and set, say to 15 cmH2O, then the ventilator will fill the lung to some volume that causes a pressure of 15 cmH2O. This is called pressure control. When the patient is

breathing on their own, such as in BiPAP or SIMV, where the pressure is set to 15 cmH2O and they take a breath, it triggers the ventilator to initiate positive pressure breath that pressurizes to 15 cm2O and then terminates the positive pressure. THESE ARE THE SAME THING, with one exception: when it is applied. In PC, the set RR dictates the 'when', but in PS, the patient is controlling their own rate, and therefore the patient controls the 'when'. In PC, we care in full CONTROL of their efforts, whereas in PS we are simply SUPPORTING it.

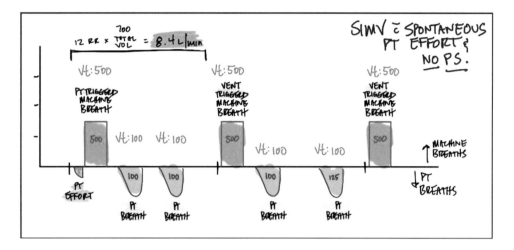

15. Please look at the graphic titled, SIMV with Spontaneous Patient Effort & No PS. You'll see in the first breath interval there is one red, upward breath- indicating a machine breath. You'll also note a small blue patient effort curve preceding this first red machine breath. This means the patient attempted to take a breath near the set time (based on the RR) and therefore the vent responded with a full machine breath- just like in A/C. Then, in that same breath interval the patient made 2 additional breath attempts. In these extra 2 breath attempts, the ventilator, being it is in SIMV mode, allowed the patient to fully take those breaths on their own power and using their own diaphragm. They can breathe whatever they can (tidal volume) under their own human faculties. In these extra breaths you see they are moving 100 mL of tidal volume each. This means that in this one breath cycle set to experience a tidal volume of only 500, they are actually experiencing 700 mL (500 mL +100 mL + 100 mL =700 mL). If their RR was set to 12, then their target minute ventilation would be 6 L/min, but they would actually be moving 8.4 L/min (700 mL x 12 RR = 8400 mL/min, or 8.4 L/min).

16. Normally, this is a good thing. As patients heal and can breathe more on their own in the ICU, the clinicians cut down the set RR and allow them to breathe more themselves. This is called weaning. To help expedite the weaning process, clinicians and engineers collaborated and invented 'pressure support.' It works EXACTLY as pressure control, except it is applied only when the patient can take a breath on their own power. Remember, the FIRST breath in each breath interval is a full, pre-set volume or pressure. In this way, SIMV ensures (or Mandates- the 'M' in SIMV) the patient receives one full breath each breath interval. Any other breath during the same breath interval is allowed, but under the power of the patient's diaphragm. In these subsequent breaths within the same breath interval, a clinician can add pressure support to assist the patient take a breath on their own. This is very useful when the patient is just beginning to heal, and their respiratory muscles are weak. As they strengthen, the clinician will reduce both RR and PS until the PS is zero and the patient is mostly breathing on their own. Then they perform an apnea test. If the patient passes the apnea test, then they are strongly considered for extubation. While this is a normal thing in the ICU, it doesn't hold much value in the typical critical care transport settings.

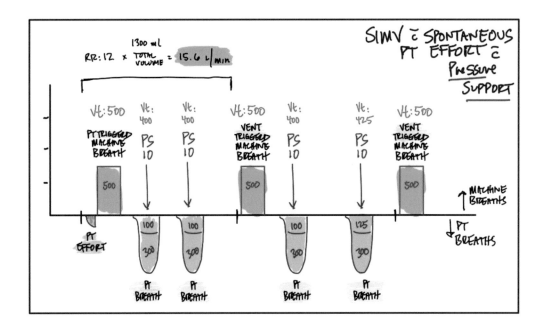

17. Look at the graphic titled, SIMV with a Spontaneous Patient with Pressure Support. Here you see 10 cmH2O of pressure support has been added (in purple). Note these are NOT involved in the machine breaths at the beginning of the breath intervals, because those are designed to be full machine breaths. Additionally, they cause an additional 300 mL of air to be drawn into the lungs per extra breath compared to the graphic, SIMV with Spontaneous Patient Effort & No PS (where 100 mL of air is inhaled per subsequent breath). This extra 300 mL each equates to an additional 600 mL PER BREATH INTERVAL as compared when NO PS was added. This results in a minute ventilation of 15.6 L/min ([500 mL + 400 mL + 400 mL] x 12 RR = 15600 mL/min, or 15.6 L/min).

18. Ultimately, SIMV is a fantastic mode, especially for weaning, however, ask yourself a question and answer truthfully before continuing: **is it our job to wean our patients off the ventilator in transport?** The answer is of course, NO. So, why would you apply pressure support to a patient in transport? I like SIMV for transporting patients, but I <u>do not</u> like SIMV with PS in transport. Looking at the 3 graphics with SIMV in the title, paralyzed patients (or otherwise apneic patients) move 6 L/min. Patients not paralyzed and over-breathing the vent without PS applied are moving a little bit more: 8.4 L/min. The patients on SIMV with PS and not paralyzed or apneic are moving an incredible 15.6 L/min!

19. The take home- If you are going to use SIMV, this author and associated experts, including physicians and respiratory therapists, suggest minimizing PS in SIMV for transport, if not eliminating it altogether.

**Pressure-Regulated Volume Control (PRVC)**

1. PRVC is a **VOLUME CONTROLED** mode. It uses an adaptive targeting scheme to target inspiratory pressure with the goal of delivering a desired minute ventilation and tidal volume. Adaptive targeting schemes use feedback methods on a breath to breath basis to discriminately adjust the pressure delivered to achieve the tidal volume target.

2. Another way to say this is PRVC benefits from the variable flow of pressure control along with the guaranteed minute ventilation of volume control. It is the best of both worlds in this capacity.

3. In this mode, you set a tidal volume and RR you want the patient to receive, thereby establishing the target minute ventilation. Additionally, you set I:E ratio, PEEP, and FiO2, along with sensitivity.

4. The ventilator takes measurements of various pressures and volumes and adjusts flow rates (called 'rise time' on most transport ventilators) to achieve the LOWEST possible pressure to ensure the set <u>TIDAL VOLUME</u>.

5. It is an incredible mode for the newbie ventilator clinician.

6. HOWEEVER, since it is a volume mode, you would want to avoid it in situations where you have a non-compliant lung, such as ARDS or acute lung injury (ALI). You'll still want to switch these patients to PRESSURE CONTROL mode in these cases, or consider the next mode: APRV if available.

## Airway Pressure Release Ventilation (APRV)

1. APRV is a very unique mode typically used on pathophysiologies resulting in oxygenation problems, such as ARDS and acute lung injury.

2. The basic concept is 2 levels of pressure throughout the ventilation cycle: one high pressure and one lower pressure. The higher pressure is experienced by the patient the majority of the time, while the lower pressure is experienced only briefly, and ultimately used as an exhalation tool.

3. Essentially, this is 2 different levels of CPAP, which already has a term: BIPAP. The higher pressure, called "P high" is set between 20-30 cmH2O (note normal PEEP, which is also CPAP, is between 3-5 cmH2O). The inspiratory time set at this pressure is called "T high." Because we must exhale air to remove CO2, then we must set a second pressure much lower to allow gas to exit the lungs. This lower pressure, called "P low" is set between 5-10 cmH2O. The inspiratory time in P low is very short and called "T low." The I:E ratio in this case is typically ranges from 2:1 to 4:1, with the larger number always being associated with T high, and the shorter time being T low.

4. During P high, air enters the lungs until a high pressure is reached and the vent keeps it there for several seconds- and typically about 4-6 seconds. After these 4-6 seconds, the ventilator switches to the P low, which causes higher pressure in the lungs than is fighting it in the vent circuit, so most of the air rushes out of the lung; essentially exhaling/ventilating the patient. Typically, within 0.5-1.0 of a second, the higher pressure is re-established and maintained for another 4-6 seconds. Basically, it's BIPAP in the intubated patient that doesn't require the patient to take breaths.

5. While this is a mode designed originally to help those patients in ARDS or acute lung injury to better oxygenate, in recent years patients with more compliant (healthy) lungs are being put to the APRV test with very positive results.

## SUMMARY OF MODES

In summary, A/C mode prevents the patient form double-stacking breaths. It does so by sensing the patient attempting to take in a breath, and before 5% of a full breath is drawn into the lungs, the vent provides an A/C breath. It does this every time the patient tries to take a breath. In SIMV, the ventilator ensures one MANDATORY breath per breath interval and other breaths can proceed under the patient's own power. On these extra breaths, PS can be added, but they can dramatically increase the minute ventilation. PS can ONLY be added in SIMV mode and CANNOT ever be added to A/C. PRVC, is a great mode for newbie clinicians, but is only good for compliant lungs. If there is ever a Pplat greater than 30, consider switching to pressure control ventilation or APRV. APRV is a mode of dueling pressures- one high and one low. It is set so the patient experiences the high pressure 2:1 to 4:1 time as much. The lower pressure is designed to allow the patient to exhale.

## Common Ventilator Settings

**Respiratory Rate:**
1. This is how often you want the ventilator to deliver a breath.
2. normal is 12 to 20 per minute for adults, 20-30 for pediatrics, and 30-40 for infants.

**I:E Ratio:**
1. This is the ratio of time for inspiration to exhalation.
2. Normally you want a 1:2 ratio unless the patient is a pediatric, has asthma, or has COPD.
3. In these special cases you want 1:4-1:6 because it allows for longer exhalation time (thus correcting air trapping).
4. Reversed I:E (2:1)- acts like constant PEEP and can be used as a powerful oxygenator.

**Breath Type:**
1. Volume Control (Tidal Volume):
   a. In volume control (VC), you set TIDAL VOLUME (Vt).
   b. Normal Vt is approximately 4-8 cc/kg and varies between institutions; based on ideal body weight.
   c. VC is very common in the pre-hospital environment and is great to control minute ventilation but is terrible for diseased lungs (like ARDS or acute lung injury– causes high PIPs).
   d. It is terrible because a diseased lung is not compliant and can be very stiff. Ventilating a diseased lung is a lot like trying to ventilate a plastic food container– it would not budge very much as a volume of gas was forced into it.
2. Pressure Control (Pressure):
   a. In pressure control (PC), you set an inspiratory pressure instead of a tidal volume.
   b. A normal starting point for PC for all ages is between 15-20 cmH2O. Most texts call for 18-22 cmH2O, but we have found 15-20 to be optimal, and will be publishing works soon to illuminate this.
   c. This is a great setting for pediatrics or people with diseased lungs, but you will have to tend minute ventilation with this type because with pressure, you cannot guarantee minute ventilation.
   d. Even though you set a PC, you can still monitor the exhaled tidal volume (Vte) to gauge how much tidal volume the patient is moving. For example, If PC is set at 20 cmH2O and the Vte is 800 cc, you can reduce the Vte to 500 cc by reducing the PC. PC is therefore tied to the Vte and can be adjusted by changing PC up or down.
   e. Using Swearingen's Vent Hero ventilator approach, he has found that 15 cmH2O is a good starting point, although it's under the 18-22 cmH2O suggested range. The reason for this is due to large tidal volumes (beyond calculated normal for patients) with 20+ cmH2O settings. This is mostly seen in healthier lungs. Best practice is to start with a pressure setting (15-20 cmH2O) and titrate that pressure setting up or down based on the measured exhaled minute ventilation (VE) and exhaled tidal volume (Vte)- to be discussed in a few pages.

**Positive End Expiratory Pressure (PEEP)**
1. PEEP is the pressure that helps to hold open alveoli.
2. Normal PEEP is 3-5 cmH2O.
3. This represents the pressure left in the lungs after exhalation and is critical to improving oxygenation.
4. PEEP helps with oxygenation by increasing the alveolar surface area and thinning out the alveolar membrane, both of which increase the speed of oxygen diffusion. Imagine blowing up a balloon– it gets bigger (more surface area) and the material becomes thinner the larger it gets (thinner membrane).

5. Another reason to do this is because when in pressure control mode, you can assume the peak inspiratory pressure (upcoming) by simply adding the PC and PEEP. If you have set the patient to 15/5. then you can assume the Peak inspiratory pressure is 25, or (20 + 5).

**Fraction of Inspired Oxygen (FiO2):**
1. This represents how much oxygen is actually being delivered to the patient.
2. It is common practice to begin at 1.0 FiO2 until you establish the patient's SpO2.
3. The goal is to wean down the FiO2 to the lowest value that will keep the SpO2 at ~95% or above.

## *Common Ventilator Measurements*

You would never put a bradycardic patient on a transcutaneous pacer and fail to 'check their pulse.' You would always check their pulse after putting them on the pacer. Right? Well, too often we fail to 'check the pulse' of the ventilator by trusting the default settings. The ventilator gives us valuable information that we can use to ensure the vent settings we have chosen are correctly being applied. Therefore, we can compare the parameters we set the vent to deliver (what we WANT going in) to what comes out of the patient's lungs (what actually REACHES the patient). When what we want going in matches what comes out of the patient's lungs, then patient-ventilator synchrony is achieved.

Once patient- ventilator synchrony is achieved, then there will be significantly fewer erroneous alarms (high minute ventilation alarm, low minute ventilation alarm, ↑ pressure alarms, etc.). Once we prevent these erroneous alarms from happening, then we can focus our time and effort towards treating and managing the patient's conditions.

**Minute Ventilation (VE)**
1. Expected: VE = RR x Vt
2. Actual (measured): VE = Vte x f
3. Minute ventilation is the amount of air that a person moves each minute, and it is a direct reflection of our offloading of $CO_2$ and a reliable estimate of pH.
4. Once you have your patient settings inputted into the ventilator, double check to make sure that the expected minute ventilation (based on your chosen settings) matches the measured minute ventilation from the patient (the real VE).
5. For example, if you set the patient to receive a tidal volume of 450cc and a respiratory rate of 10/min, then the expected minute ventilation should be 4.5 L/min. If the ventilator reports 8L/min, then you know there is a patient - ventilator dys-synchrony.
6. Any mismatch between your expected minute ventilation and the measured (true) minute ventilation that the ventilator reports should be investigated. See below.

**Frequency (f)**
1. This describes how many breath cycles (breaths) are occurring each minute. This is the true respiratory rate. This should match your set RR on the vent.
2. If your expected minute ventilation is higher than the measured minute ventilation, then first check frequency.
3. A high frequency represents a patient who is over breathing the vent or breathing faster than the rate that you set. These patients typically need sedation.

**Exhaled Tidal Volume (Vte)**
1. This describes the actual volume of air that exits the patient's lungs and is a true representation of the actual tidal volume. This should match TV.
2. If you set the ventilator to deliver a tidal volume of 450cc and the ventilator reports that your Vte is 325cc, then you would have evidence to explain a low minute volume.

3. For example, you set the ventilator to deliver 450cc at a rate of 10/min; therefore, you expect a minute ventilation of 4.5 L/min. If the ventilator reports that your frequency is 10 and your Vte is 325cc, then the ventilator will also report a minute ventilation of 3.25 L/min. This is because the ventilator calculates minute ventilation based on frequency (f) and exhaled tidal volume (Vte).

### Peak Inspiratory Pressure (PIP)

1. Normal: < 35 cmH2O
2. As mentioned previously, this is the highest pressure achieved measured during inhalation. So, when all the inspired air is still in the chest, that highest pressure is known as the peak inspiratory pressure.
3. This is a direct reflection of airway resistance and can tell us a great deal of the patency of the lower airways.
4. You can set an alarm for both a high and low PIP- these are called your high pressure and low-pressure alarms, respectively.
5. Low pressure alarms can be caused by a leak, a ruptured ETT pilot bulb, disconnected vent tubing, extended patient, and vent tubing that is not correctly connected to the ventilator itself.
6. High pressure alarms can be caused by secretions and in the airway, bronchospasms, kinking of the ET tube, stepping on the vent tubing, and tension pneumothorax.
7. Use the D.O.P.E. acronym to troubleshoot any high-pressure alarms (dislodgement, obstruction, pneumothorax, equipment). If you fail to identify the reason for the high-pressure alarm using this acronym, then proceed to check a plateau pressure.

### Plateau Pressure (Pplat)

1. Normal: < 30 cmH2O
2. Plateau pressure reflects the compliance, or elasticity, of the lungs. It represents the pressures within the alveoli.
3. As a healthy person, you want good compliant and elastic lungs. People with ARDS or acute lung injury can develop stiff, rigid , non-elastic lungs. This rigidity prevents good compliance and thus their lungs are not elastic but rather are stiff, like a wooden box.
4. What would happen if you tried to force air into a wooden box? Most likely you would reach high pressures fast. This is what happens in ARDS and acute lung injury patients. Their lungs are not compliant, and as we try to ventilate their lungs we reach high pressure is very quickly.
5. Therefore, plateau pressure is a good way to identify the compliance of the lungs.

### PIP and Pplat

1. These two metrics are very important in helping us to understand why a high-pressure alarm is going off.
2. If you have a high-pressure alarm and you have not found any cause of the increased pressure using the DOPE acronym, then you should obtain a plateau pressure.
3. If your PIP is high and your plateau pressure is normal, then it is in airway resistance problem: this usually means secretions or bronchospasm- treat with suctioning and/or bronchodilators.
4. If your PIP and your plateau pressure are both high, then you most likely have a compliance problem: this usually indicates ARDS or acute lung injury- treat by switching to pressure-controlled ventilation IMMEDIATELY (if you not already).

## INITIATING MECHANICAL VENTILATION

### *Ensure Perfusion*

1. Once you have set the ventilator to ventilate your patient, you will need two specific vital signs to guide you to make changes on the ventilator (pulse oximetry and EtCO2).

2. To trust these two vital sign parameters, you need to have a perfusing blood pressure. A perfusing blood pressure is one that is delivering oxygen to the distal tissues (skin, brain, heart, lung, liver), or anywhere where arteries turn into capillaries.

3. As you are approaching applying the mechanical ventilator, it is important to identify if you have a blood pressure high enough to produce a radial (or other distal pulse in an extremity) pulse. The presence of a radial pulse indicates the heart is pushing blood with enough pressure behind it to deliver the blood to the distal tissues, thus perfusing those tissues.

4. If a patient has frank hypotension or has a borderline BP without a distal pulse, then you need to address it immediately so that when you are ready to apply the ventilator to the patient, you will be able to trust the vitals (O2 saturations and EtCO2).

5. You typically will arrive on scene where care has already been established, and with-it IVs (or multiple). Simply ask them to give you an appropriate size fluid bolus for that patient in order to increase BP.

6. There will be times where you will not be able to get the blood pressure up significantly to produce a distal pulse. In these cases, you will just have to shoot blindly, so to speak. In low perfusion states, your pulse oximetry reading will likely be low– because monitoring devices clip on the finger, and if perfusion isn't high enough to get to the fingertip, then the reading will be low.

7. Your EtCO2 will most likely be falsely low because without that adequate perfusion, oxygen is not being delivered to the tissues. When tissues go without oxygen for any length of time, they begin building up acids. Acids then are converted quickly into CO2 for discard via exhalation. However, without adequate blood pressure and perfusion, carbon dioxide cannot be picked up from the tissues to be taken to the lungs for exhalation.

8. In summary, without a blood pressure to produce adequate perfusion, oxygen isn't being delivered (causing acidosis) and CO2 isn't being picked up from the tissues (giving a falsely low EtCO2 in the serum because all the built up CO2 is stuck in the cells). This causes low SpO2 and low EtCO2 until perfusion is restored– then more reliable values are displayed.

### *Targeted Minute Ventilation and Acidosis*

1. You need to know what minute ventilation your patient requires. If your patient is acidotic and you set the overused vent settings of RR12 and TV 500 on your ventilator, then you could kill them.

2. Most acidotic patients are trying to off load acid out of their body by exhalation. One major mechanism this is achieved by is to breathe faster (think of Kussmaul's in a DKA patient) to get rid of excess acid. Breathing faster means they are increasing their minute ventilation (minute ventilation = RR x tidal volume) to keep up with their body's acid production.

3. Normal minute ventilation (VE) = 100 mL/kg/min for adults, 200 mL/kg/min for pediatrics, and 300 mL/kg/min for infants.

4. If a patient is acidotic or potentially acidotic, with the ventilator we need to target a minute ventilation greater than the highest normal value for that age range. For this reason, we suggest these acidotic starting points: 120 mL/kg/min for adults, 240 mL/kg/min for pediatrics, and 360 mL/kg/min for infants.

5. If an adult patient is breathing fast (>30/min), there is an acidotic problem, and it would be unsafe to slow their RR or reduce the TV. An adult patient breathing over 30/min is a physiologic reflex to remove acid. This isn't direct evidence of acidosis (like a low pH would be), but it SUGGESTS a potential for acidosis.

6. If their EtCO2 is higher than 45 mmHg, especially if it is significantly higher (>50 mmHg), then it is suggestive that an underlying acidosis is present. This also isn't a direct indication of acidosis, but a strong likelihood.
7. If you set a higher VE and the patient isn't acidotic, then you'll know quickly by monitoring for a lowering EtCO2(EtCO2 is a good estimation of pH most of the time).
8. On the other hand, if your patient is acidotic and you apply the ventilator using only a normal minute ventilation for their age, then you could severely exacerbate their acidosis, which could kill them.
9. <u>Swearingen's Rule</u>: If a patient is not suspect for acidosis, start the patient on a normal minute ventilation. If the patient IS suspect for acidosis use: 120 mL/kg/min for adults, 240 mL/kg/min for pediatrics, and 360 mL/kg/min for infants.
10. If any of these questions answer with "yes", then apply **Swearingen's Rule**:
    a. pH < 7.35?
    b. RR > 30/min? (or > 10 over highest normal for age)
    c. EtCO2 > 45 mmHg?

## *Minute Ventilation Centered Calculations*

1. I'll be bold. Stop guessing. By this, I mean target a specific minute ventilation for the patient instead of simply putting them on the default ventilator settings  RR 12 and 500 tidal volume.
2. By assessing for acidosis or potential acidosis and by applying Swearingen's Rule, you can arrive at minute ventilation higher than normal minute ventilation, therefore combating any acidosis.
11. For normal pH status patients, use 100 mL/kg/min for adults, 200 mL/kg/min for pediatrics, and 300 mL/kg/min for infants.
3. If they are acidotic then add 1-2 L/min, or use 120 mL/kg/min for adults, 240 mL/kg/min for pediatrics, and 360 mL/kg/min for infants.
4. Once you determine your targeted minute volume for your patient, you need to calculate the patient's ideal body weight (IBW). It is important to use IBW and not actual body weight. Please see the picture below.

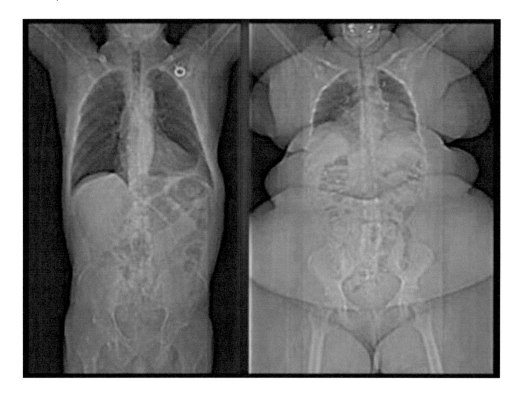

5.  The chest walls of both patients are very similar in size; however, they drastically vary in actual body weight. In pharmacology, certainly use actual body weight since there is approximately 1 mile of vasculature in each pound of fat tissue. But, when calculating ventilator volumes (tidal volume), use the IBW.
6.  IBW (Devine) Formula: (2.3)(# inches over 5 feet) + (50 for men or 45.5 for women)
7.  Next calculate the ideal tidal volume (ITV) based on IBW. The result of the 5-8 cc/kg x IBW is the ITV.
8.  Divide the targeted minute ventilation by the ITV. Since minute ventilation is the product of respiratory rate and tidal volume, if we use ITV and targeted minute ventilation, we can derive the respiratory rate. Therefore, you can arrive at appropriate minute ventilation, respiratory rate, and ideal tidal volume which is patient specific. No guessing involved- you're simply calculating and selecting the appropriate respiratory rate from ITV and the targeted minute ventilation.
9.  Example 1: you have a 6'4'' male who just got intubated and you need to apply the ventilator. The patient's vitals are BP 70/50, HR 112, RR 24, pulse oximetry 88% and EtCO2 of 55.
    a.  The BP is low; therefore, an aggressive fluid bolus should be administered. A normal saline bolus of 500cc– 1000cc would be a good start.
    b.  The patient is 6'4''. To calculate the IBW, you need to figure out the number of inches higher than 60 inches the patient is. Just remember that 5 feet is 60 inches, so subtract 5 feet from however tall your patient is. In this case, 6 feet subtracted from 6'4'' is 1 foot 4 inches. One foot is 12 inches. Therefore, 6'4'' is 16 inches above 60 inches. (2.3)(16) + 50 = 86.8. Rounding up, the patient's ideal body weight is 87 kg.
    c.  The patient has evidence of potential acidosis (high EtCO2). Remember, this isn't at all a direct indication of acidosis, but it is a suggestion. Since this is an adult, the normal minute ventilation is 4-8 L/min. Applying Swearingen's Rule, 120 mL/kg/min for this patient. So, the target minute ventilation, based on our approach, is 10400 mL/min, or 10.4 L/min.
    d.  Normal tidal volume is 4-8 cc/kg. Multiply your calculated IBW of 87 by 5, 6, 7 or 8. In this example, let's use 6 cc/kg since it in in the middle. The result of 6 cc/kg x 87 kg = 522 cc, also called the ideal tidal volume (ITV).
    e.  Recall our targeted minute ventilation is 9000 cc. Divide this 9000 cc by our IDV of 609 cc: 10400/ 522 = 19.9, or about 20. This 20 represents the respiratory rate we need to set with our ITV to achieve our target minute ventilation of 10,400 cc. This works because minute ventilation = RR x Vt.
    f.  Next choose and apply the non-calculated ventilator settings (I:E, PEEP, FiO2) based on clinical presentation.
    g.  This method intelligently redesigns the vent approach.

## *Apply the Calculated Settings*

1.  Now you can apply the mechanical ventilator with the initial settings you have calculated. Use all the provided information to begin applying the mechanical ventilator. Use the example data from the above section.
2.  Choose volume ventilation or pressure ventilation.
3.  Choose the mode (assist control or SIMV).
4.  Choose initial settings:
    a.  Respiratory Rate (RR): 20/ min (from example 1)
    b.  Tidal volume (Vt): 522 cc (from example 1)
    c.  I:E Ratio: 1:2 (no evidence of asthma/ COPD/ bronchospasm, and not a pediatric)
    d.  PEEP: 5 cmH2O (3-5 cmH2O is normal, so we chose 5 cmH2O here because it's the high end of normal)
    e.  FiO2: 1.0 (good to start at 1.0 and wean down later).

## *Ensure the initial settings match the measured data from the ventilator*

1.  Consider a hypoglycemic patient who you treated with dextrose. Would you ever administer dextrose to a patient and FAIL to check their blood sugar after? Of course you wouldn't. My

question, then, is why on earth would you set a ventilator up and not read the data the ventilator measures from the patient?

2. It is important to ensure that your initial vent settings match what is coming out of the patient (which is what the vent measures). It is as easy as matching the settings with the monitored data from the vent.

3. If you set the ventilator and fail to 1) check the monitored data from the vent and 2) fail to do something to correct any desynchrony, then you will hear multiple alarms. These alarms will take your attention away from your patient when you could have easily prevented it by synchronizing the patient and vent.

4. Review the table on the next page. You'll note that several vent setting parameters (Vt, RR, VE) do not match the values for the first three monitored vent data parameters. (Vte, f, VE-actual) therefore, this patient does not present with patient– ventilator synchrony.

5. Ensure your settings MATCH the data that the ventilator is reporting.

### CHECK Minute Ventilation (VE)

1. The SET minute ventilation (VE) must closely match (within 10% of your setting) your targeted minute ventilation

2. If your patient is acidotic or potentially acidotic, then you need a higher than normal minute ventilation: > 8 L/min for an adult, > about 4 for a pediatric, and > 1-2 for an infant. These are guidelines, and your VE choices should always be driven by EtCO2.

3. If your patient is NOT acidotic, then applying a VE within the normal age range of minute ventilation for your patient is a great starting point. Again, your VE choices should always be driven by EtCO2.

4. So, if you set the ventilator to deliver a RR of 12 and a tidal volume (Vt) of 500, then you are targeting a minute ventilation of 6 L (12 x 500cc = 6000cc, or 6 L).

5. If you obtained the measured (or actual) minute ventilation from the ventilator (VE) and it was 4 L, then you would know there was a discrepancy that needs to be addressed.

### CHECK Respiratory Rate (RR)

1. The SET RR should match (f).

2. If you have a high frequency (f), that likely means either
   a. the patient also has spontaneous respiratory effort, or
   b. the vehicle/ aircraft vibrations are causing the ventilator to trigger.

3. For spontaneous breaths– sedate and/or paralyze the patient. In doing so you are CONTROLING their respirations and not letting them spontaneously breathe. You can positively impact their physiology by being in control of their ventilation and oxygenation, so be sure to stay in control.

4. For vibrations– REDUCE the sensitivity on your ventilator. A low sensitivity means it is easy for the patient (or vehicle vibrations) to trigger a breath. A HIGH sensitivity means it is harder to trigger a breath. "H" for High and Hard to trigger.

### CHECK Tidal Volume (Vt)

1. The SET Vt should match Vte

2. When you set a tidal volume (Vt), you are asking the ventilator to deliver a chosen volume specific to your patient's size and pathophysiology.

3. If you decide that the patient needs 500cc for their Vt, then you also need to check to make sure that volume makes it into the patient's lungs.

4. To make sure the patient is receiving this volume of 500 cc, you look to the exhaled tidal volume (Vte), which describes the total volume that was exhaled. This represents the ACTUAL tidal volume the patient received.

5. Vte will never be greater than the Vt set on the vent, but it may be lower. A lower Vte relative to the Vt means either:

a. Air Trapping- present if AutoPEEP (obtained from an expiratory hold maneuver) is not zero.

b. Air Leak: Air leaks can be determined by a flat (unfilled) pilot balloon on a tracheal tube; or bubbling/ gurgling around a placed tracheal tube

c. Dead space: Dead space can occur when there is a much larger vent circuit than designed for the patient. Remember, transport vents have been calibrated based on averages– averaged adults, peds, and infants. Sometimes the averages will be off, and you'll have dead space.

6. To correct this LOW Vte, we need to fix air-trapping, any leaks in the system, or increase the Vt setting to a higher value to correct for dead space. This would allow enough volume reaching the patient, and thus our Vte will be increased to closer to what we originally wanted as the tidal volume. If 500cc set, and 200cc reaches the patient, then go up on your setting to ~300 to make up the difference. If you ensure these increases do not raise your PIP over 35 cmH2O, then it is a safe solution.

7. In the end, the REAL Vt is the Vte because it represents the volume the patient actually receives.

**PPI vs. Pplat**

There are two important pressures to be aware of and monitor: peak inspiratory pressure (PIP) and plateau pressure (Pplat). You can conceptualize PIP by considering the magnitude the energy the breath possesses. As air is pushed into the lung, the energy can be categorized as kinetic and static.

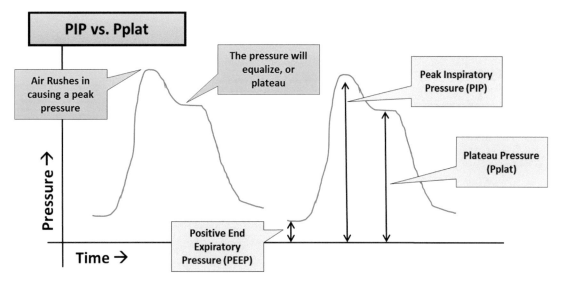

Once air is in the lung and not moving, that would be the static component of the pressure. When the air is in transit to the lung, that represents its kinetic component. Basically, plateau pressure is simply the static component, whereas PIP is both the static and kinetic component. As you can see above, the PIP is the highest pressure possible as air rushes into the lung. Then, as this high pressure equalizes, or plateau, we get a glimpse of how "elastic" the lung is. A healthy lung is nice and elastic, and therefore this plateau pressure will be under 30 cmH2O. Plateau pressures higher than 30 cmH2O represent DISEASED lungs or lungs actively being damaged. If lungs are being damaged dude to a high Pplat- <u>**SWITCH TO PRESSURE CONTROL IMMEDIATELY**</u>!

Once your vent settings are set and you have made sure the settings closely match the measured vent data parameters, then next you need to evaluate for pressures to ensure they are safe for the patient.

**CHECK Peak Inspiratory Pressure (PIP)**
1. The PIP should always remain under 35 cmH2O.
2. Technically, most mechanical ventilation literature states it can be 40 cmH2O, but the MeduPros.com and Vent Hero methods build in a safety buffer, so we say stop making changes that will increase PIP once you get to the 35 cmH2O pressure ceiling.

**CHECK Plateau Pressure (Pplat)**
1. The Pplat should always remain under 30 cmH2O.
2. Technically, most mechanical ventilation literature states it can be 35 cmH2O, but the MeduPros.com and Vent Hero methods build in a safety buffer, so we say stop making changes that will increase PIP once you get to the 30 cmH2O pressure ceiling.

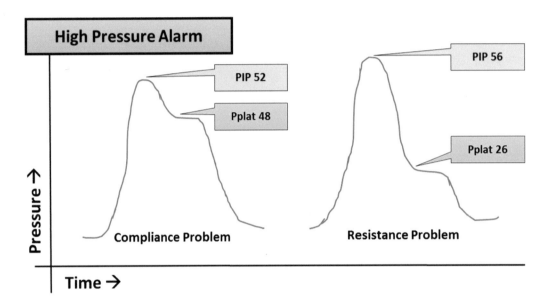

When you have a high-pressure alarm sound, it is important to identify if it is a compliance problem or an airway resistance problem. **REMEMBER**:

    a. a high PIP and normal Pplat = airway resistance problem;
    b. Both a high PIP and a high Pplat = a compliance (diseased lung) problem.

Typically, we treat airway resistance problems with suctioning and bronchodilators, while we treat compliance problems by <u>switching to pressure control (PC) ventilation IMMEDIATELY</u> because we are damaging lung tissue with each breath at plateau pressures greater than 30 cmH2O.

## Adjusting the Mechanical Ventilator

First off, ensure you have adequate perfusion and blood pressure. Without this, the two parameters you'll use to drive changes on the ventilator (pulse oximetry/ EtCO2) will not be accurate. You cannot trust your EtCO2 or your SpO2 if you have a significantly low blood pressure (best indicated by an absence of a radial pulse).

**EtCO2**
1. The only effective means for changing exhaled carbon dioxide is to enhance or reduce minute ventilation.
2. Therefore, changing respiratory rate and tidal volume (or pressure control if in PC type ventilation) are the only two ways to effectively change your EtCO2.

     a. Increasing RR/TV/PC → a reduction of EtCO2

     b. Decreasing RR/TV/PC → a surplus of EtCO2

**SpO2**

1. The only effective means for improving pulse oximetry is to increase either FiO2 or PEEP.
2. Increasing the FiO2 adds more oxygen molecules into the lungs, therefore they diffuse faster into the alveolar capillary membrane (Fick's Law).
3. Increasing PEEP is like blowing more air into a balloon. Air blown into a balloon results in thinner walls of the balloon and more surface area of the balloon. Therefore, when you apply more PEEP, you effectively thin the alveolar capillary membrane as well as increase the surface area of the alveolar capillary membrane thus improving perfusion and oxygenation (yes, that is Fick's Law again).
4. The only problem with adding peep is that when you add more than 8 cm andH2O of PEEP, you reduce cardiac output (and blood pressure) by tamponading off the lung vasculature and right side of the heart.
5. Additionally, by squeezing the lung vasculature, a backflow occurs like CHF where blood can back up into the system {including the cranium} which can lead to an increased ICP. This is controversial in the literature, but I wanted you to be aware of it.
6. Be cautious with applying more than 8 cmH2O to hypertensive patients and neuro patients.
7. However, consider this example. A patient requires 9 of PEEP to achieve oxygen saturations of 95%. Once you achieve these saturations, the blood pressure drops from 110/70 to 88/60. You may be tempted to reduce the PEEP knowing it most likely caused the drop in BP. I'd STRONGLY encourage you to keep the PEEP and support BP with fluids/ pressors. The PEEP is actually oxygenating the patient– don't remove it. Protect it with fluids/ pressors.

     a. Increasing FiO2 → improved SpO2

     b. Increasing PEEP → improved SpO2

**Don't be afraid of the ventilator.**

1. It can be a scary piece of equipment if you do not practice it- SO PRACTICE!
2. But if you realize that setting up a ventilator is as simple as applying normal ranges for the patient's age (unless they're acidotic) or targeting minute volume, double checking to making sure that what is going into the patient is actually coming out of the patient (ventilator pulse check), and then simply make changes based on EtCO2 and SpO2 measurements, then this becomes a very approachable skill.
3. The key is practice, practice, practice. Be sure to practice this skill repeatedly. Consider how you would set up a ventilator on every single patient regardless of whether they actually need mechanical ventilation or not. #alwaysready.

# PART 7: RESPIRATORY MANAGEMENT QUESTIONS

1. A 61 kg patient with altered mental status is intubated and has the following ventilator settings: A/C 11, Vt 460, FIO2 100%, PEEP 4. His vital signs are BP 124/76, HR 70, SPO2 98%, ETCO2 52. The next most appropriate action is to?

     a. Reduce RR

     b. Increase PEEP

     c. Increase Vt

     d. Decrease FiO2

2. A patient has been intubated for an altered mental status. He has the following clinical findings: SIMV 12 (f 24), Vt 390, FIO2 100% PEEP 4. The vital signs are BP 118/68, HR 64, SPO2 98%, and EtCO2 30. Which of the following is the most appropriate action?
   a. Increase their RR
   b. Administer versed
   c. Manually bag patient
   d. Reduce their FiO2

3. While caring for a patient who is mechanically ventilated and on positive end-expiratory pressure (PEEP), it is important to understand how PEEP works. Which of the following statements is TRUE regarding PEEP?
   a. It occurs at the beginning of a machine breath
   b. It decreases the functional residual capacity (FRC)
   c. It causes an increased venous return
   d. It may increase intrathoracic pressure

4. Your partner tells you they have set up your additive type ventilator on pressure control ventilation at 18/4 on 100% oxygen with normal I:E. This information tells you what about your patient?
   a. Their PIP is 24 and PEEP is 4
   b. The pressure control is 18
   c. The minute ventilation is 4L
   d. The I:E is either 1:4 or 1:5

5. You are currently setting the mechanical ventilator for your asthma patient who was recently intubated. You choose to apply the SIMV mode. You know that this mode will do which of the following?
   a. Allow the patient to breathe on their own
   b. Synchronize with each inhaled breath
   c. Require a paralytic be administered early
   d. Causes PEEP to rise with each breath

6. Potential hazards of positive-pressure mechanical ventilation are pneumothorax, subcutaneous emphysema, and which of the following?
   a. under-oxygenation
   b. cardiac tamponade
   c. decreased cardiac output
   d. widening pulse pressures

7. On your way to an interfacility transfer, you receive word that your respiratory failure patient has the following ABG: pH 7.22/ pCO2 47/ HCO3 29/ pO2 82/ BE 0. Interpret these findings.
   a. Respiratory acidosis
   b. Metabolic acidosis
   c. Respiratory alkalosis
   d. Metabolic alkalosis

8.  You are dispatched to a local hospital where your patient has the following ABG: pH 7.33/ pCO2 45/ HCO3 20/ pO2 83/ BE 1. Interpret these findings.
    a.  Respiratory acidosis
    b.  Metabolic acidosis
    c.  Respiratory alkalosis
    d.  Metabolic alkalosis

9.  The patient you are transporting to the regional hospital presents with the following ABG: pH 7.47/ pCO2 25/ HCO3 25/ pO2 89/ BE 1. Interpret these findings.
    a.  Respiratory acidosis
    b.  Metabolic alkalosis
    c.  Metabolic acidosis
    d.  Respiratory alkalosis

10. As you are packaging your patient, the RN returns with the following ABG: pH 7.46/ pCO2 44/ HCO3 43/ pO2 87/ BE 2. Interpret these findings.
    a.  Metabolic alkalosis
    b.  Respiratory alkalosis
    c.  Metabolic acidosis
    d.  Respiratory acidosis

11. A chronically ill patient has the following ABG: pH 7.29/ pCO2 49/ HCO3 30/ pO2 98/ BE 1. What degree of compensation is present here, if any?
    a.  This is a MIXED problem
    b.  Fully compensated
    c.  This is an ACUTE problem
    d.  Partially compensated

12. You are orienting a new employee and mention an ABG that you recently had on a flight: pH 7.35/ pCO2 50/ HCO3 29/ pO2 87/ BE 1. What degree of compensation is present here, if any?
    a.  This is an ACUTE problem
    b.  Partially compensated
    c.  Fully compensated
    d.  This is a MIXED problem

13. You are noticing a change in the patient's status. Upon and arterial blood draw and analysis, you obtain the following ABG: pH 7.21/ pCO2 61/ HCO3 22/ pO2 120/ BE 0. What degree of compensation is present here, if any?
    a.  This is a MIXED problem
    b.  This is an ACUTE problem
    c.  Partially compensated
    d.  Fully compensated

14. As you are looking over your intubated patient's chart, you notice the following ABG: pH 7.32/ pCO2 46/ HCO3 20/ pO2 87/ BE 0. What degree of compensation is present here, if any?
    a. Partially compensated
    b. This is an ACUTE problem
    c. This is a MIXED problem
    d. Fully compensated

15. After establishing your initial vent settings and one vent change, you notice the SpO2 is 88%. Which of the following is the best management for this patient?
    a. Increase PEEP
    b. Increase rate
    c. Increase the TV
    d. Increase the PC

16. You are examining a patient before you begin the packaging process and notice that their EtCO2 is 49 mmHg. How would you best correct this problem?
    a. Change FiO2 from 1 to 0.7
    b. Change Vt from 600 to 450
    c. Change PEEP from 5 to 3
    d. Change RR from 12 to 16

17. You're transporting a motor vehicle collision patient from the scene to a level one trauma center. The accident happened approximately 1 hour ago, and the patient was just extricated 10 minutes ago. The ambient temperature is near freezing. Which of the following findings would you most likely see with this patient?
    a. Profound hypotension from the ambient temp
    b. Slurring of the QRS evident on the 12 lead ECG
    c. Left shift of oxyhemoglobin disassociation curve
    d. Significant DIC from being entrapped for 50 min

18. Your intubated patient is on a mechanical ventilator, and you notice the following findings: HR 101, SpO2 94%, MV 3.5 L/min, EtCO2 55, and a Vte of 450 cc. What do these values tell you about the oxyhemoglobin disassociation curve?
    a. There is a shift to the left
    b. There is a shift to the right
    c. Reduction in oxygen supply
    d. Reduction in oxygen demand

19. Originally, the ABG on your respiratory distress patient was as follows: 7.32/ CO2 49/ HCO3 22. At this time, the potassium was 4.5 mmHg. The new ABG is as follows: 7.22/ CO2 59/ HCO3 21. Which of the following potassium values would be correct following this change?
    a. 5.1 mmol/L
    b. 3.9 mmol/L
    c. 4.8 mEq/L
    d. 4.2 mEq/L

20. You're transporting a trauma patient to a trauma center. Earlier, they had oxygen saturations of 100% on room air, but now their oxygen saturation is 90%. What would you expect their PaO2 is at this time?
    a. 80 mmHg
    b. 70 mmHg
    c. 60 mmHg
    d. 50 mmHg


21. You are treating a patient with severe shortness of breath with wheezing. Currently, their oxygen saturation is 88% and they have the following arterial blood gas data: 7.31/ CO2 56/ HCO3 23. What is the next most appropriate treatment to perform on this patient?
    a. Intubation
    b. Magnesium
    c. Terbutaline
    d. Epinephrine


22. A patient with acute respiratory distress syndrome is being transported to an ICU. You have them on the mechanical ventilator as follows: PC 20, PEEP of 20, RR 14, FiO2 of 1.0 on assist control. The patient's SpO2 is still incredibly low. Which of the following could improve the patient's oxygen saturations?
    a. Reduce PEEP
    b. Increase MV
    c. Raise the TV
    d. Reverse I:E


23. Look at the provided chest x-ray [Appendix E; CXR #2; ]. What are the arrows pointing to?
    a. A collapsed lung
    b. Wide mediastinum
    c. Cardiac tamponade
    d. Cardiomegaly


# PART 8: RESPIRATORY MANAGEMENT RATIONALES


1. (C) This patient has an increased EtCO2 (52 mmHg) and to correct this problem we need to increase his minute ventilation. We could either increase RR or increase Vt. There is no option to increase RR, but there is an option to increase Vt, therefore, it is the correct answer.

2. (B) This patient is over breathing the vent (note his (f) is more than the set rate of 12) so they have blown off a lot of EtCO2 (30 mmHg). To fix this problem we need to sedate the patient which will reduce the frequency, and thus the minute ventilation). This will in turn allow the EtCO2 to rise toward normal. Increasing the RR to match the (f) is a practice that should never happen. All that does is cover up the issue and fails to address the underlying problem. The only other way to correct this is to increase the SENSITIVITY should the patient be paralyzed.

3. **(D)** If you increase PEEP you are risking increasing the intrathoracic pressure, which could reduce the venous return to the heart. If this occurs, simply correct it with a fluid bolus and replace the preload.

4. **(B)** The verbal shorthand "18/4" is telling you that the pressure control (PC) is set at 18 and the PEEP is set at 4. You add these numbers together to get 22, so the PIP is 22. The ventilator is set to deliver 18 cmH2O into the patients lungs which is on top of the 4 cmH2O of PEEP that was left over from the last breath for a total of 22 cmH2O. Normal I:E is 1:2, so the I:E option is incorrect. We do not have the information to know the minute ventilation, so that option is also wrong.

5. **(A)** This mode allows for spontaneous breaths. Some spontaneous breaths can happen unassisted, and some are assisted (depending on where in the respiratory cycle the patient attempts a breath). This mode does not synchronize to the patient with each breath, so that option is wrong. It also doesn't require a paralytic, nor does it automatically increase PEEP, so both those answers are also wrong.

6. **(C)** Positive pressure ventilation (PPV) forces air into a lung that normally pulls air into itself with negative pressure. This is foreign to our physiology and can be detrimental if used incorrectly. Any increase in intrathoracic pressure, such as the increase that occurs with PPV, there is a reduction in venous return to the heart, thus reducing preload. This reduction in preload translates into lower cardiac output. PPV allows for increased oxygenation (with PEEP and FiO2), so that option is incorrect. It also will not inherently cause a cardiac tamponade, so that option is also incorrect. Widening pulse pressure is a sign of cardiac tamponade, and we just said that PPV doesn't cause this condition.

7. **(A)** Step 1– first part- is pH acidotic or alkalotic? Step 2– the culprit- which sub-parameter match's the pH- if PaCO2 matches then its "respiratory" as middle name and if HCO3 matches then the middle name is "metabolic". Step 3- ID level of compensation- acute (if pH and one sub-parameter match and the other sub-parameter are NORMAL), Mixed (all parameters either acidic or alkalotic), Partially compensated (if 3 No Rule present), and Fully compensation (if pH is normal and both sub-parameters are abnormal).

8. **(B)** Step 1– first part- is pH acidotic or alkalotic? Step 2– the culprit- which sub-parameter matches the pH- if PaCO2 matches then its "respiratory" as middle name and if HCO3 matches then the middle name is "metabolic". Step 3- ID level of compensation- acute (if pH and one sub-parameter match and the other sub-parameter are NORMAL), Mixed (all parameters either acidic or alkalotic), Partially compensated (if 3 No Rule present), and Fully compensated (if pH is normal and both sub-parameters are abnormal).

9. **(D)** Step 1– first part- is pH acidotic or alkalotic? Step 2– the culprit- which sub-parameter matches the pH- if PaCO2 matches then its "respiratory" as middle name and if HCO3 matches then the middle name is "metabolic". Step 3- ID level of compensation- acute (if pH and one sub-parameter match and the other sub-parameter are NORMAL), Mixed (all parameters either acidic or alkalotic), Partially compensated (if 3 No Rule present), and Fully compensated (if pH is normal and both sub-parameters are abnormal).

10. **(A)** Step 1– first part- is pH acidotic or alkalotic? Step 2– the culprit- which sub-parameter matches the pH- if PaCO2 matches then its "respiratory" as middle name and if HCO3 matches then the middle name is "metabolic". Step 3- ID level of compensation- acute (if pH and one sub-parameter match and the other sub- CONTINUED) parameter is NORMAL), Mixed (all parameters either acidic or alkalotic), Partially compensated (if 3 No Rule present), and Fully compensated (if pH is normal and both sub-parameters are abnormal).

11. **(D)** Step 1– first part- is pH acidotic or alkalotic? Step 2– the culprit- which sub-parameter matches the pH- if PaCO2 matches then its "respiratory" as middle name and if HCO3 matches then the middle name is "metabolic". Step 3- ID level of compensation- acute (if pH and one sub-parameter match and the other sub-parameter are NORMAL), Mixed (all parameters either acidic or alkalotic),

Partially compensated (if 3 No Rule present), and Fully compensated (if pH is normal and both sub-parameters are abnormal).

12. **(C)** Step 1– first part- is pH acidotic or alkalotic? Step 2– the culprit- which sub-parameter matches the pH- if $PaCO_2$ matches then its "respiratory" as middle name and if $HCO_3$ matches then the middle name is "metabolic". Step 3- ID level of compensation- acute (if pH and one sub-parameter match and the other sub-parameter are NORMAL), Mixed (all parameters either acidic or alkalotic), Partially compensated (if 3 No Rule present), and Fully compensated (if pH is normal and both sub-parameters are abnormal).

13. **(B)** Step 1– first part- is pH acidotic or alkalotic? Step 2– the culprit- which sub-parameter matches the pH- if $PaCO_2$ matches then its "respiratory" as middle name and if $HCO_3$ matches then the middle name is "metabolic". Step 3- ID level of compensation- acute (if pH and one sub-parameter match and the other sub-parameter are NORMAL), Mixed (all parameters either acidic or alkalotic), Partially compensated (if 3 No Rule present), and Fully compensated (if pH is normal and both sub-parameters are abnormal).

14. **(C)** Step 1– first part- is pH acidotic or alkalotic? Step 2– the culprit- which sub-parameter matches the pH- if $PaCO_2$ matches then its "respiratory" as middle name and if $HCO_3$ matches then the middle name is "metabolic". Step 3- ID level of compensation- acute (if pH and one sub-parameter match and the other sub-parameter are NORMAL), Mixed (all parameters either acidic or alkalotic), Partially compensated (if 3 No Rule present), and Fully compensated (if pH is normal and both sub-parameters are abnormal).

15. **(A)** The only settings that can effect a change in $SpO_2$ is increasing or decreasing PEEP and/ or $FiO_2$.

16. **(D)** The only settings that can change $EtCO_2$ is TV, RR, and pressure control. Increasing TV, RR, and PC will REDUCE $EtCO_2$ while decreasing TV, RR, and PC will all ELEVATE $EtCO_2$.

17. **(C)** With this patient, the lower temperature will shift the oxyhemoglobin disassociation curve to the left, along with a high affinity (stickiness) for oxygen by the red blood cell. This results in decreased release of oxygen once the red blood cell is passing the tissues. This means that the AC to saturation is high, but oxygen is just not released from the red blood cell at the level of the tissues. Therefore, the tissues become hypoxic, acidic, and can die. Slurring does not happen on the QRS because of cold temperatures, and Osbourne wave does. Hypotension just does not occur because it's cold, and DIC does not occur just because a patient is entrapped.

18. **(B)** The oxyhemoglobin disassociation curve speaks to the affinity, or stickiness, of oxygen to the red blood cell. It does not discuss oxygen supply or demand. The real question here is, is it a left or a right shift? Remember that increased $CO_2$ (as well as increased acid, temperature, & DPG) indicate a shift to the right.

19. **(A)** Every change in pH of 0.1, the potassium changes 0.6 in the opposite direction. Therefore, if pH is 7.32 and changes to 7.22 (a reduction), then the potassium will increase. If it started out at 4.5 mmol/L, then it would be 5.1 mmol/L after the change in pH.

20. **(C)** If the monitored $SpO_2$ is 90%, then the expected $PaCO_2$ is 60 mmHg. If the monitored $SpO_2$ is 80%, then the expected $PaCO_2$ is 50 mmHg. If the monitored $SpO_2$ is 70%, then the expected $PaCO_2$ is 40 mmHg.

21. **(A)** Once the $CO_2$ gets above 55 mmHg and the [H remains acidic, then respiratory failure is present. The other medications are all appropriate but at this point, the patient needs to be intubated.

22. **(D)** Reversing the I:E ratio will put the patient and maximal PEEP. This will help to maximize their oxidation ability. Increasing the minute ventilation will not help and increasing the tidal volume will essentially increase the minute ventilation, so these two selections are incorrect. Reducing PEEP will worsen oxygenation, so it is an incorrect answer is well .

23. **(A)** This x– ray indicates a collapsed lung or pneumothoracies.

# CHAPTER 3: CARDIAC MANAGMENT

## PART 1: SYSTEMIC CARDIAC REVIEW

### INTRODUCTION

Ultimately, we want to know that the heart is adequately propelling blood forward through our vasculature. That's why we conduct a cardiac assessment. Therefore, we need to take measurements of multiple parameters to know that this forward pumping is occurring adequately. Once we know these measurements, then we can act. For example, if BP is low, then we can give fluids, administer an inotrope, or give a pressor; if the heart is beating too slow, we can apply electrical therapy to increase rate. The BIG PICTURE is to determine if the cardiovascular system is operating adequately, and if not, then to remedy the problem.

### *FORWARD FLOW AND PREVENTING ACIDOSIS*
1.  To be able to assess and manage complicated cardiac problems, we need to understand its components: electrical and mechanical (the pump and flow).
2.  These components drive blood forward and with it, nutrients to tissues and cells. Additionally, the blood's forward flow through the venous system picks up cellular 'trash' for disposal ($CO_2$ and lactic acids).
3.  Our job as critical care transport clinicians will essentially be to simply prevent acidosis. As normal metabolism progresses, sugar and oxygen are utilized to make energy, heat, water, and carbon dioxide.
4.  If we do not provide adequate oxygen to our patients or if we fail to ensure perfusion (transporting oxygen to the cells/ picking up metabolic trash like $CO_2$), then acidosis occurs.
5.  Consider a cold classroom. If a teacher does not turn on the heat inside a classroom in a winter, then you may not be able to focus on the lessons of the day. Most likely, you would be too focused on your ensuing hypothermia and how to stay warm. This same thing happens in the body when acid surrounds it bathes our cells. Our cells fail to do their job: nervous tissue cannot conduct electricity, cardiac tissue cannot pull blood anymore, liver tissue cannot clear out toxins, and our kidneys cannot concentrate urine. Over time, this results in total systemic collapse and death.
6.  In the critical care transport setting, you will be asked to manage difficult cases, but a systematic approach will help you identify the information that will assist you in making clinical decisions.

### *THE CONDUCTIVE SYSTEM*
1.  The conduction system is composed of the SA node, the AV node, and the conductive tissue pathways which produce electrical impulses.
2.  The heart contracts in response to electrical stimuli produced by the SA node, the AV node, the bundle of HIS, Purkinje fibers, and even in the myocytes. Automaticity– myocytes produce own stimulus when HR is too low).
3.  We can measure this flow of electricity as it progresses down this conduction system by viewing an ECG.
4.  In a healthy heart, the SA node generates an electrical impulse and it travels to the AV node: this results in atrial depolarization, we recognize this as the P– wave on the ECG.
5.  The stimulus then spreads through the bundle of His producing ventricular depolarization: we recognize this as the QRS complex on the ECG.

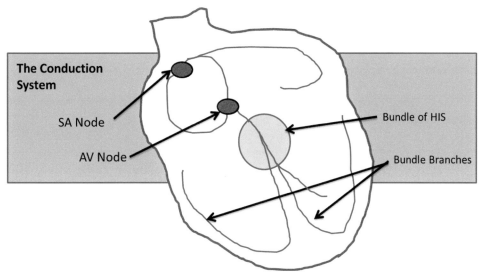

The Conduction System

SA Node

AV Node

Bundle of HIS

Bundle Branches

6. The atria are repolarized as the ventricles are Depolarized, so there isn't a clear atrial repolarization waveform on the ECG. It is "buried" behind the big QRS waveform.
7. The T wave represents ventricular repolarization.
8. It is important to identify the normal morphology (shape) of the ECG. Different conditions will cause the ECG to vary in appearance, and we can recognize these patterns, identify a pathophysiology, and then choose the appropriate treatment based on the pathophysiology.
9. The PRIMARY pacemaker is the SA node, and it fires at 60-100 times/min.
10. Secondary pacer sites:
    a. AV Junction: 40-60 times/min
    b. Purkinje System: 20-40 times/min

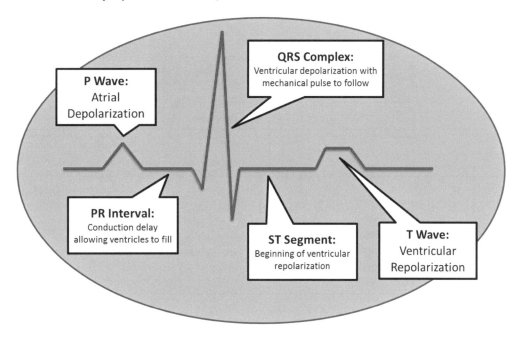

P Wave: Atrial Depolarization

QRS Complex: Ventricular depolarization with mechanical pulse to follow

PR Interval: Conduction delay allowing ventricles to fill

ST Segment: Beginning of ventricular repolarization

T Wave: Ventricular Repolarization

## THE CARDIAC PUMP

1. The CARDIAC CYCLE comprises one complete phase of atrial contraction, ventricular contraction, atrial relaxation and ventricular relaxation.
2. Both atria contract simultaneously, and the ventricles also contract simultaneously immediately after the atria do.
3. The term systole (which means contraction), can be used to describe a specific chamber of the heart, but often it is generally referring to VENTRICULAR contraction.
4. The term diastole (which means relax), can be used to describe any specific chamber of the heart, but, like "systole," it is generally used to describe VENTRICULAR relaxation.
5. The cardiac pump is composed of the muscular chambers (atria and ventricles) and valves and functions to keep blood moving forward.
6. Pump Physiology:

   **INITIAL VALVE STATUS:** AV Valves OPEN; Semilunar Valves CLOSED
   a. AV Valves: Mitral and Tricuspid.
   b. Semilunar Valves: Pulmonic and aortic
   c. Blood passively enters the atria and flows into the ventricles.
   d. Atrial depolarization occurs (noted by p-wave on the ECG).
   e. Atrial contraction follows moments later, pushing, even more, blood into the ventricles on top of the passive filling. This extra "push" is called the ATRIAL KICK. This extra blood in the ventricles increases the ventricular stretch, and when this happens, there is greater contractility. Just like jumping on a trampoline makes you go higher into the air, more ventricular stretch allows the ventricle to contract more forcefully.

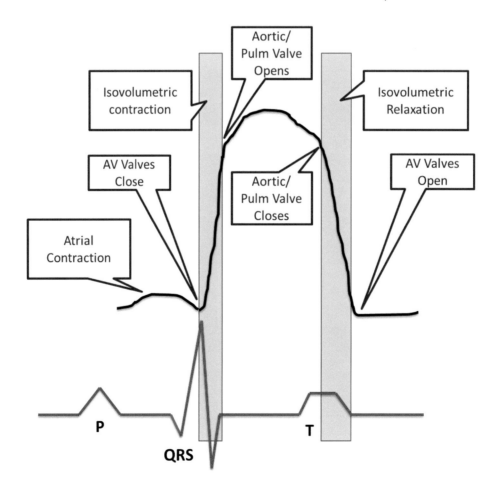

     f.    As the ventricles fill, pressure increases. At the same time pressure in the atria decreases Once ventricular pressure is higher than atrial pressure, the AV valves close. This closure represents the S1 heart tone, or the "**lub**".

**VALVE STATUS: ALL CLOSED.**

     g.    The ventricles depolarize, which is evident by the QRS on the ECG.

     h.    Ventricular contraction begins moments later, but it is an ISOVOLUMETRIC CONTRACTION, meaning there is not a volume change since all valves are closed, and there isn't flow between the chambers for a brief moment. Contraction is happening and getting stronger, but no fluid is moving. In this isovolumetric contraction, there is a rapid rise in ventricular pressure.

     i.    Once the pressure in the ventricles become higher than the pressures in the lungs and the aorta, the SEMILUNAR VALVES (the aortic and pulmonic valves) abruptly open, and blood rushes the lungs and into the aorta.

**VALVE STATUS: CLOSED AV, OPEN semilunar valves**

     j.    At this point, blood is being pushed out of the ventricles, and the pressure in the ventricles is falling. At the same time, the atria are receiving blood from the central venous system and the pulmonary vasculature.

     k.    Once there is greater pressure in the aorta and pulmonary artery, the semilunar valves close. This represents the S2 heart tone, or the "**dub**".

**VALVE STATUS: ALL CLOSED.**

     l.    With all the valves closed again, the ventricle begins to relax and creates a lowering ventricular pressure without the flow of blood (or volume), and this is called: ISOVOLUMETRIC RELAXATION.

     m.    At the same time, atrial pressures increase from passive filling from the vena cava and pulmonary veins.

     n.    Once atrial pressures are higher than ventricular pressures, the AV valves reopen.

**VALVE STATUS: Semilunar valves CLOSED; AV valves OPEN.**

     o.    Passive ventricular filling occurs as blood arrives from the vena cava and pulmonary veins into the atria and is funneled past the AV valves and into the ventricles.

     p.    Then, the entire cycle repeats.

7. Pump pathophysiology may result from valvular disease, injured or infarcted myocardium, or traumatized vascular structures.

## BLOOD FLOW

1. Normal physiology depends on the forward flow of blood. In diseased states, we will use therapies to improve the forward flow of blood. Therefore, the foundation of all cardiac management is to maintain the effective forward flow of blood.

2. **Path of Unoxygenated Blood Flow**: Superior Vena Cava & Inferior Vena Cava → R Atrium → Tricuspid valve → R Ventricle → Pulmonic Valve → Pulmonary Artery to lungs (gets oxygenated)

3. **Path of Oxygenated Blood Flow**: Pulmonary Veins → L Atrium → Mitral Valve → L Ventricle → Aortic Valve → Aorta → Coronary Arteries (during diastole) → Body

## CARDIAC OUTPUT

1. The volume of blood (in liters) ejected by the heart each minute.

2. Normal:
     a.    Adults 4-8 L/min
     b.    Peds 1-3 L/min
     c.    Infants 0.8-1 L/min

3. Formula: CO = HR x SV

**HEART RATE**

1. This means that any medicine or procedure that ↓ HR will generally REDUCE the CO.
2. Any medicine or procedure that ↑ HR will generally ELEVATE the CO.

**Stroke Volume**

1. The stroke volume (SV) is the amount of blood pumped out of the heart in a single BEAT.
2. Normal:
    a. Adults 60-100 mL/beat
    b. Peds 15-50 mL/beat
    c. Infants 5-15 mL/beat
3. Major Factors:
    a. There are three factors that affect the amount of blood ejected out of the heart with each beat: preload, afterload, and contractility.
    b. Preload:
        i. This represents the fluid returning to the atria (thus ventricles) before ventricular contraction.
        ii. Anytime we are administering a fluid bolus, or challenge, to a patient to replace intravascular volume, we are replacing lost preload.
    c. Contractility:
        i. This is the amount of force generated by the contracting ventricle.
        ii. According to **Frank– Starling mechanism**, the more a ventricle is filled with blood, the stronger the contraction of that ventricle. The more the myocytes stretch, the more powerful the contraction.
        iii. This means that any medicine or procedure that ↓ CONTRACTILITY will REDUCE the CO.
        iv. Any medicine or procedure that ↑ contractility will ELEVATE the CO.
    d. Afterload:
        i. This directly represents the pressure the heart must pump against to eject blood into the aorta or lungs.
        ii. High systemic (SVR)or high pulmonary (PVR) blood pressure makes it more difficult for the heart to pump blood into those areas.
            1. SVR- systemic vascular resistance
            2. PVR- pulmonary vascular resistance
    e. When conceptualizing preload and afterload, one way is to consider the 'water hose' analogy. If the faucet is barely on, then only a small amount of water is flowing (poor preload) indicating, a lower pressure. However, if you put your thumb on the end of the hose and partially cover the opening, then water flows out violently in a powerful stream (increased afterload).
    f. AFTERLOAD Goes Both Ways…
        i. Decreases in afterload with failing heart will improve CO.
        ii. An exception to this rule that reducing afterload improves CO is when pressors are used **_AND_** there is sufficient volume in the vasculature.
        iii. When the 'tank is full' and a pressor is added, it will indeed increase the afterload, thus make it harder to advance blood into the arterial tree. However, the hope and goal is that this price is worth the increase in preload this causes.
        iv. With increased afterload (and with a 'full tank') it influences blood in the venous system to be pushed into the right atria, therefore increasing preload.
        v. This occurs from the increased pressure in the arterial tree pushing blood forward into the venous system.

# CO = HR x Preload x Contractility x (-Afterload)

1. You can see here that we added preload, afterload, and contractility into the CO = HR x SV equation since SV will change based on these three factors.
2. Therefore, we can rely on the following therapeutic mechanisms:
   a. To ↑ cardiac output: ↑ HR, preload, or contractility.
   b. To ↑ cardiac output: ↓ afterload (with a fluid overloaded heart).
   c. To ↑ cardiac output: ↑ afterload (with a normal heart strength).
   d. To ↓ cardiac output: ↓ HR, preload, or contractility.
   e. Atropine and beta 1 agonists will ↑ HR; while beta blockers and calcium channel blockers will ↓ HR.
   f. Isotonic fluids and increasing blood pressures will ↑ preload; while hypotension and/ or hypovolemia will ↓ preload.
   g. Improving preload and inotropes will ↑ contractility; while reduced preload will ↓ contractility.
   h. Any medication where VASODILATION is a direct effect or a side effect will ↓ afterload; however, any medication where VASOCONSTRICTION is a direct effect or a side effect will ↑ afterload.
3. You can see here why it is important to understand medication mechanisms. If you know the mechanism, then you can apply it to pathophysiology, and change these parameters to improve your patient's cardiac output.

### Mean Arterial Pressure (MAP)
1. Mean Arterial Pressure:  [systolic BP  +  (2 x diastolic BP)/3]
2. Normal: > 60-70 mmHg
3. The MAP is so important to critical care medicine. It is accepted throughout the literature that MAP is the perfusion pressure that allows blood pumped from heart to reach the distal tissues and organs.
4. If MAP falls below the normal value for too long, then hypoxia is triggered in distal tissues which later can lead to acidosis, coma, and death.

# PART 2: THE CARDIAC ASSESSMENT

## INTRODUCTION

The cardiac assessment is complex because it has so many components: general assessment, 3– lead monitoring, 12– lead monitoring, hemodynamic monitoring and management, balloon pump monitoring and management, among others. This section will cover a general cardiac examination with advanced assessments later in the chapter. If at any point during the initial assessment that you identify a life threat, correct it immediately. Do not wait to continue the initial assessment.

## Initial Assessment

1. As you approach the patient, look at their body position, work of breathing and skin condition and color.
   a. Their body position alone often provides valuable information: tripod means they are short of breath/ hypoxic, laying on the ground with weak muscles may indicate what the patient is in extreme hypoxia.
   b. Normal respiratory effort indicates that the patient is receiving adequate oxygen, but labored respirations often indicates hypoxia.
   c. Normal skin color indicates adequate perfusion, but pale or mottled skin can indicate poor perfusion.
2. Assess Mental Status
   a. AVPU: Awake– eyes open spontaneously; Verbal- arouses to stimulation by voice; Painful– purposeful movements to painful stimuli; Unresponsive- no response to any stimuli
   b. GCS:
      i. Eye Opening: Spontaneous (4); to speech (3); to painful stimuli (2); no opening at all (1)
      ii. Verbal Effort: normal conversation (5); confused (4); inappropriate words (3); incomprehensible sounds (2); no verbal effort (1)
      iii. Motor Effort: follows commands (6); localizes pains (5); withdraws from pain (4); decorticate posturing (3); decerebrate posturing (2); no motor effort (1)
3. Airway: Ensure a patent airway.
4. Breathing and Respiratory Effort: Note rate, quality (normal or labored), and rhythm (normal or abnormal respiratory patterns).
5. Circulation:
   a. Ensure the patient has a pulse and note the rate, strength (normal, bounding, or weak), and quality (regular or irregular).
   b. Compare central to peripheral pulses.
   c. Obtain and assess heart rate, blood pressure, pulse oximetry, cardiac monitoring, and labs/ images, if available.
6. Focused Cardiac Assessment
   a. Consider Chief Complaint
      i. Chest Pain: Indicates potential myocardial ischemia/ injury (but absence does not rule an MI out!)
      ii. Burning/ Tearing Back Pain: Indicates dissecting aneurysm
      iii. Palpitations: Indicates a dysrhythmia
   b. Assess the Patient's History
      i. Orthopnea: Indicates left sided heart failure
      ii. Paroxysmal Nocturnal Dyspnea: Indicates left sided heart failure
      iii. Medications indicating Coronary Artery Disease (CAD): anticoagulant/ antiplatelet; beta blockers; calcium channel blockers; nitrates
      iv. Medications indicating hypertension (HTN): beta blockers; calcium channel blockers; ACE inhibitors, serotonin reuptake inhibitor (SRIs)
      v. Medications indicating congestive heart failure (CHF): digitalis or other inotropes; diuretics
   c. Assess for body style:
      i. Obese: indicates a risk factor for acute coronary syndromes (ACS)
      ii. Cachectic: indicates poor nutrition and possible electrolyte problems
      iii. Barrel Chest: Indicates the patient likely has COPD
   d. Assess Head to Toe:
      i. Tripod: indicates hypoxia and potential ACS
      ii. Cool, moist skin: Indicates poor cardiac output

        iii.    Sticky mucus membranes: Indicates poor cardiac output

        iv.    Delayed capillary refill: Indicates poor cardiac output

        v.    JVD: Indicates right-sided heart failure

        vi.    Bruits: Indicates arterial stenosis

        vii.    Clubbing: Indicates COPD

        viii.    Hepatojugular Reflex: Indicates right-sided heart failure

        ix.    Ascites: Indicates possible right sided heart failure

        x.    Pulmonary edema: Indicates left sided heart failure

        xi.    Pedal edema: Indicates right-sided heart failure

e.    Assess Vital Signs

        i.    Mental status change: Indicates hypoxia from poor brain perfusion; hypoglycemia; electrolyte disturbances

        ii.    Bradycardia: Indicates prolonged hypoxia or beta blocker/ narcotic/benzodiazepine OD/ inferior wall AMI

        iii.    Tachycardia: Indicates hypoxia, low cardiac output, hypovolemia, pain/anxiety, trauma

        iv.    Dramatic increase in EtCO2 during CPR: Indicates ROSC (Return of Spontaneous Circulation)

        v.    Low BP (< 90mmHg): Indicates blood loss, dehydration, uncompensated shock, sedation/ nitrates/ pain med OD, Tension pneumothorax, cardiac tamponade

        vi.    High EtCO2: Indicates low tidal volume, slow RR, respiratory acidosis

        vii.    Low EtCO2: Indicates high tidal volume, fast RR, respiratory alkalosis; POOR PERFUSION

        viii.    Low SpO2: Indicates low oxygen at the capillary beds, hypovolemia, pain/anxiety, falling cardiac output

f.    Assess 12 Lead ECG.

g.    Assess Hemodynamic Monitoring

h.    Assess Labs and Images.

i.    Assess Previous Treatments

j.    Medications: make sure any infusions are appropriate and infusing correctly

        i.    Devices/ Procedures: Ensure any applied medical devices/ procedures were appropriately conducted and ensure their continued maintenance throughout transport.

        ii.    Continue patient monitoring as appropriate.

# PART 3: THE 12-LEAD ASSESSMENT

## INTRODUCTION

The 12 lead ECG is a staple assessment and can help confirm suspicions of myocardial ischemia or infarction. Anytime you assess a 12 lead ECG, you should always do so in a SYSTEMATIC manner- do it the same way each and every time.

## ABCS OF ECGS

This is my method to approach the morphologies of the 12 lead ECG in alphabetical order: axis, blocks, periCarditis (use the 'C' in pericarditis, not the 'P'), drug effects, electrolyte abnormalities, "Funny" waves, general impression, hypertrophy, and infarcts.

## AXIS

1. Axis is essentially a representation of the electrical direction within the heart.
2. Typically, the flow of electrical current begins at the SA node and progresses down the conduction system toward the apex (bottom tip) of the heart.
3. Normal axis is measured in the frontal plane and is best conceptualized by visualizing a circle with zero degrees beginning at the 3 o'clock position.
4. Moving from this zero in a clockwise direction, we arrive at 90 degrees (at 6 o'clock position), and to 180 degrees (at 9 o'clock position). Beginning at the 3 0'clock position and moving counter-clockwise, we arrive at –90 degrees (at 12 o'clock position ) and then on to –180 degrees (at the 9 o'clock position).
5. By assessing the axis, you can identify hemiblocks and potential early signs of cardiac ischemia.
6. Ischemia = poor blood flow = no oxygen to conductive tissue and myocardium = hemiblocks occur = axis becomes abnormal

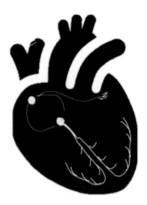

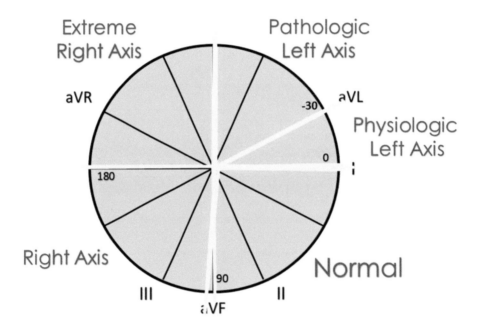

7. Measurement Method: You can identify axis by the measurements printed on the ECG. This information is typically found on the top left of the printed ECG and labeled as either "R" or "QRS".
   a. Normal axis: 0– 90 degrees
   b. Right axis deviation: 90– 180 degrees
   c. Extreme right axis deviation: -90- -180 degrees
   d. Physiologic left axis deviation: 0 to –30 degrees
   e. Pathologic left axis deviation: -30 to –90 degrees
8. Lead I/ aVF Method:
   a. An alternative method is to look at Lead I and aVF for positive and negative QRS deflections on the ECG.
   b. A POSITIVE QRS deflection is one that most of the ECG looks UPRIGHT.

c.    A NEGATIVE QRS deflection is one that the majority of waveform looks DOWNWARD.

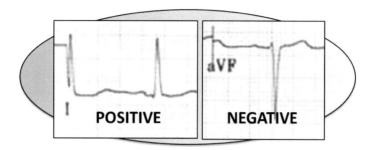

d.    Findings and Interpretation:
     i.    ↑ Lead I and ↑ aVF = Normal Axis
     ii.   ↑ Lead I and ↓ aVF = Left Axis Deviation
          1.   To identify if it is pathological, look at lead II.
          2.   If it's NEGATIVE, then the axis is pathologic. (pathologic left axis deviation).
          3.   If it's POSITIVE, then the axis is physiologic (physiologic left axis deviation).
     iii.  ↓ Lead I and ↑ aVF = Right Axis Deviation
     iv.   ↓ Lead I and ↓ aVF =  Extreme Right Axis Deviation
e.    In the previous figure, Lead I is POSITIVE, and aVF is NEGATIVE; therefore, this ECG is representative of a left axis deviation. We now need to determine if Lead II is positive or negative:

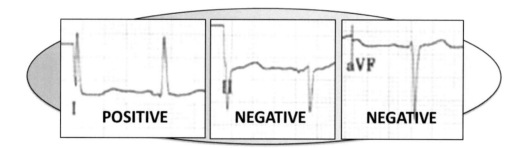

f.    By examining Lead II, we see that it is NEGATIVE, and therefore, this ECG is representative of pathologic left axis deviation, and thus, could be an early sign that there are coronary artery occlusion and myocardial ischemia.

9.   Axis Etiologies:
     a.   Pathologic Left Axis: This is caused by inferior AMI, left bundle branch block, left anterior hemiblock or left ventricular hypertrophy.
     b.   Right Axis Deviation: This is caused by left posterior hemiblock, or right ventricular hypertrophy (right sided heart failure and/ or cor pulmonale).
     c.   Extreme Right Axis Deviation: This is caused by ventricular arrhythmia; therefore, a wide and fast QRS complex is most likely ventricular tachycardia.

## BLOCKS

1. A block is simply a disruption in the conductive tissue (most likely from myocardial ischemia) where the electrical pulse is not allowed to progress down the conduction system of the heart normally. It is like a roadblock.
2. Once the electrical pulse hits the "road block", the impulse must find a way around the "roadblock". When the impulse goes "off road", we can detect this on a 12 lead ECG.
3. Axis is one way to identify quickly if a particular block is occurring. A second way to identify a block is to look at the width and direction (upward or downward deflections) in V1. There are other ways to identify blocks; however, we will look at these two methods.

### Axis: Method

    a. Beyond the Bundle of His along the conductive tissue, we find our bundle branches.

    b. The left bundle branch splits into two parts:

    c. Left anterior fascicle

    i. Left posterior fascicle

    d. When one of these two are blocked, it is called a "HEMIBLOCK" (see the top of next page).

    e. If you have pathologic left axis deviation, then you have a left anterior hemifascicular block (left anterior hemiblock).

    f. If you have a right axis deviation, then you are likely witnessing a left posterior hemifascicular block (left posterior hemiblock).

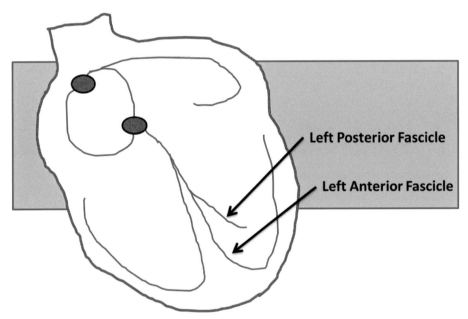

### V1 Method

1. A block is something that slows down, or blocks completely, the normal conduction of the heart.
2. The ECG Paper reads from left to right.
3. We know that the QRS complex should be less than 120milliseconds, therefore, a wide QRS complex indicates a blockage in the conduction system.
4. One method of identifying this phenomenon is to look at the lead V1 on the 12 lead ECG.
5. 120 milliseconds is equivalent to 3 small boxes on the ECG paper, thus looking for the late conduction from a block is as simple as counting more than three boxes.
6. Criteria:

    a. Wide complexes in V1 (greater than 3 small boxes on the ECG tracing, or >120ms) indicate a bundle branch is blocked.

b. Left Turn:
   i. Starting at the ST segment, trace the ECG backward to the J point.
   ii. If at the J point (and still tracking backward on the ECG) the deflection goes DOWNWARD, then there is a LEFT bundle branch block.

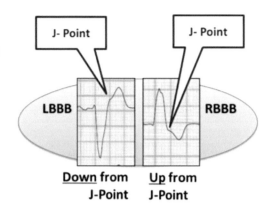

c. If you are turning left in your car, you push the turn signal down to indicate left, just like you do in V1: if you have a downward deflection from the J point in V1, it is a LEFT bundle branch block.
   i. Right Turn:
   ii. Starting at the ST segment, trace the ECG backward to the J point.
   iii. If at the J point (and still tracking backward on the ECG) the deflection goes UPWARD, then there is a right bundle branch block.
   iv. If you are turning RIGHT in your car, you push the turn signal up to indicate right, just like you do in V1: if you have an upward deflection from the J point in V1, it is a RIGHT bundle branch block.

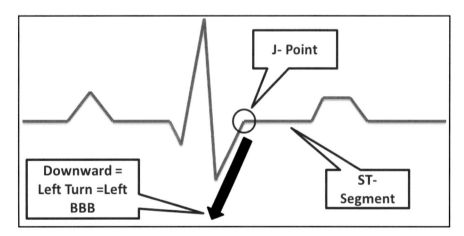

7. Blocks can be categorized according to where they fall in the conduction system: sinoatrial area (SA), the atrioventricular area (AV), and the intraventricular area (IV).
    a. SA blocks: sinus arrest, sinus pause, or sinus block
    b. AV blocks: first-degree, second-degree type I, second-degree type II
    c. IV blocks: hemiblocks (fascicular blocks), bundle branch blocks
8. Don't let "fascicular" confuse you. Fascicular just means a portion of the conduction system.
    a. If you have a left anterior hemiblock, then you have a fascicular block.
    b. If you have a first-degree heart block and a left anterior hemiblock, then you have a BIFASCICULAR block.
    c. Any combination of 3 different blocks is termed a TRIFASCICULAR block.

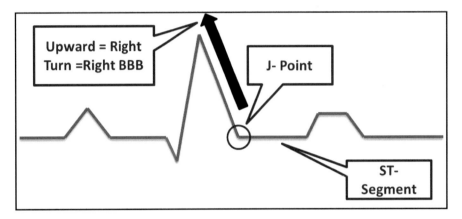

## PERI*CARDITIS*

1. Pericarditis can mimic an acute myocardial infarction (AMI), so it is important to be able to distinguish AMI from pericarditis quickly.
2. Pericarditis is an inflammation of the pericardial sac which can be caused by infection, chest trauma, AMI, drugs, and autoimmune disorders.
3. Features of Pericarditis:
    a. Global ST– Segment Elevation:
        i. We will later review the various AMI patterns, such as II, III, and aVF for an inferior wall AMI.
        ii. Pericarditis has global ST elevation or said another way, almost every 12 leads show ST– elevation patterns.
    b. PR Depression: With pericarditis, some of the leads will reflect a depressed PR segment, which is an angled (normally) PR under the isoelectric line.
    c. Notching: With pericarditis, in some leads you may note a notching on the right side of the QRS complex. If this is observed, then you'll have another piece of evidence supporting pericarditis.

d. Scooping and Upward Concave ST Segment: With pericarditis, in some leads you may also see an upward scooping pattern of the ST segment.

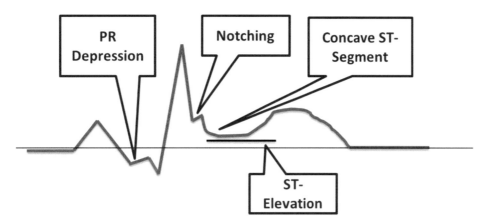

4. It is important to take into consideration all the pieces of information that may support either a

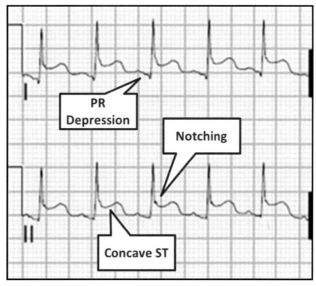

pericarditis field diagnosis or an AMI.
5. Hint: ST segment elevation in both leads I and II is indicative of pericarditis.
    a. ST Elevation in leads I and aVL = high lateral AMI pattern
    b. ST elevation in II, III, and aVF = inferior AMI pattern
    c. Leads I and II look at opposite sides of the heart.
    d. So, unless they are have a remarkably huge AMI, then the presence of ST elevation in lead I and lead II indicates PERICARDITIS. This is a quick trick to differentiate AMI vs. pericarditis.

## DRUG EFFECTS

### Digitalis
1. Almost every medication has the potential to change the ECG, however, digitalis is one of the few with SPECIFC ECG changes.
2. Digitalis is a medication administered to improve contractility in heart failure patients.
3. 12 Lead Presentation: It looks like a soup ladle or Hockey stick.
4. Digitalis may also cause a variety of cardiac dysrhythmias.
5. Management:

i. REVERSAL: Digibind (6 vials for chronic OD, and 10 for acute).
ii. MAINTAIN POTASSIUM: Target 4 mEq/L. If hyperkalemic, then provide standard therapy (calcium, dextrose & insulin, bicarb, albuterol, Kayexalate)
iii. BRADYCARDIA: atropine, pacing, dopamine, or epinephrine.

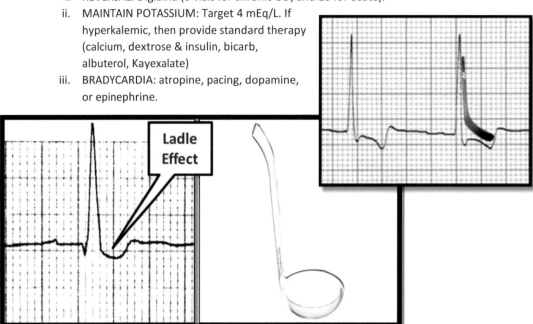

**Ladle Effect**

## TCA Overdose
1. Tricyclic Antidepressants are sodium channel blockers, so an overdose represents sodium channel blockade.
2. These can present with:
    i. Tachycardia
    ii. Prolonged PR & QRS
    iii. R wave in aVR
    iv. Right Axis Deviation
    v. AMS
    vi. Seizures
3. Management:
    i. AMS: RSI the patient for airway protection.
    ii. RECENT INGESTION: Activated charcoal can be considered if it was within 30 minutes.
    iii. HYPOTENSION:IV normal saline (for sodium) and pressors if needed.
    iv. SODIUM REPLACEMENT: Sodium bicarb
    v. SEIZURES: 3% saline, benzodiazepines, phenytoin or phosphenytoin. Use the 3% saline first.

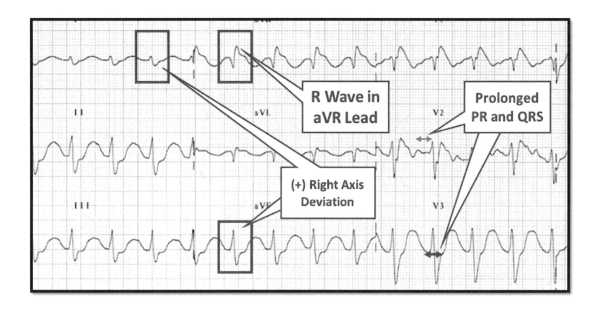

## ELECTROLYTE EFFECTS

### Hyperkalemia

1. Tall, PEAKED T waves are characteristic.
2. Usually occurs at or above 5.5 mEq/L
3. Gets taller and wider as K+ continues to increase
4. PATHOLOGIC: when T wave is 2/3 the height of R wave
5. As K+ continues to rise, the QRS will widen and take a sine wave pattern.
6. Management: provide standard therapy (calcium, dextrose & insulin, bicarb, albuterol, Kayexalate

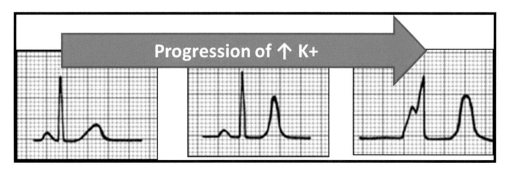

### Hypokalemia

1. The presence of U waves is characteristic.
2. Occurs with:
3. ST segment depression
4. Low T wave amplitude
5. Progressively growing and prominent U wave with worsening hypokalemia.
6. QU interval is long (>450 ms).

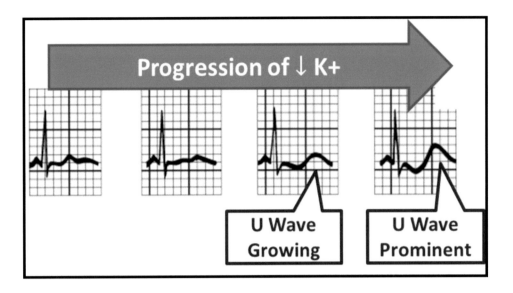

7. Management:
    i. 10 mEq of K+ should increase serum K+ by 0.1
    ii. Must mix with a minimum of 100mL for each 10 mEq to not damage blood vessels
    iii. **Peripheral:** 10 mEq/L/hr until K+ is > 3.5
    iv. **Central:** Up to 10-40 mEq/L/hr
    v. Consider replacing Magnesium also!

**Hypercalcemia**
1. Tall, wide, and ROUND T waves
2. Occurs with:
    a. $Ca^{2+}$ > 13 mg/dL
    b. Short QRS
    c. Widening QRS
3. Management: 2-3 L of isotonic crystalloid

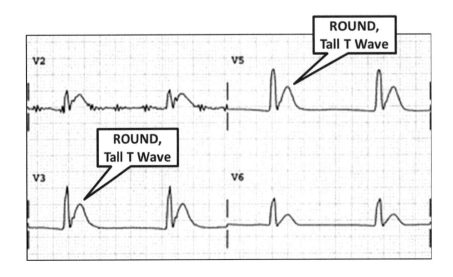

**Hypocalcemia**

1. Presentation:
   a. Main presentation is PROLONGED QT INTERVAL.
   b. Serum $Ca^{2+}$ < 8.5 mg/dL
   c. Chvostek's Sign and Trousseau's Sign present
2. Management
   a. Calculate corrected serum calcium:
   b. [(Normal albumin- serum albumin) x 0.8] + serum $Ca^{2+}$
   c. 1-2 grams over 15 minutes

**Hypernatremia**

1. Presentation:
   a. Serum Na+ > 145 mmol/L (critical is about 155 mmol/L)
   b. Chvostek's Sign and Trousseau's Sign present
2. Management
   a. Calculate corrected serum calcium:
   b. [(Normal albumin- serum albumin) x 0.8] + serum $Ca^{2+}$
   c. 1-2 grams over 15 minutes

**Hypocalcemia**

1. Presentation:
   a. Main presentation is PROLONGED QT INTERVAL.
   b. Serum $Ca^{2+}$ < 8.5 mg/dL
   c. Chvostek's Sign and Trousseau's Sign present
2. Management
   a. Calculate corrected serum calcium:
   b. [(Normal albumin- serum albumin) x 0.8] + serum $Ca^{2+}$
   c. 1-2 grams over 15 minutes
   d.

## *FUNNY WAVES*

1. There are several miscellaneous 12 lead ECG waveforms that are worth noting, so they will be discussed here.
2. Waveforms to discuss: Delta Wave, Notching, Osborne Wave, Pathologic Q wave, and Sine Waves.

### Delta Wave

1. Typically seen in Wolf-Parkinson-White (WPW) syndrome
2. An accessory pathway called the Bundle of Kent allows impulses to bypass the AV node to get to the ventricles
3. Bypassing the AV node can cause SVT or A-Fib which then can lead to hemodynamic instability
4. Two Major Electrophysiological Events Occur in WPW:
    i. PR interval shortened to <120ms
    ii. QRS widens to >100ms

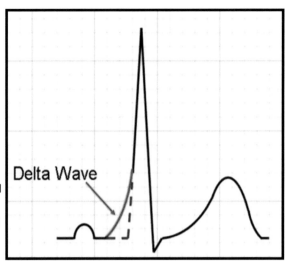

### QRS Notching

1. Almost always a benign (non-AMI) cause of ST elevation
    i. Early repolarization
    ii. Pericarditis
2. HINT: QRS Notching WITH ST elevation is 'almost 100%' NEGATIVE for infarction. So, if you have ST elevation and you have notching with it, then look around for other evidence of PERICARDITIS, because it is most likely NOT an AMI.

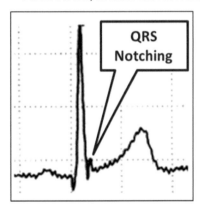 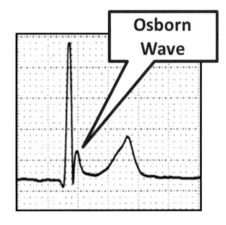

### Osborn Wave (pictured above right)

1. This interesting waveform is seen in hypothermic patients: < 90°F.
2. It is a positive deflection at the J point (can be negative in aVR and V1)
3. It is also called a J wave
4. Studies have reflected that Osborn wave prominence is proportional to degree of hypothermia
5. Hypothermia seen with bradycardia and QT prolongation

**Pathologic Q Waves**

1. Usually, Q waves represent septal innervation
2. Q waves can be pathological after significant myocardial damage, thus indicate an old infarction
3. Two Major Criteria in Identifying a Pathologic Q-Wave:
   a. > 0.03 of a second
   b. > 1/3 the height of the R wave

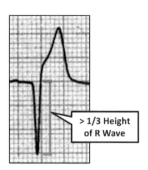

> 1/3 Height of R Wave

**Sine Wave**

1. Typically, a sign of GRAVE conduction pathology
2. Seen in severe hyperkalemia
3. Bizarre, wide QRS should prompt a conduction delay pathology

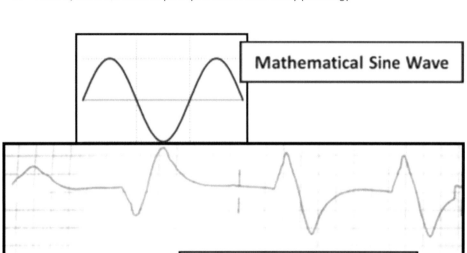

Mathematical Sine Wave

ECG Sine Wave

## GENERAL IMPRESSION

Always decide on a general impression, which considers the all the information relative to the patient's condition.

## HYPERTROPHY

1. Hypertrophy is a thickening (from excessive growth) of a chamber of the heart
2. It is caused by an increased workload; thus the heart works harder and gets bigger– just like at the gym. However, unlike at the gym, ventricular hypertrophy is usually associated with significant myocardial disease– which isn't a good thing.
3. With larger cardiac muscle mass comes higher voltage and waveform morphology changes

**Left Atrial Enlargement (LAE)**

1. Results in prolonged electrical conduction and "M" shaped P wave as the large left atria slows conduction as the impulse propagates (shown as the 'dip' in the "M" shape).
2. When the atria are the same size and strength, you won't see the "M" shape.
3. Typically, this is caused by severe mitral valve disease.
4. This is also known as: P-mitrale.
5. To positively identify left atrial enlargement (LAE) on a 12 lead ECG, either you must observe a P– wave > 0.12 of a second or observe an "M" shaped P wave. These observations must occur in leads I or II.

6. Note: there are multiple criteria for identifying morphologies not only with hypertrophy but also with almost any ECG morphology. Here we present one method. Use either this method or one you are more familiar with using.

**Right Atrial Enlargement (RAE)**
1. The characteristic finding is tall, peaked P waves.
2. RAE is caused by conditions which increase the pressures incurred by the RA
    a. COPD
    b. PE
3. This is also known as P- pulmonale
4. To positively identify right atrial enlargement (RAE) on a 12 lead ECG, either you must observe a tall, peaked P-wave higher than 2.5mm high in either lead I or II.

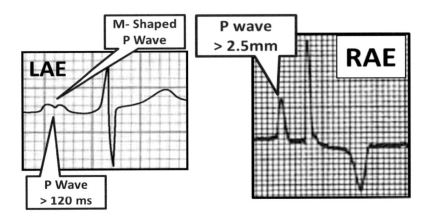

**Biatrial Enlargement**
1. As the name implies, biatrial enlargement is where BOTH atria are enlarged.
2. To identify this morphology, you will need to recognize a biphasic P wave (phase 1 and phase 2).
3. A biphasic P wave looks like a sine wave, but isolated to just the P wave itself:
4. Biatrial Enlargement (BAE) Criteria:
    i. Lead II: Evidence of either P mitral or P pulmonale, **AND...**
    ii. V1: Evidence of a biphasic P wave

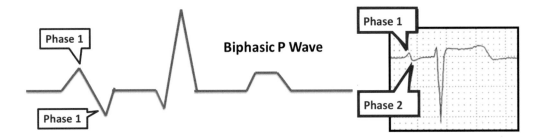

**Left Ventricular Hypertrophy (LVH)**
1. Left ventricular hypertrophy is an enlarged left ventricle that occurs when it has to pump against increasing resistance.
2. This resistance can come in the form of a diseased aortic valve, or chronic hypertension.
3. We have looked at simple PQRST waveform names, but now lets dig a little deeper into wave nomenclature.

4. To be able to identify left ventricular hypertrophy, we must have a clear understanding of wave nomenclature on the ECG.
    a. Q wave: first negative deflection
    b. R wave: first positive deflection that crosses or begins at the isoelectric line
    c. S: negative deflection following the R or Q wave.
    d. Not every QRS complex has a Q, R, and/or S.
    e. Capitalized letters are reserved for bigger waves while lowercase letters are reserved for smaller waves.
    f. Additionally, there can the prime, noted (') waveforms that results from multiple R or S waves.
    g. The ultimate goal is to name each portion of the QRS complex.
5. There are multiple criteria to identify left ventricular hypertrophy, like most ECG morphologies and waveforms. In this case, only one criterion has to be met to be able to field diagnose the patient was left ventricular hypertrophy, not multiple.
6. Remember, the QRS complex is sometimes referred to as the "R" complex.
7. Left Ventricular Hypertrophy Criteria (LVH)
    a. Take the Deepest S (look in V1 or V2 and add it to the tallest R (look in V5 or V6); if the sum is larger than 35mm, then LVH is present.
    b. Look in aVL. If the aVL R wave is larger than 11mm, then LVH is present.

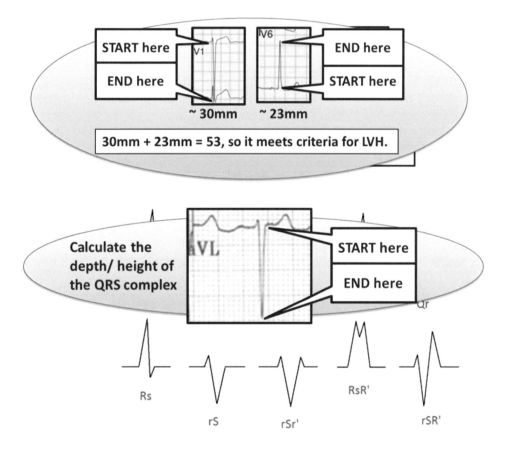

**Right Ventricular Hypertrophy (RVH)**
1. Enlargement of the right ventricle can occur from pulmonary hypertension, pulmonary embolism, scoring of the lungs, and anything that will increase pressure in the lung vasculature.
2. All of these conditions create a situation where the right ventricle has to work harder to pull blood into the pulmonary vasculature, therefore the right ventricle enlarges.
3. Right Ventricular Hypertrophy Criteria
   a. Look in V1 or V2: if the R wave is taller than the S wave, then RVH is present.
   b. This is called the R:S Ratio

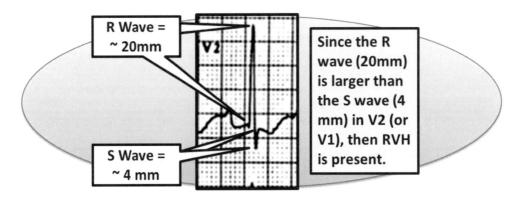

## *ACUTE MYOCARDIAL INFARCTION (AMI)*

1. It is imperative that you can identify not only the location of an infarction on a 12 lead tracing, but also recognize which coronary artery is occluded.
2. The location and size of and infarction depends on which artery is blocked, and where along its course the blockage occurs.
3. Acute myocardial infarctions begin as an ischemic problem. For whatever pathophysiology, oxygen is not being delivered to the heart muscle, therefore it goes into anaerobic metabolism, creates copious amounts of acid, and begins to shut down the heart's normal activities.
4. The progression of ischemic heart disease generally begins with ischemia (lack of oxygen), is followed by injury (minor myocardial damage), and finally ends with infarction (death of the cardiac tissue).
5. In general, if the infarction is occurring at the anterior, lateral, or septal walls, then it is involving the left ventricle and is most likely fed by the **left coronary artery** or one of its branches.
6. Inferior wall infarctions are typically the result of the **right coronary artery** being occluded.
7. There are two different categories of acute myocardial infarctions: ST– elevation myocardial infarction (STEMI) and non ST– elevation myocardial infarction (NSTEMI).
8. The AMI patterns we will discuss will be characteristic of ST elevation, which is indicative of infarction.
9. It is important to understand that the heart is not two dimensional, but three dimensional. It can be helpful to think of it as a sphere, with a left side and a right side, a front and the back, and a top and bottom.
10. The ST elevation patterns we will discuss identify infarction to one side of the sphere, or heart. It is important to know that reciprocal depression can occur on the opposite side of the heart, which can also be helpful in identifying the myocardial region where the infarction is taking place.

11. It is important to remember that a single lead with ST elevation is not enough to diagnose myocardial infarction. There must be at least 2 occurrences of ST elevation next to one another (contiguous) to be able to identify it as true infarction.

12. For example, if there was ST elevation in V1 and V5, and no other evidence of ST elevation throughout the ECG, and those are noncontiguous and therefore that cannot be defined as a myocardial infarction.

13. However, elevation in V3 and V4 meet the criteria of being contiguous (next to one another) and would indicate an inferior myocardial infarction.

14. Additionally, if there is ST elevation beginning in lead V1 and progressing to lead V5, then this indicates a larger infarction involving the septal, interior, and a portion of the lateral walls of the left ventricle.

15. It is common to merge names of the major areas should ST elevation be involved in multiple contiguous locations of the heart.

16. For example, the above example of V1 through V5, the current nomenclature would most likely be anterioseptal AMI with lateral involvement. This is because both the anterior and the septal leads are fully involved, and there is some lateral involvement.

17. Another example would include ST elevations in V5, V6, II, III, and aVF. This is called an inferiolateral AMI because there is inferior and lateral ST elevation changes.

18. When you have multiple leads with ST elevation, it is important to rule out pericarditis. Please see prior 12 lead assessment on pericarditis.

19. When assessing for ST-elevation myocardial infarction (STEMI), it is important to take everything into account. Be sure to use not only ST elevation changes but also, reciprocal changes to build a body of evidence to support your field diagnosis. Additionally, laboratory values should be utilized as well as the clinical picture and physical exam.

20. Myocardial infarction should never be diagnosed based on a 12 lead ECG alone. The full clinical picture, including labs, and serial ECGs, should be utilized to get an accurate and global picture of the heart.

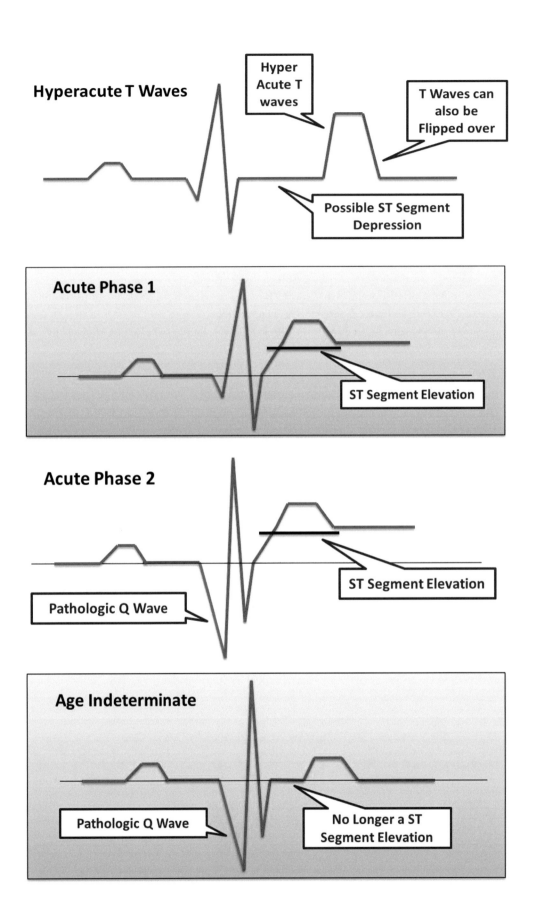

**Inferior AMI**

1. Leads: II, III, aVF (see below)
2. Reciprocal Leads: I, aVL
3. Main Coronary Artery:  RCA (Right Coronary Artery)

| I | aVR | V1 | V4 |
| --- | --- | --- | --- |
| II | aVL | V2 | V5 |
| III | aVF | V3 | V6 |

Inferior AMI

**Anterior AMI**

1. Leads: V3, V4 (see below)
2. Reciprocal Leads: Posterior leads (V8, V9)
3. Main Coronary Artery:  LAD (Left Anterior Descending)

| I | aVR | V1 | V4 |
| --- | --- | --- | --- |
| II | aVL | V2 | V5 |
| III | aVF | V3 | V6 |

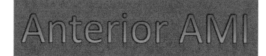

Anterior AMI

**Septal AMI**

1. Leads: V1, V2 (see below)
2. Reciprocal Leads: None
3. Main Coronary Artery:  LAD (Left Anterior Descending)

| I | aVR | V1 | V4 |
|---|-----|----|----|
| II | aVL | V2 | V5 |
| III | aVF | V3 | V6 |

**Septal AMI**

**Lateral and High Lateral AMI**
1. Leads: V5, V6 and Lead I, aVL (see below)
2. Reciprocal Leads: II, III, aVF
3. Main Coronary Arteries:  LAD (Left Anterior Descending)  and LCx (Left Circumflex)

| I | aVR | V1 | V4 |
|---|-----|----|----|
| II | aVL | V2 | V5 |
| III | aVF | V3 | V6 |

**Lateral AMI**

| I | aVR | V1 | V4 |
|---|-----|----|----|
| II | aVL | V2 | V5 |
| III | aVF | V3 | V6 |

**High Lateral AMI**

**Sgarbossa Criteria**

1. An in-vogue test question topic currently in the critical care certification circles is the Sgarbossa Criteria. This is a method of identifying an ST elevation AMI when a left bundle branch block is present.

2. Traditionally, when a left bundle branch block (LBBB) was discovered, it occurs with some ST elevation, so that elevation could not be trusted in the diagnosis of infarction.

3. However, recall that as the myocardium is deprived of oxygen for an extended length of time, it will begin to fail. Muscle begins to pump poorly, and conductive tissue doesn't conduct the electrical impulses well– so blocks occur.

4. **Sgarbossa Criteria**:
   a. ST elevation ≥1 mm in any lead with a positive QRS complex (i.e., concordance): apply 5 points
   b. ST depression ≥1 mm in lead V1, V2, or V3: apply 3 points
   c. ST elevation ≥5 mm in a lead with a negative (discordant) QRS complex: apply 2 points
   d. **Modified Smith's Rule** (ST Depression): If the DEPTH of ST depression divided by the height of R wave is > 0.25, then AMI is present.
   e. **Modified Smith's Rule** (ST Elevation): If the HEIGHT of ST elevation divided by depth of S wave is > 0.25, then AMI is present.

5. Normally, when a left bundle branch block (LBBB) occurs the ST segments should be either isoelectric or go in the opposite direction (disconcordant) of the dominant portion of the QRS complex. So typically, in V1 the QRS is mainly negative, and the ST segment is elevated, which is a normal finding in LBBB. So basically, in an LBBB that is not occurring with an ST elevation AMI, the QRS complex goes one way, and the ST elevation goes the opposite way (this is disconcordance).

6. Two of the three of Sgarbossa's criteria are based on this QRS and ST elevation "same side" concept. The first criterion says any ST elevation with a positive QRS meets criteria. The second criterion says any ST depression in V1-V3, which is normally QRS– negative leads any way (same side), meets criteria.

7. The third criterion is different but also has proven to identify AMI in the presence of LBBB. The third criterion says that is there is ST elevation in ANY lead > 5 mm with a NEGATIVE QRS (opposite side), then criteria is met.

8. Point values are added for each criterion found. Criteria 1 earns 5 points per occurrence, criteria 2 earns 3 points per occurrence, and criteria 3 earns 2 points per occurrence. Three (3) points total means there is a 98% chance there is an AMI with the observed LBBB.

9. So, bottom line– if you find JUST ONE of criteria 1 or 2, then an AMI is happening with the LBBB.

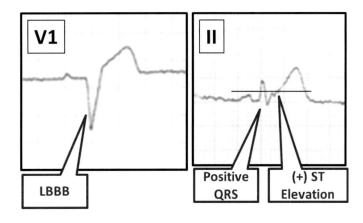

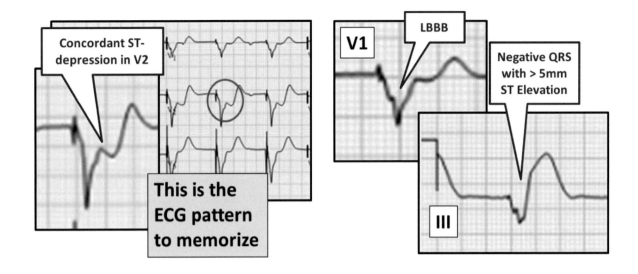

# PART 4: ASSESSMENT OF HEMODYNAMICS

## INTRODUCTION

Assessing for hemodynamic status will not be conducted on every patient but can be very helpful and useful when the information is available. Hemodynamics is an important part of cardiovascular physiology dealing with the forces the pump (the heart) must develop to circulate blood through the cardiovascular system.

Hemodynamic monitoring is based on the invasive measurement of systemic; pulmonary arterial and venous pressures; and cardiac output. Since organ blood flow cannot be directly measured in clinical practice, arterial blood pressure is used, despite limitations, as an estimate of the adequacy of tissue perfusion. Classic hemodynamic monitoring is achieved through the Swan– Ganz catheter, which is a catheter designed to be placed in the pulmonary artery. The catheter is placed into the femoral vein and fed through the venous system to the vena cava, the right atrium, the right ventricle, and into the pulmonary artery.

There are some technologies that use algorithms to assess these values such as the Flo Trac and bioimpedance devices. In this section we will focus on the assessment component of hemodynamics. More in- depth pathophysiology and management for conditions associated with these assessments will be covered later in this text.

## WATER PIPE CONCEPT

1.  To understand and to use information gained from the hemodynamic assessment, an intuitive concept must be developed and fortified. To achieve this let's take a look at some pipes.
2.  Water flows through these pipes from A through D. Throughout this piping there are red shut off valves, which are labeled A, B, C, and D.

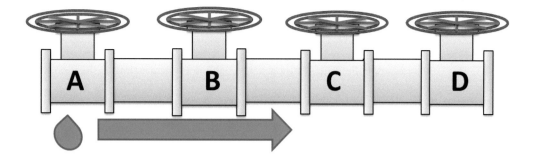

3. The water pressure is currently even throughout these four valves and throughout the entire piping system. But what would happen if we tightened valve C? If you put a squeeze on valve C, then the pressure in A and B would increase. This occurs because there is a constant flow through the system, so when we apply "squeeze" to valve C, pressure behind that portion of the piping develops a backward pressure.

4. Alternatively, if a valve is loosened, that pressure decreases. This simple concept of increasing pressure occurs behind where a "squeeze" is being applied, and a decreasing pressure in front where the pipes will be "loosened" is the foundation needed to understand hemodynamics. The key is always understanding how the 'squeeze' or 'loosening' occurs and applying it backward. Remember, hemodynamics describes a forward flow of blood.


## VESSEL CONCEPT

1. Let's consider in other and more specific set of piping:

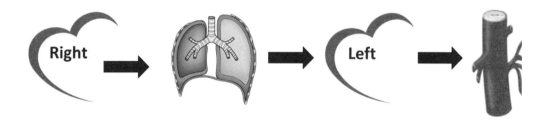

2. Recall that blood flows into the right atria and ventricle (preload), and then flows into the pulmonary system (pulmonary vascular resistance), and then flows into the left side of the heart, and then is pushed into the arterial system (afterload). The amount of blood pumped into the system is called cardiac output.

3. Each section of the above can be assessed to identify specific pathological conditions. It is important to know each of these parts.

## HEMODYNAMIC PARAMETERS

### Central Venous Pressure (CVP)

1. Normal: 2-6 mmHg
2. CVP is the pressure of the fluid returning to the right atrium and estimates the fluid status of the right side of the heart.
3. HIGH CVP: Circulatory overload (over infusion of IV fluids, worsening CHF); venous congestion (PEEP, right ventricular failure, tamponade); poor contraction of the right ventricle (infarct, pericarditis); high pulmonary vascular resistance (pulmonary edema, COPD).
4. LOW CVP: hemorrhage, third spacing, extreme vasodilation (shock, venous- specific vasodilator medications)
5. Generally speaking, any condition that reduces the volume of fluid return back to the heart will lower CVP. Any condition that prevents the forward flow of blood from the right side of the heart into the lungs will increase CVP.

### Right Ventricular Pressure (RVP)

1. Normal: 25-30 mmHg systolic, 0-5 mmHg for diastolic
2. RVP is the pressure that the right ventricle is producing.
3. HIGH SYSTOLIC: Pulmonary hypertension, pulmonary stenosis.
4. HIGH DIASTOLIC: Right ventricular failure, pericarditis, and tamponade.
5. Generally speaking, the pressures within the right ventricle also depends on what is in front of it. Recall the valves: in the case of pulmonary hypertension, there is "squeeze" occurring in the pulmonary vascular system, therefore the pressures in the right ventricle are higher. Flow moves forward, if there is a squeeze applied, then a back pressure occurs
6. Once a Swan– Ganz catheter has been inserted, pressure monitoring begins at the right ventricle. It is also very important to note that you should keep the catheter advancing because the right ventricle is very easily irritated by the catheter itself and can lead to PVCs and other arrhythmias.

### Pulmonary Artery Pressure (PAP)

1. Normal: 15-30 mmHg (systolic); 5-10 mmHg (diastolic); the mean is < 20mmHg
2. PAP is the pressure in the pulmonary artery itself. Right ventricular and pulmonary artery systolic pressures should be the same, but the pulmonary artery diastolic pressure will be different.
3. HIGH PAP: Left ventricular failure, peripheral vascular disease (hypertension, embolism, edema), tamponade.
4. LOW PAP: Volume depletion, drugs and medications, aspiration, pulmonary stenosis.
5. Generally speaking, if this number is high, consider the patient "wet" on the left side, and if this parameter is low, then you can consider the patient "dry" on the left side.

### Pulmonary Capillary Wedge Pressure (PCWP)

1. Normal: 4-12mmHg
2. PCWP represents the fluid status of the left side of the heart. It is achieved by inflating and occluding a tiny balloon in the pulmonary artery and measuring pressures between the balloon on the left side of the heart. This balloon is the characteristic feature of these Swan– Ganz catheter.

3. HIGH PCWP: Left ventricular failure (audible S3 sound probably present), tamponade, pulmonary edema, mitral valve stenosis or insufficiency, fluid overload.
4. LOW PCWP: Hypovolemia, afterload reduction cause by vasodilators.
5. Generally speaking, a high afterload will cause the PCWP to increase because of the inability to flow easily forward. Medications administered to reduce afterload (vasodilators) will reduce PCWP. If this number is high, consider the patient "wet" on the left side, and if this parameter is low, then you can consider the patient "dry" on the left side.
6. PAP can be used to estimate PCWP during transport.

### Systemic Vascular Resistance (SVR)

1. Normal: 800-1300 dynes/sec/cm3
2. SVR is the resistance or pressure; that must be overcome by the left ventricle to produce forward blood flow.
3. HIGH SVR: Hypovolemia, hypothermia, vasopressors, hypertension, cardiogenic shock, massive pulmonary embolism, cardiac tamponade.
4. LOW SVR: Vasodilator therapy, early septic shock.
5. Remember: a low SVR indicates a decreased afterload. Therefore, the patient is peripherally dilated; while a high SVR means an increased afterload, indicating the patient is peripherally constricted.
6. Generally speaking, the SVR is how we compensate for varying fluid states. Our body increases SVR when we have low blood volume, and we can increase SVR by giving vasopressors. We lower SVR when we give vasodilators.

### Cardiac Output (CO)

1. Normal: 4-6 L/min
2. CO represents the amount of blood ejected by the heart into systemic circulation each minute. Remember this equation: CO = Heart Rate x Stroke Volume. Also recall that stroke volume is determined by preload (CVP), contractility, and afterload (SVR).
3. HIGH CO: Pulmonary edema, early sepsis, increased metabolic state (fever, tachycardia, burn), mild hypertension with widened pulse pressure.
4. LOW CO: Too much PEEP, infarction, decreased stroke volume (dehydration, diuresis, infarction) valve disease poor filling of the left ventricle, hypotension, tamponade.
5. One Possible Assessment Technique
6. This technique provides a template to look for common conditions and is a good method to begin learning how to evaluate hemodynamics.

## HEMODYNAMIC ASSESSMENT

### Asses Fluid Status

1. It is important to identify whether the patient's fluid status is normal, fluid over– loaded, or hypovolemic.
2. High CVP= wet system

      a. Seen with ascites, JVD, and peripheral edema

      b. Requires meds to improve forward blood flow

3. High PCWP (left side) = wet lungs

      a. Seen with pulmonary edema

      b. Requires meds to improve blood flow, like dobutamine) and meds to reduce afterload (like vasodilators)

4. Low CVP= dry system

      a. Seen in hypovolemia (from dehydration or hemorrhage)

      b. Treatment typically requires liters of isotonic fluids and sometimes blood

5. Low PCWP= dry lungs

      a. Seen in hypovolemia (from dehydration or hemorrhage)

      b. Treatment typically requires liters of isotonic fluids and sometimes blood

## Shock Profiles

Shock occurs for various reasons, and we can identify these reasons based off hemodynamics alone. Most of these conditions require more information than the values of these parameters. You must look at the entire picture.

### Hypovolemic Shock

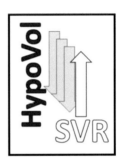

1. Caused by too little fluid in the system– loss can be from dehydration or bleeding
2. CVP is low (inadequate fluid in the system)
3. PCWP is low (inadequate fluid in the system)
4. CO is low (inadequate fluid in the system).
5. SVR is HIGH. This is because the body will compensate for the low fluid status with vasoconstriction.
6. So, looking at the logo for this profile on the previous page, all the components of this profile are low, EXCEPT SVR. This is the characteristic profile for hypovolemic shock.

### Cardiogenic Shock

1. Cardiogenic shock occurs when the heart has been damaged so badly that pumping capacity is compromised, and  forward blood flow is significantly reduced, thus causing a backup of blood and increasing pressures.
2. CVP is high. This is because of the backup of forward flow.
3. PCWP is high. This is because of the backup of forward flow.
4. CO is low. This is because the heart is damaged and cannot push blood forward, therefore; a reduced amount of blood is pumped out.
5. SVR is HIGH (or normal). This is because meds may be on board to increase contractility (like Dobutamine), but it could be normal.
6. So, looking at the logo for this profile on the previous page, all the components of this profile are high, EXCEPT CO, which is low. This is the characteristic profile for cardiogenic shock.

**Distributive Shock– General**

1. Distributive shock is characterized by a very low SVR, which causes difficulty in distributing blood to the tissues (due to the low pressure caused by vasodilation).

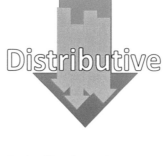

2. CVP is low or normal. If low, it's because most of the blood volume are in the dilated vascular system.
3. PCWP is low or normal. This is because most of the blood volume are in the dilated vascular system.
4. CO is low. This is because most of the blood volume are in the dilated vascular system.
5. SVR is low. This is because most of the blood volume are in the dilated vascular system.
6. So, looking at the logo for this profile on the previous page, the central characteristic is that all the parameters are an LOW.
7. All forms of distributive shock all have low SVR, but the different forms all have something else that is characteristic. More on this upcoming.

**Septic Shock**

1. Septic shock is a complication caused by an infection where toxins can trigger a full-body inflammatory response.
2. CVP is normal or low. This is because most of the blood volume are in the dilated vascular system.
3. PCWP is normal or low. This is because most of the blood volume are in the dilated vascular system
4. CO is HIGH. This is because the body is trying to compensate by pumping out copious amounts of blood.
5. SVR is LOW. This is because whatever bacteria causing the sepsis is releasing toxins that cause massive vasodilation. Yes, bacteria poop causes vasodilation– write that down.
6. Pair this information with temperature– fever supports the diagnosis of sepsis.
7. So, looking at the graphic for septic shock profile on the previous page, the two characteristic parameters are a low SVR and a high CO, and in the presence of fever.
8. It should be noted that a septic shock is a form of distributive shock.

**Neurogenic Shock**

1. Neuro shock is characterized by a very low SVR from cut spinal nerves which normally tell the blood vessels to squeeze.
2. Without that nervous control, massive vasodilation occurs. This causes difficulty in distributing blood to the tissues (due to the low pressure caused by vasodilation).
3. CVP is low or normal. If low, it's because most of the blood volume are in the dilated vascular system.
4. PCWP is low or normal. This is because most of the blood volume is in the dilated vascular system.
5. CO is low. This is because most of the blood volume is in the dilated vascular system.
6. SVR is characteristically LOW. This is because most of the blood volume is in the dilated vascular system.
7. So, looking at the logo for this profile, the central characteristic is all the parameters are an LOW.

8. LOW HR: Neurogenic shock is also associated with bradycardia because with cut spinal nerves (adrenergic nerves) there is uncontested vagal stimulation. Said another way, since the sympathetic nerves are cut, and then the parasympathetic nervous system predominates, which means slower HR and lower BP.

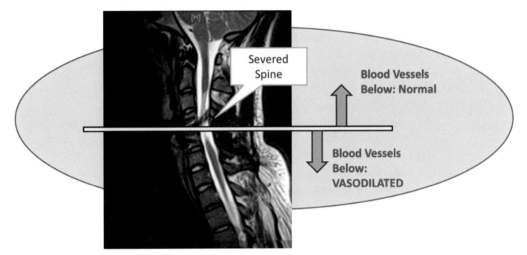

## Condition Profiles

### Cardiac Tamponade & Tension Pneumothorax
1. CVP is high. This is because there is global pressure on the heart from the tamponade.
2. PCWP is high. This is because there is global pressure on the heart from the tamponade.
3. CO is low. This is due to the compression of the heart muscle preventing adequate pumping.
4. SVR is high (or normal). This is because there is global pressure on the heart from the tamponade.
5. So, this should resemble cardiogenic shock. The difference is the cause– cardiogenic shock is caused by a primary pump failure, but tamponade is typically caused by secondary heart failure induced by a traumatic event.

### Pulmonary Embolism
1. CVP is high. This is because the PE in the lungs blocks forward flow.
2. PCWP is normal to low. This is because the PE affects the vasculature behind the lungs, thus, CVP and right ventricular pressures elevate, and the PCWP is normal to low.
3. CO is normal to low. This is because the PE will cause a back pressure, and not affect the PCWP or CO much.
4. SVR is normal or low. This is because the PE will cause a back pressure, and not affect the PCWP or CO much.
5. Another hemodynamic parameter that would be helpful in this case is the pulmonary vascular resistance because the PE increases the vascular pressure in the lungs.
6. This is also the profile for right sided heart failure.

## GENRAL MANAGEMENT STRATEGIES

### Hypovolemic shock
1. Correct with copious amounts of fluid (liters and liters if needed). Fluid resuscitation endpoint is either normalized CVP, PCWP, and CO; or pulmonary edema.
2. Vasopressors are a last resort and ONLY after adequate fluid resuscitation.

### Cardiogenic shock

1. Improve CO with inotropes (increases contractility); avoid fluid (will worsen fluid overload); reduce afterload (vasodilators).
2. Dobutamine is great in this scenario because it increases contractility AND causes vasodilation– its win-win.

### Distributive shocks

1. General: Vasopressors to improve afterload (SVR).
2. **Anaphylaxis**: Epinephrine- improves low SVR via vasoconstriction and reduces the effects of histamine (which caused the vasodilation in the first place).
3. **Sepsis**: Lots of fluid to replace the fluid that is third spacing from vasodilation  (low SVR, edematous extremities). Pressors to improve SVR (norepi used in the ICU).
4. **Neurogenic**: vasopressors to correct the low afterload (SVR). Typically, this won't require much fluid resuscitation, but then again, a little fluid resuscitation is usually good.
5. Remember, hemodynamics simply represent flow through the heart. If there is a blockage for any reason, influence the system at that point to improve flow. For example, if afterload is too high and not allowing blood flow, then reduce afterload with a vasodilator. If the system has low volume (dry), then add fluid. Keep it simple.

## PART 5: ASSESSMENT OF IABP COUNTERPULSATION

## INTRODUCTION

This assessment  will be supplemented by a full management section in Part 9. The intra– aortic balloon pump (IABP) is a device that is designed to increase myocardial oxygen supply and to improve cardiac output. The catheter and balloon are fed up the femoral artery and placed in the aorta above the renal arteries and about 1-2 cm from the subclavian artery. On x-ray, this level is at the 2nd or 3rd intercostal space.

The IABP works by a balloon inflating within the aorta while the heart is in relaxation. This inflation slams blood into the coronary arteries, thus increasing myocardial oxygen. The balloon deflates the moment before ventricular contraction. Deflation of the balloon during this time creates a cavity in the aorta thus reducing afterload, which improves cardiac output.

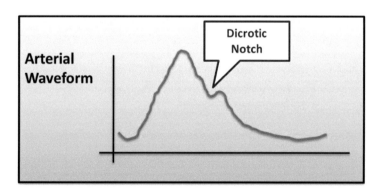

Most systems are programmed to inflate in the middle of the T wave on the ECG and to deflate just before the QRS complex. It is the job of the transport clinician to observe the timing and to make adjustments based on timing. The target for the inflation point is the **Dicrotic notch,** which signifies the opening of the aortic valve. You will need to be able to identify if the timing for inflation and deflation is on target, early, or late. The  worst timing error is EARLY INFLATION.

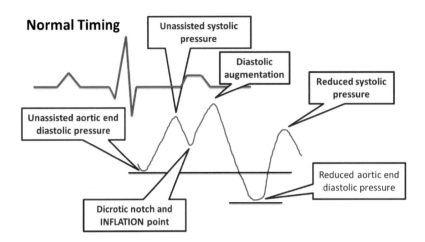

### Early Inflation

1. Key Feature: inflation begins before the dicrotic notch
2. This causes premature closure of the aortic valve as the inflating balloon pushes blood backwards towards the head and forces the open aortic valve closed.
3. It increases myocardial oxygen demand and significantly increases afterload.

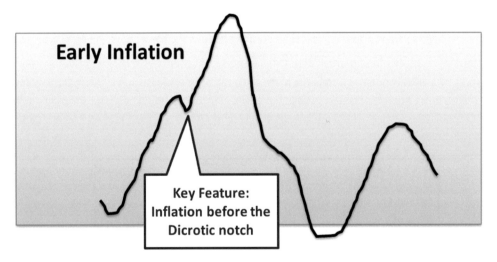

## Late Inflation

1. Key Feature: a clear view of the dicrotic notch with balloon inflation after the dicrotic notch.
2. This results in suboptimal coronary artery perfusion. This occurs because every second that passes beyond the dicrotic notch without balloon inflation results in progressively reduced oxygenation

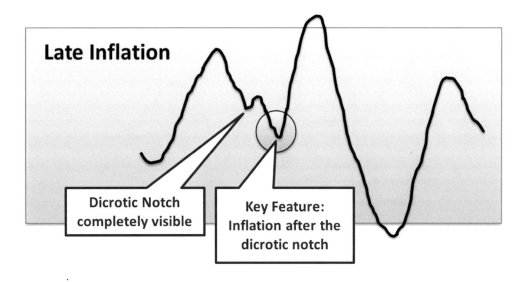

## Early Deflation

1. Key Feature: Sharp drop after diastolic augmentation with a potential rise in aortic end–diastolic pressure. U– shaped end– diastolic curvature.
2. This causes sub– optimal coronary artery perfusion and also creates the potential for retrograde blood flow from the coronary arteries back into the aorta. This occurs because the balloon deflation creates a suction effect.

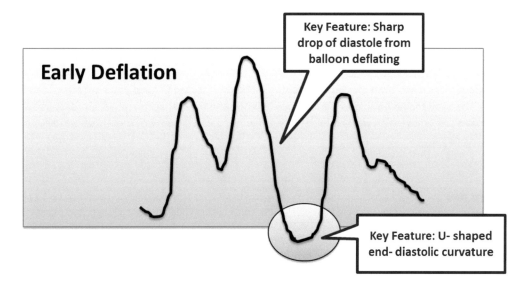

### Late Deflation

1. Key Feature: Widened diastolic augmentation and raised assisted end– diastolic pressure.
2. This prevents the beneficial effects of balloon deflation because the balloon is still inflated (late deflation) and the heart has to pump against the still inflated balloon.

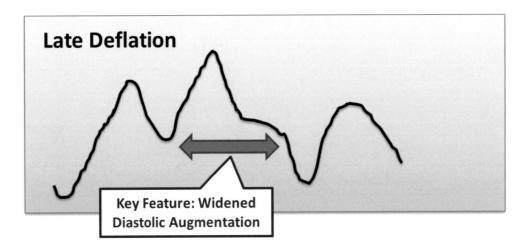

# PART 6: CARDIAC CONDITONS

## INTRODUCTION

You will be exposed, repeatedly, to moderately complex respiratory conditions, and at times, you will be forced to contend with a highly complex medical situation. Fix what you can fix and treat what you can treat. Use medical control if needed.

Consider using a system I use to study where I know the 3 domains of a medical condition: Pathophysiology, Assessment (S/S), and Management, or PAM for short. If you know the pathophysiology of a condition, you should be able to describe the signs and symptoms, as well as how to manage the condition. Similarly, if you are provided with a series of treatments, you should be able to backtrack (usually with a little history) what the pathophysiology is and therefore how to identify it. Finally, if someone gives you a set of signs and symptoms, then you should be able to identify the condition and the management. So, you see, from any of these domains are known, then you should be able to figure out the other two. Therefore, we will study the content in this way.

## CONDITIONS

### Acute Coronary Syndrome

1. Patho: narrowing lumen of the coronary arteries → reduced blood flow to myocardium → hypoxic myocardium → myocardial ischemia → myocardial injury → myocardial death → arrhythmia
2. S/S: history of chest pain or atypical MI symptoms; (+) ST elevation on 12 lead ECG; elevated troponin T and CK-MB levels; presence of pathologic Q waves (indicates cardiovascular disease history)

3. MGT: Oxygen, Nitrates (use cautiously with right sided infarctions), aspirin, analgesic (morphine or fentanyl). Also, consider beta blockade, heprinization, calcium channel blockers, fibrinolytics, and cath lab needs.

## Aortic Aneurysm

1. Patho: Force of blood impacts aortic wall--> weakens the media layer--> unglues the layers of the aorta--> this area pooches out
2. S/S: chief complaint of abdominal pulsations, back pain, throbbing pain (late sign), abdominal bruits, widening mediastinum on x-ray, confirms CT or MRI and image showing the abdominal aortic aneurysm. Hypotension is the hallmark sign of rupture.
3. MGT: keep patient calm, in the absence of hypotension, time to be taken to evaluate via CT or MRI- consultation needed with the surgeon; in the presence of hypotension: crystalloid infusion and PRBCs is warranted— IMMEDIATE SURGERY REQUIRED. Keep blood pressure slightly sub-normal.

## Aortic Dissection

1. Patho: Force of blood impacts aortic wall--> weakens the media layer--> unglues the layers of the aorta--> this area pooches out--> the intima tears away from media--> blood accumulates between them--> can tear all the way back to the heart--> regurgitation and coronary blood flow affected. Commonly classified on the DeBakey scale and Stanford scales (Stanford A = DeBakey types I and II, Stanford B = DeBakey type III).
2. S/S: Constant moderate to severe back pain, tearing pain, an urge to defecate, pain unrelieved by position change, wide mediastinum on x-ray.
3. MGT: in the absence of hypotension, evaluate via CT or MRI- consultation needed with the surgeon; in the presence of hypotension: crystalloid infusion and PRBCs is warranted— IMMEDIATE SURGERY REQUIRED.

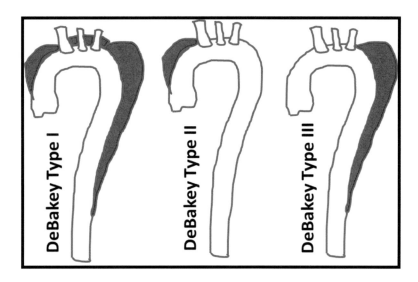

## Cardiogenic Shock

1. Patho: Heart injured/ Dz--> weakened pump--> failure to maintain tissue perfusion--> anaerobic metabolism--> global acidosis--> dysrhythmias--> death.

2. S/S: Pale/cool skin, week/thready pulse, reduced urine output, AMS, hypotension, hemodynamic profile (CVP↑/PCWP↑/CO↓/SVR↑).
3. MGT: 12 lead, fluid challenge, avoid pulmonary edema, improve cardiac output (increase contractility- Dobutamine; reduce afterload-vasodilators). The patient may require IABP or a ventricular assist device (VAD).
4. It is important to note that if the cause of shock is due to a right ventricular infarction, the hemodynamic parameters will change to (CVP↑/PCWP↓ or norm/CO↓/SVR↑). These patients will need lots of volume Fluid. You should also consider avoiding dopamine because it will increase the pulmonary vascular resistance.

## Cardiomyopathy

1. Patho: Dilated- stretched myocardium--> poor pump; hypertrophic- poor filling--> poor EF, restrictive-scar tissue--> poor elasticity .
2. S/S: Chest pain, fatigue, weakness, pale/cool skin, week/thready pulse, reduced urine output, AMS, hypotension, valvular problems, S3 and S4 can potentially be heard, cardiomegaly on x ray (looks spherical), ejection fraction < 45%.
3. MGT: DILATED: heart failure management (CPAP, nitrates, loop diuretics, morphine, ACE inhibitors, inotropes), HYPERTROPHIC/ RESTRICTIVE: negative inotropes like calcium and beta blockers

## Congestive Heart Failure (CHF)

1. Patho: Injury/ disease causing poor pumping ability of the heart--> blood backs up in systemic or pulmonary circuit--> Left side- rales; Right side- edema, hepatojugular reflex, JVD, and ascites.
2. S/S: 1-2 word dyspnea, JVD, ascites, pedal edema, hepatojugular reflux, pulmonary edema, pink/ frothy sputum, (+) BNP, hemodynamic profile like that of cardiogenic shock (CVP↑/PCWP↑/CO↓/SVR↑).
3. MGT: Improve oxygenation (add FiO2 or PEEP), decrease myocardial workload (decrease afterload with vasodilators; improve contractility with positive inotropes), and by decreasing preload (vasodilators and diuretics to remove fluid from the system).

## Endocarditis

1. Patho: bacterial infection--> inflammation of the inner lining of the heart, the valves or chambers; found commonly in IV drug users.
2. S/S: Fever, chills, sweats, anorexia, weight loss, malaise, HEART MURMUR (valve damage and ruptured chorea tendonae), anemia, microscopic hematuria
3. MGT: IV antibiotics (penicillin, vancomycin, cephalosporin), fluids, anticoagulants

## Hypertensive Emergencies

1. Patho: Acute increase in BP--> danger of end- organ damage.
2. S/S: Diastolic pressure > 140mmHg with end– organ damage; altered level of consciousness, seizures, blindness, neurologic deficits
3. MGT: Lower blood pressure in a gradual, controlled manner within 30 to 60 minutes; FSBG, transport only (if 20-30 min from ER), labetalol/ nitro (if long transport time).

## Pericarditis

1. Patho: infection and inflation to the pericardium
2. S/S: Sub- sternal chest pain, manifests as a sharp, pleuritic pain that worsens with inspiration or cough; this pain goes away when the patient leans forward, and worsens when they lay down supine; elevated erythrocyte sedimentation rate (indicates infection); pericardial changes on the ECG (PR depression, global ST elevation, notching, and concave upward ST segment).
3. MGT: Oxygenation, ventilation and perfusion support. NSAIDs and steroids, in addition to antibiotics

## ST Elevation Myocardial Infarction (STEMI)

1. Patho: plaque ruptures--> floats down and occludes a coronary vessel--> ischemic myocardium--> myocardial injury/death
2. S/S: Sub- sternal chest pain or atypical MI symptoms; (+) ST elevation on 12 lead ECG; elevated troponin T and CK-MB levels; the presence of pathologic Q waves (indicates cardiovascular disease history).
   i. (I) Inferior: ST elevation in II, III, and aVF
   ii. (S) Septal: ST elevation in V1 and V2
   iii. (A) Anterior: ST elevation in V3 and V4
   iv. (L) Lateral: ST elevation in V5 and V6
   v. (T) High Lateral: ST elevation in Lead I and aVL
   vi. ISALT is a good acronym. T = top= high lateral AMI.
3. MGT: Oxygen, ASA, NTG, morphine/ fentanyl, Heparin or Lovenox, beta blockers, PCTA

## Non- ST Elevation Myocardial Infarction (NSTEMI)

1. Patho: unstable angina (>20 min) caused by a narrowing of the arteries overtime
2. S/S: unstable angina (>20 min), ST-segment depression with CP, (+) elevated troponin/ CK.
3. MGT: Oxygen, ASA, NTG, morphine/ fentanyl, heparin or Lovenox, beta blockers, PCTA
4. The shock states are added to this portion of the cardiac chapter due to their close affiliation with hemodynamics.

## Hypovolemic Shock

1. Patho: Shock that occurs as a result of a large amount of fluid displaced from the circulatory system. This can occur from dehydration or hemorrhage. There are 4 classes of blood loss:
   a. Class I: 0-15% of blood lost from body: mild tachycardia and maybe increased pulse pressure
   b. Class II: 15-30% of blood lost: increase in renin, decrease in urine output, increase in ADH, leading to: tachycardia, tachypnea, decrease in PP, cool clammy skin, delayed cap refill, anxiety
   c. Class III: 30-40% of blood lost: risk of major organ failure, renal failure, mental status changes, leading to: tachycardia, tachypnea, systolic drop, and oliguria
   d. Class IV: >40% of blood lost: multiple organ failures, almost always irreversible, leading to: loss of consciousness, cold pale skin, tachycardia, narrowed pulse pressure, very low systolic
2. S/S: History; exam; hemodynamic monitoring, ABG, CBC, CMP with electrolytes, U/A, lactate, SvO2, 12-lead, type-cross and screen, hemodynamic profile ( CVP↓/PCWP↓/CO↓/SVR↑)
3. MGT: ABCs, Fluid resuscitation, correct hypovolemia (crystalloids and blood then pressors), restore tissue perfusion, minimize fluid losses

## Septic Shock

1. Patho: Infection based (typically Gram negative ) systemic vasodilation, usually happens when infection symptoms go unnoticed, immunodeficient patients
2. S/S: systemic vasodilation, maldistribution of blood, and myocardial depression. Overwhelming immune response to bacteria, low TPR, increased permeability, edema, hypotension, purpura and petechial, hemodynamic profile (CVP↓/PCWP↓/CO↑/SVR↓).
3. MGT: two blood cultures to diagnose, maintenance of body systems (Fluid replacement and O2), antibiotic and stabilization of cardiac function (hemodynamics)

## Anaphylactic Shock

1. Patho: Severe allergic response, causing release of histamine, vasodilation, hypotension, systemic capillary permeability, fluid loss out of tissue

2. S/S: Severely leaky capillaries: vasodilation and hypotension down to dangerous levels, hemodynamic profile (CVP↓/PCWP↓/CO↓/SVR↓).
3. MGT: Fluid replacement may require 10's of liters to replace lost fluid, treatment for allergic reaction (epinephrine, diphenhydramine, solu-medrol).

### Neurogenic Shock

1. Patho: Trauma → damaged autonomic nerves → loss of vasomotor tone → vasodilation → low systemic vascular resistance
2. S/S: DECREASED heart rate that will NOT GO UP (bradycardia), imbalance of para/sympathetic control, massive systemic dilation (vasodilation), hemodynamic profile (CVP↓/PCWP↓/CO↓/SVR↓).– with BRADYCARDIA– commit this to memory.
3. MGT: Spinal precautions; support hemodynamics (fluids then pressors).

# PART 7: CARDIAC LAB VALUES

## INTRODUCTION

The cardiovascular system is composed of the heart, blood vessels, and the blood; therefore, there are numerous laboratory studies that could be included in this section. We have selected a few to discuss now, and others will be revealed in the chapters where they are most pertinent. While some may be repeated, I'll try to keep this to a minimum. Please note that both the U.S. units and international units (SI) will be presented if available. Not all lab values will have both. Focus on what applies to you.

## LAB VALUES

### Red Blood Cells (RBCs)

1. This describes the number of red blood cells in our blood.
2. Normal: 3.5-5.5 [x 103/mL]
3. HIGH: dehydration, high altitude, chronic hypoxia
4. LOW: anemia (almost all forms), hemodilution, chemotherapy

### White Blood Cells (WBCs)

1. This describes the number of white blood cells in our blood. It is the white blood cell's job to defend us from foreign invaders.
2. Normal: 4– 11 [x 103/mL]
3. HIGH: infection, inflammatory disease, anemia, burns, cancer
4. LOW: Sepsis, B12 deficiency, aplastic anemia, liver disease
5. Critical Values: < 0.5 or > 50.

### Platelets (Plts)

1. Platelets are cell remnants that play a fundamental role in hemostasis. Too few platelets and excessive bleeding can occur, too many platelets can cause blood clots to form and cause stroke, myocardial infarction, and pulmonary embolism.
2. Normal: 150-400 [x 109/L]
3. HIGH: Anemia, acute blood loss, preeclampsia, infection
4. LOW: DIC, HIV, blood transfusion, chemotherapy
5. Critical Values: < 50 or > 1000

## Hematocrit (Hct)

1. The hematocrit is the proportion of blood volume that is made up of red blood cells. It gives an indication of oxygen caring capacity.
2. Normal:
   a. Male: 40-50 [%]
   b. Female: 35-45 [%]
3. HIGH: Dehydration, burns, CHF, COPD
4. LOW: Hemorrhage, hemodilution, iron deficiency, malnutrition
5. Critical Values: <15 or >60 %

## Hemoglobin (HGB)

1. Hemoglobin is the iron-containing oxygen transport protein in the red blood cells. A hemoglobin value that is too low is anemia. Typically the value is 3 times that of the hemoglobin level. [HCT = 3 x HGB]
2. Normal: (US)
   a. Male: 13-17.5 [g/dL]
   b. Female: 12.1- 15.7 [mmol/L]
3. Normal: (SI)
   a. Male: 13-17.5 [g/dL]
   b. Female: 12.1– 15.7 [mmol/L]
4. HIGH: Dehydration, burns, CHF, COPD
5. LOW: Hemorrhage, hemodilution, iron deficiency, malnutrition
6. Critical Values: <5 or >20 g/dL

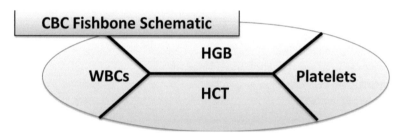

## Potassium

1. Potassium is a cation mostly in the intracellular fluid. The most common cause of hyperkalemia is renal dysfunction. The most common cause of hypokalemia is vomiting and diarrhea.
2. Normal: 3.5-5.5 [mEq/L]
3. HIGH: acidosis, chronic renal failure, massive tissue damage, ACE inhibitors
4. LOW: Diarrhea, diuretics, low potassium intake, salicylates
5. Critical Values: <3 or >6

## Sodium

1. Sodium is a cation primarily found in the extracellular fluid. It plays a role in blood pressure, fluid balance, nerve impulse conduction, and acid-base balance.
2. Normal:
   a. US: 135-145 [mEq/L]
   b. SI: 135-145 [mmol/L]
3. HIGH: Dehydration, diabetes, pregnancy, hyperaldosteronism
4. LOW: diarrhea, vomiting, fluid replacement with D5W, too much free water, hyperthyroidism, CHF, ACE inhibitors
5. Critical Values: <120 or >155

## Chloride

1. Chloride is an anion found primarily in extracellular fluids and is an essential component in maintaining acid-base balance, transmitting nerve impulses, and in regulating fluid plus shifts in and out of the cell.
2. Normal:
   a. US: 98-107 [mEq/L]
   b. SI: 98-107 [mmol/L]
3. HIGH: diarrhea, dehydration, excessive fluid resuscitation with normal saline, renal failure, respiratory acidosis
4. LOW: Diaphoresis, diuretics, SIADH, adrenal insufficiency, bicarbonates
5. Critical Values: <80 or >115

## Bicarbonate

1. Serum bicarbonate is important in identifying acid-base abnormalities.
2. Normal: 22-26 [mEq/L]
3. HIGH: Compensatory respiratory acidosis, metabolic alkalosis, vomiting, Cushing's disease
4. LOW: Chronic diarrhea, compensatory respiratory alkalosis, ketoacidosis, renal failure, volume overload
5. Critical Values: <15 or >40

## Blood Urea Nitrogen (BUN)

1. BUN is a byproduct of protein metabolism produced by the liver. As we make urine and excrete it, we get rid of BUN and keep it balanced. This is not the most sensitive of tests because there must be 50% of renal destruction before the BUN elevates.
2. Normal:
   a. US: 5-20 [mg/dL]
   b. SI: 1.8-7.1 [mmol/L]
3. HIGH: Chronic renal failure, dehydration, GI bleed, shock
4. LOW: Hemodilution, liver failure
5. Critical Values: >99 mg/dL

## Creatinine

1. Creatinine is produced at a consistent rate in the body, therefore urinary excretion must occur to keep this metabolite balanced. It is a great indicator of real function.
2. Normal: (US)
   a. Male: 0.6-1.2 [mg/dL]
   b. Female: 0.8-1.4 [mg/dL]
3. Normal: (SI)
   a. Male: 46-92 [mmol/L]
   b. Female: 61-107 [mmol/L]
4. HIGH: Acute tubular necrosis, congestive heart failure, dehydration, pre-eclampsia, rhabdomyolysis
5. LOW: Decreased muscle mass (young, old patients), myasthenia gravis
6. Critical Values: >5 mmol/L

## Glucose

1. Glucose is a simple sugar that is the main source of energy for our body. High blood glucose can damage organs over time (diabetes), while low blood sugar may cause brain damage and is a true medical emergency.
2. Normal:
   a. US: 65-100 [mq/dL]

        b.   SI: 3.8-5.8 [mmol/L]
3. HIGH: Diabetes mellitus, Cushing's syndrome, stress, catecholamine administration
4. LOW: Malnutrition, alcohol ingestion, insulin overdose, hypothyroidism
5. Critical Values: < 65 or >125 mmol/L

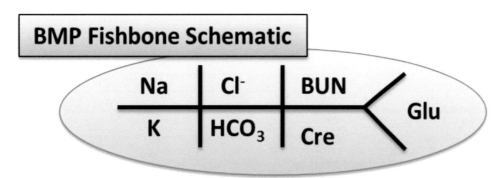

## Troponin T
1. Troponin is a protein in cardiac muscle that provides high specificity.  Elevation of Troponin T is seen 5 hours post MI, and peaks between 24 and 36 hours.
2. Normal: < 0.1 [ng/mL]
3. HIGH: Anything the damages cardiac muscle (cardiac trauma, myocardial infarction, cardiomyopathy, cardiac surgery)
4. LOW: None.

## Creatine Kinase (CK-MB)
1. This is a marker for cardiac ischemia.  It rises at 5 hours post myocardial infarction, and peaks between 18 and 36 hours.
2. Normal: 0-5 [ng/mL]
3. HIGH: Anything that damages cardiac muscle (cardiac trauma, myocardial infarction, cardiomyopathy, cardiac surgery)
4. LOW: None

## Myoglobin
1. Myoglobin is a protein found in cardiac and skeletal muscle.  An elevation of myoglobin by 25% within 90 minutes of angina is consistent with myocardial infarction.
2. Normal: < 0.09 [mg/mL]
3. HIGH: Anything the damages cardiac or skeletal muscle
4. LOW: None

## B– type Natriuretic Peptide (BNP)
1. BNP this secreted by the ventricular myocardium and acts as a vasodilator when the heart senses volume overload.  Additionally, it attempts to suppress the renin-angiotensin system to decrease sympathetic tone (blood pressure).
2. Normal:
        a.   US: < 100  [pq/mL]
        b.   SI: < 347 [pmol/L]
3. HIGH: Acute coronary syndrome, chronic renal failure, congestive heart failure, coronary artery disease, left ventricular dysfunction, pulmonary embolism, atrial fibrillation.
4. LOW: None.

# PART 8: CARDIAC PHARMACOLOGY

## INTRODUCTION

One of the most important concepts in pharmacology is understanding the mechanism by which medications work. If we see that blood pressure is low, then we need to choose a medication which will raise blood pressure. There are multiple ways which this can be done. Understanding pharmacological mechanisms will give you the tools to successfully use the following information, both in the field and on your critical care certification exams.

## SYMPATHETIC VS. PARASYMPATHETIC

The autonomic nervous system has two branches: sympathetic and parasympathetic. The sympathetic branch increases blood pressure, increases heart rate, increases myocardial contractility and increases bronchial dilation. The parasympathetic branch drops blood pressure, decreases heart rate, reduces myocardial contractility, and causes bronchospasm. So yes, these nervous systems are the exact opposite.

The sympathetic and the parasympathetic nervous systems are constantly in a tug of war battle depending on our external environment. If we are in no danger, the "feed or breed" system takes over (parasympathetic nervous system). If we're terrified and feeling like we are in danger, then the "fight or flight" system takes over (sympathetic nervous system).

We will not discuss the parasympathetic receptors; however, it is important that you understand the sympathetic nervous system receptors. I am not talking about an in depth understanding; rather I am talking about the useful knowledge set on these receptors.

The Sympathetic Receptors include:

- Alpha 1: Causes vasoconstriction → blood pressure ↑
- Beta 1: Increases HR & contractility → ↑ cardiac output
- Beta 2: Causes bronchodilation → improves airflow to lungs

One way to remember the difference between the beta receptors is to think "one heart, two lungs". Beta 1 affects the heart while beta 2 affects the lungs. Simple. You're welcome.

These receptors also have other functions, but it is important to develop a working knowledge of this information so that you can use it in the field or on a critical care certification exam. Therefore, we will focus on these main effects of the alpha and beta receptors.

### Agonists vs. Antagonists

Agonists: an agonist stimulates the receptor to do what it was designed to do. For example, a beta 2 agonist causes bronchodilation, and an alpha 1 agonist causes vasoconstriction.

Antagonists: an antagonist blocks a particular sector so that the OPPOSITE of what that receptor was designed to do actually happens. For example, a beta blocker will slow heart rate, reduce contractility, and potentially could cause bronchospasm. This occurs because it blocks the normal functions of the beta receptor; therefore, the opposite effect occurs. Understanding what the receptors do, as well as the difference between agonists versus antagonists, will help you successfully manage your patient in the field, in addition to successfully answering critical care certification exam questions.

## AUTONOMIC MEDICATIONS

### Dopamine
1. Class: Vasopressor, Sympathomimetic
2. Mechanism: stimulates the beta and alpha receptors resulting in increased contractility and myocardial workload, as well as peripheral vasoconstriction.
3. Indications: hypotension, low cardiac output, poor perfusion
4. Contraindications: Uncontrolled tachycardia, ventricular irritability, hypertension
5. Hemodynamics: (~ CVP/ ~PCWP/↑CO/↑SVR); dopamine will also slightly increase pulmonary vascular resistance.
6. **NOTE: The (~) sign indicates that a parameter will most likely be normal, but could be a little high or low. Mostly normal.**
7. Dose:
    a. Renal Dose: 2-5 mg/kg/min
    b. Beta Dose: 5-10 mg/kg/min
    c. Alpha Dose: 10-20 mg/kg/min
    d. With the renal dosing, you'll have reduced cardiac output, but as you get into the beta (increase heart rate in contractility), and the alpha (vasoconstriction) doses, cardiac output increases.
8. Remember always to FILL THE TANK before adding a pressor. The pressor does no good if you have not adequately fluid resuscitated your patients.

### Levophed
1. Class: Vasopressor, Sympathomimetic
2. Mechanism: strongly stimulates the alpha 1 receptors in addition to stimulating some beta receptors. This results in significant venous and arterial vasoconstriction.
3. Indications: hypotension, low cardiac output, poor perfusion
4. Contraindications: Uncontrolled tachycardia, ventricular irritability, hypertension
5. Hemodynamics: (↑CVP/ ↑PCWP/↑CO/↑SVR); dopamine additionally will slightly increase pulmonary vascular resistance.
6. Dose: 1-30 mg/min (typical therapeutic use is ~8-12 mg/min )

### Epinephrine
1. Class: Vasopressor, Sympathomimetic, bronchodilator
2. Mechanism: Markedly stimulates both the alpha and beta receptors resulting in significant increases in heart rate, blood pressure, and cardiac output.
3. Indications: hypotension, low cardiac output, poor perfusion, pulseless ventricular tachycardia, ventricular fibrillation, pulseless electrical activity
4. Contraindications: Hypertension, tachycardia, acute coronary syndromes, hypersensitivity
5. Hemodynamics: (↑CVP/ ↑PCWP/↑CO/↑SVR).
6. Dose: 1-30 mg/min
    a. Hypotension, adults:1- 4 mg/min
    b. Anaphylaxis, adults: 0.1-0.5 mg SQ/IM
    c. Hypotension, pediatric: 0.1- 1.0 mg/min
    d. Anaphylaxis, pediatrics: 0.01 mg/kg IM

### Phenylepherine
1. Class: Vasopressor, Sympathomimetic
2. Mechanism: Strongly stimulates the alpha 1 receptor but does not increase in HR/ contractility.
3. Indications: hypotension

4. Contraindications: Hypertension, tachycardia, acute coronary syndromes, hypersensitivity
5. Dose:
    a. (Adult): 0.75 mcg/kg over 2-3 minutes for loading.
    b. (Adult): 50 mcg/min
    c. Peds: 5-20 mcg/kg; maint. 0.1-0.5 mcg/kg/min
6. Hemodynamics: (↑CVP/ ↑PCWP/↑CO/↑SVR).

## Vasopressin

1. Class: Anti– Diuretic Hormone, Vasopressor
2. Mechanism: Retains water within the vasculature system and at higher doses than are endogenous within the body, it produces vascular smooth muscle contraction (vasoconstriction), thus blood pressure elevates.
3. Indications: hypotension, low perfusion, anti– diuretic to combat diabetes insipidus.
4. Contraindications: Hypertension, tachycardia, acute coronary syndromes, hypersensitivity
5. Hemodynamics: (~CVP/ ~PCWP/~CO/↑SVR).
6. Dose: 10 units IV


# INOTROPIC AGENTS

## Dobutamine:

1. Class: Positive Inotrope, Sympathomimetic
2. Mechanism: highly stimulates beta 1 receptors, but also reduces afterload.  By increasing contractility and decreasing SVR, it makes for a fantastic medication for heart failure patients.
3. Indications: Congestive heart failure, poor cardiac output
4. Contraindications: acute coronary syndrome, tachycardia, hypertension, hypersensitivity
5. Hemodynamics: (~ CVP/ ~PCWP/↑CO/↓SVR); Note that Dobutamine reduces SVR and Dopamine increases SVR.
6. Dose: 2-20 mg/kg/min

## Amrinone:

1. Class: Inotrope
2. Mechanism: causes the release of calcium, which improves myocardial contractility. Additionally, it causes direct arterial vasodilation. Improved contractility increases cardiac output; vasodilation reduces afterload.
3. Indications: congestive heart failure.
4. Contraindications: hypotension, valvular disease
5. Hemodynamics: (~CVP/ ↓PCWP/↑CO/↓SVR).

## Milrinone:

1. Class: Inotrope
2. Mechanism: causes the release of calcium, which improves myocardial contractility. Additionally, it causes direct arterial vasodilation. Improved contractility increases cardiac output; vasodilation reduces afterload.
3. Indications: congestive heart failure.
4. Contraindications: hypotension, valvular disease
5. Hemodynamics: (~CVP/ ↓PCWP/↑CO/↓SVR).
6. Dose:
    a. Loading dose (adult): 50 mg/kg over 10 minutes
    b. Maintenance dose (Adult): 0.375- 0.75 mg/kg/min

## VASODILATORS

### Nitroglycerin:
1. Class: Nitrate Vasodilator
2. Mechanism: relaxes vascular and coronary vascular bed, thus decreasing systolic and diastolic blood pressure and improved coronary blood flow.
3. Indications: hypertension, ischemic chest pain, AMI
4. Contraindications: hypotension, hypersensitivity
5. Hemodynamics: (~CVP/ ↓PCWP/↑CO/↓SVR).
6. Dose: 5-50 mg/min
7. Start low (~ 15 mg/min) and titrate up as needed.

### Nitroprusside:
1. Class: Nitrate Vasodilators
2. Mechanism: relaxes vascular and coronary vascular bed, thus decreasing systolic and diastolic blood pressure and improved coronary blood flow.
3. Indications: hypertension, ischemic chest pain, AMI
4. Contraindications: hypotension, hypersensitivity
5. Hemodynamics: (~CVP/ ↓PCWP/↑CO/↓SVR).
6. Dose: 0.5-10 mg/kg/min

### Hydralazine
1. Class: Vasodilator
2. Mechanism: Direct acting arterial vasodilator, but has little effect on venous system.
3. Indications: PIH, eclampsia, CHF, pulmonary hypertension
4. Contraindications: acute coronary syndromes, valvular disease, AMI, hypersensitivity
5. Hemodynamics: (↑CVP/ ↑PCWP/↓CO/↑SVR).
6. Dose: 5-40 mg over 2-3 minutes

### Nicardipine
1. Class: Antihypertensive, Calcium Channel Blocker
2. Mechanism: Relaxes myocardial tissue and vascular smooth muscle.
3. Indications: hypertensive emergencies, CHF, pulmonary hypertension
4. Contraindications: advanced aortic stenosis, hypersensitivity
5. Hemodynamics: (↓CVP/ ~PCWP/↓CO/↓SVR).
6. Dose:
7. Adult: 5 mg/hr initially; increase by 2.5 mg/hr q 15 minutes (max of 15 mg/hr)
8. Peds: 1-3 mg/kg/min


## CARDIOPROTECTIVE MEDICATIONS

### Labetalol:
1. Class: Beta Blocker
2. Mechanism: Causes non-selective beta blockade.  Non-selective means that both beta receptors are blocked, thus, HR, AV conduction, and contractility will all be reduced, and bronchospasm is a possibility.  Additionally, it partially blocks alpha 1, so vasodilation occurs.
3. Indications: hypertensive crisis
4. Contraindications: asthma, hypotension, bradycardia, cardiac failure, high degree heart block.
5. Hemodynamics: (↓CVP/ ↓PCWP/↓CO/↓SVR).
6. Dose:

a. 20 mg IV over 2 minutes; may repeat 40-80 mg q 10 minutes; max of 300 mg
b. Maintenance infusion: 2 mg/min

### Esmolol

1. Class: Beta Blocker
2. Mechanism: Causes non-selective beta blockade. Non-selective means that both beta receptors are blocked, thus HR, AV conduction, and contractility will both be reduced, and bronchospasm is a possibility.
3. Indications: hypertensive crisis, hypertension associated with aortic aneurysms
4. Contraindications: acute coronary syndromes, valvular disease, AMI, hypersensitivity
5. Hemodynamics: ($\downarrow$CVP/ $\downarrow$PCWP/$\downarrow$CO/$\downarrow$SVR).
6. Dose: 500 mg/kg/min for 1 minute, then 25 mg/kg/min maintenance infusion; max of 300 mg/kg/min.

### Metoprolol

1. Class: Beta Blocker
2. Mechanism: SPECIFIC Beta 1 blocker, therefore, HR, contractility, and AV conduction are reduced, but there is no effect on bronchial smooth muscle.
3. Indications: AMI, hypertension.
4. Contraindications: bradycardia, cardiac failure, hypotension, high degree AV block, valvular disease
5. Hemodynamics: (~CVP/ ~PCWP/$\downarrow$CO/~SVR).
6. Dose: 5 mg slow IV initially; repeat up to 3 times at 5-minute intervals

### Aspirin:

1. Class: Platelet Aggregate Inhibitor, analgesic, anti-pyretic
2. Mechanism: reduces the synthesis of clotting factors VII, IX, and X, which prevents the platelets from sticking together$\rightarrow$ makes blood thinner and easier to pump.
3. Indications: AMI, angina.
4. Contraindications: allergy, bleeding tendencies, severe anemia, pregnancy
5. Hemodynamics: (~CVP/ ~PCWP/~CO/~SVR).
6. Dose: 162– 324 mg PO

## ACE INHIBITORS

### Enalapril:

1. Class: ACE Inhibitor
2. Mechanism: Blocks angiotensin converting enzyme from converting angiotensin I into angiotensin II (a very potent vasoconstrictor), which results in lower blood pressure. It also will lower PCWP.
3. Indications: hypertension, used with Lasix in CHF exacerbation, AMI
4. Contraindications: pre-existing hypotension, cardiogenic shock, hypersensitivity.
5. Hemodynamics: ($\downarrow$CVP/ $\downarrow$PCWP/$\downarrow$CO/$\downarrow$SVR).
6. Dose:
   a. Adults: 1.25 mg IV over 5 minutes; may repeat q 6 hours
   b. Peds: 5-10 mg/kg q 8 hours

## ANTICOAGULANTS

### Heparin

1. Class: Anticoagulant

2. Mechanism: Blocks the conversion of both prothrombin → thrombin and fibrinogen → fibrin, therefore, it prevents future clots from forming. It does not dissolve existing clots.
3. Indications: AMI, PE, A-fib, DIC
4. Contraindications: bleeding tendencies, thrombocytopenia (low platelets in the blood), intracranial hemorrhage
5. Hemodynamics: (~CVP/ ~PCWP/~CO/~SVR).
6. Dose:
   a. Adults: 5000 units IV bolus; then maintenance infusion of 1000 units/hr
   b. Peds: 50 units/kg IVP initially; maintenance infusion 50-100 units/kg IVP q 4 hours

## Lovenox:

1. Class: Anticoagulant, Low molecular weight heparin
2. Mechanism: Blocks the conversion of both prothrombin → thrombin, therefore, it prevents future clots from forming. It does not dissolve existing clots.
3. Indications: AMI, DVT
4. Contraindications: Bleeding tendencies, hypersensitivity
5. Hemodynamics: (~CVP/ ~PCWP/~CO/~SVR).
6. Dose: 1 mg/kg SQ; may repeat q 12 hours

## Integrillin:

1. Class: Anti-thrombotic, Glycoprotein IIB/IIIA Inhibitor
2. Mechanism: Inhibits platelet aggregation by preventing the binding of fibrinogen (Von Willebrand factor) thus making clotting time longer.
3. Indications: AMI, cardiac procedures
4. Contraindications: Bleeding tendencies, anemia, thrombocytopenia, hypersensitivity
5. Hemodynamics: (~CVP/ ~PCWP/~CO/~SVR).
6. Dose: 180 mg/kg initially; maintenance infusion: 2 mg/kg/min

# FIBRINOLYTICS

## Reteplase (rt-PA)

1. Class: Fibrinolytic
2. Mechanism: Causes the release of plasminogen, which is then converted into plasmin. Plasmin destroys fibrin (the clot's glue) therefore the clot breaks up, and blood flow is restored.
3. Indications: Active AMI
4. Contraindications: bleeding tendencies, uncontrolled hypertension
5. Hemodynamics: (~CVP/ ~PCWP/~CO/~SVR).
6. Dose: 10 units IVP over 2 minutes; repeat in 30 minutes

## Alteplase (t-PA):

1. Class: Fibrinolytic
2. Mechanism: Causes the release of plasminogen, which is then converted into plasmin. Plasmin destroys fibrin (the clot's glue) therefore the clot breaks up, and blood flow is restored.
3. Indications: Active AMI, ischemic stroke, acute PE
4. Contraindications: bleeding tendencies, uncontrolled hypertension
5. Hemodynamics: (~CVP/ ~PCWP/~CO/~SVR).
6. Dose:
   a. AMI
      i. If >65 kg; 15 mg IVP over 2 minutes, followed by 50 mg IV over the next 30 minutes, followed by 35 mg IV over the next 60 minutes.

ii. If < 65 kg; 15 mg IVP over 2 minutes, followed by 0.75 mg/kg IV over the next 30 minutes, followed by 0.5 mg/kg IV over the next 60 minutes.

b. Ischemic Stroke: 0.9 mg/kg IV (max 90 mg) with first 10% of dose given over 1 minute

c. Pulmonary Embolism: 100 mg over 2 hours

## Tenecteplase (TNKASE)

1. Class: Fibrinolytic
2. Mechanism: Causes the release of plasminogen, which is then converted into plasmin. Plasmin destroys fibrin (the clot's glue) therefore the clot breaks up, and blood flow is restored. The advantage over other fibrinolytics: one-time dose.
3. Indications: Active AMI
4. Contraindications: bleeding tendencies, uncontrolled hypertension, stroke, classic relative and absolute contraindications
5. Hemodynamics: (~CVP/ ~PCWP/~CO/~SVR).
6. Dose:
   a. < 60 kg = 30 mg over 5 seconds
   b. 60– 70 kg = 35 mg over 5 seconds
   c. 70– 80 kg = 40 mg over 5 seconds
   d. 80– 90 kg = 45 mg over 5 seconds
   e. 90 kg = 50 mg over 5 seconds

# ANTIDYSRYTHMICS

## Lidocaine

1. Class: Antidysrhythmic Class IB
2. Mechanism: Suppresses the automaticity of ischemic ectopic locations in the myocardium (reduces the fibrillation threshold). It additionally raises the ventricular fibrillation threshold.
3. Indications: ventricular tachycardia, ventricular fibrillation, PVCs, wide– complex tachycardias
4. Contraindications: bradycardia with ventricular ectopy, hypersensitivity
5. Hemodynamics: (~CVP/ ~PCWP/~CO/~SVR).
6. Dose:
7. Adults: 1– 1.5 mg/kg over 3 minutes; repeat q 5 minutes; maintenance infusion: 1– 4 mg/min
8. Peds: 0.5– 1 mg/kg over 3 minutes; maintenance infusion: 20-50 mg/kg/min.

## Procainamide

1. Class: Antidysrhythmic Class IA
2. Mechanism: Slows conduction through the myocardium, which suppresses ectopy throughout the heart.
3. Indications: Second line for ventricular tachycardia, ventricular fibrillation, PVCs, wide– complex tachycardias
4. Contraindications: bradycardia with ventricular ectopy, hypersensitivity
5. Hemodynamics: (~CVP/ ~PCWP/↓CO/~SVR).
6. Dose: 20 mg/min loading infusion up to 17 mg/kg (max dose), or until the cessation of ectopy, hypotension, or lengthening QT interval.

## Amiodarone

1. Class: Antidysrhythmic Class III
2. Mechanism: Blocks sodium and potassium channels, increases the duration of impulses, relaxes smooth muscles, and acts as an alpha and beta blocker→ therefore, we have slower HR, conduction, contractility, and blood pressure (BP is only minorly affected– not potent).

3. Indications: Initial treatment for ventricular tachycardia, ventricular fibrillation, PVCs, wide–complex tachycardias
4. Contraindications: bradycardia with ventricular ectopy, hypersensitivity
5. Hemodynamics: (~CVP/ ~PCWP/↓CO/~SVR).
6. Dose: 150 mg IV bolus over 10 minutes; maintenance infusion: 1 mg/min over the next 6 hours; then 0.5mg/min over the next 18 hours.

## Atropine

1. Class: Anticholinergic
2. Mechanism: Blocks the parasympathetic receptors (slow system) and speeds up the heart
3. Indications: bradycardia, organophosphate poisoning
4. Contraindications: hypersensitivity
5. Hemodynamics: (~CVP/ ~PCWP/↑CO/~SVR).
6. Dose:
7. Adults: Cardiac- 1 mg IV q 3-5 minutes; organophosphate poisoning– 2-3mg IV bolus and repeat until the poisoned patient's secretions dry up.
8. Peds: 0.01-0.03 mg/kg IV push.

## Adenosine

1. Class: Antidysrhythmic Class IV-Like
2. Mechanism: Blocks potassium channels which slow conduction (slows HR) and stops reentry pathways (resets SVT).
3. Indications: SVT
4. Contraindications: High degree AV block, sick sinus syndrome
5. Hemodynamics: (~CVP/ ~PCWP/~CO/~SVR).
6. Dose: 6 mg rapid IV push with 10cc NS flush; second and third doses– 12 mg rapid IV push with 10cc NS flush to a max of 30 mg.

## Magnesium Sulfate

1. Class: Electrolyte, Muscle relaxant
2. Mechanism: decreases the excitability of muscles, therefore, relaxes skeletal and smooth muscle: reduces BP, relaxes uterine contractions, bronchodilates, slows HR.
3. Indications: ventricular tachycardia refractory to other treatments, eclampsia, tocolysis for pregnancy
4. Contraindications: Bradycardia, hypotension, heart block
5. Hemodynamics: (↓CVP/ ↓PCWP/↓CO/↓SVR).
6. Dose:
   a. Adults: 1-2 g administered IV over 10-20 minutes
   b. Peds: 25-50 mg/kg IV or IM

## Diltiazem

1. Class: Calcium Channel Blocker
2. Mechanism: Blocks calcium channels which cause a reduced conduction velocity through the conduction system. Additionally, it decreases contractility and afterload.
3. Indications: A-fib/ A-flutter with rapid ventricular response, SVT refractory to adenosine
4. Contraindications: Bradycardia, hypotension, heart block
5. Hemodynamics: (↓CVP/ ↓PCWP/↓CO/↓SVR).
6. Dose: 0.25 mg/kg IVP over 2 minutes; if no response, administer 0.35 mg/kg over 2 minutes; maintenance infusion: 5-15 mg/min.

# PART 9: CARDIAC DEVICE MANAGEMENT

## PULMONARY ARTERY CATHETER MANAGEMENT

### GENERAL

1. The PA catheter provides hemodynamic information that cannot be obtained by simple physical assessment. PA catheters are designed to determine precise hemodynamic measurements of stroke volume, cardiac output, intracardiac and pulmonary artery pressures, estimates of systematic and pulmonary vascular resistance, and mixed venous oxygenation data from its blood sampling ability.

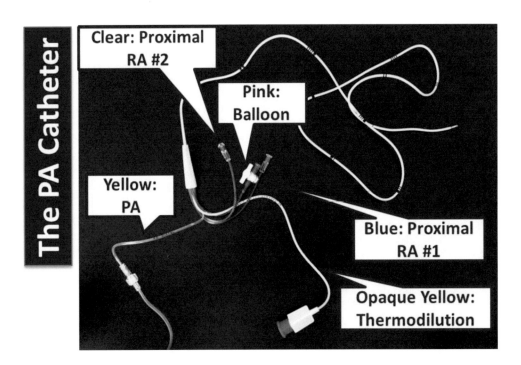

2. The PA catheter is also helpful in determining the etiology of various pathophysiologies. Such conditions include the etiology of shock, the differentiation between mechanisms of pulmonary edema (cardiogenic versus noncardiogenic), pulmonary hypertension, and the diagnosis of multiple cardiac abnormalities such as mitral regurgitation and cardiac tamponade.
3. It can be used in the management of patients with conditions where hemodynamic stability is important for improving an outcome or guiding therapy decisions (renal failure, sepsis, burns).
4. Minor complications include insertion and maintenance of the catheter problems (infection, ventricular fibrillation), inaccuracies in the measurements. And difficulties in interpreting PA catheter parameters.
5. Major complication: pulmonary artery rupture. This has a very high mortality rate. Fortunately, this is a rare occurrence when the procedure is performed correctly.
6. Look back to review the various pressures the PA catheter will experience on its way from insertion to the pulmonary artery (see Part 4, Assessment of Hemodynamics of this chapter).

7. It is important to know where the catheter is relative to the pressure waveform.

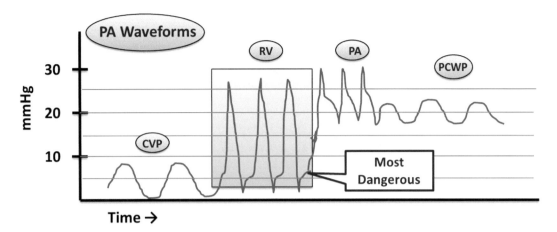

## CATHETER MIGRATION

1. This is a common and DEADLY complication of PA monitoring.
2. The most important waveform is the right ventricular waveform. If you notice this waveform, the heart could start producing some significant PVCs and could progress to ventricular fibrillation.
3. The best course of action that has been identified in the literature is to withdraw the catheter back into the right atrium (RA). In the RA, the waveform is exactly like the CVP. So, as you withdrew, it would look like the tall right ventricular (RV) waveform that is ~ 30/10 mmHg, to the low pressure (2-6 mmHg) of the RA waveform (if RA and CVP are exactly the same).
4. PARAMEDICS! I NEED YOUR ATTENTION! On your critical care certification exams, you must answer RV migration questions with the following: advance the catheter back into the PA. Sorry, but these exams have the correct answers as marked as ADVANCE, now withdraw. In real life, withdraw. On the exam, ADVANCE (FOR PARAMEDICS ONLY).
5. The below waveform is a real example. Notice the tall waves the corresponding higher pressures AND lower pressures. The PA placement would also have these systolic pressures of about 46mmHg, however the PA diastolic pressures would be more like 20 mmHg. Here the diastolic pressures are about 8 mmHg, and this is the RV pressures. That is how you tell– RV pressures have lower diastolic pressures, and the PA has higher diastolic pressures. As the PA catheter warms to that of the body it is in, it will get more flexible and can migrate– always be looking for this during transport.
6. Dampening
7. The pressure monitoring device/ monitor and its set up (transducer, pressure bag, etc) requires a consistent flow of clean data. To keep data clean, be sure to have shorter tubing sets (less

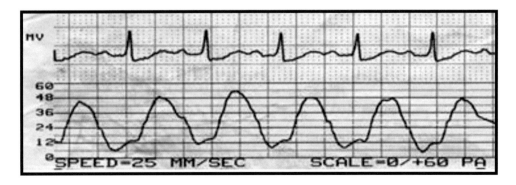

chance for kinks) and use the fewest number of stopcocks possible (less chance of air getting into system).

## DAMPINING WAVEFORM

1. The pressure monitoring device/ monitor and its set up (transducer, pressure bag, etc) requires a consistent flow of clean data. To keep data clean, be sure to have shorter tubing sets (less chance for kinks) and use the fewest amount of stopcocks possible (less chance of air getting into system).
2. If you experience waveform problems like the ones displayed here to the right. Follow these steps:
   a. Check for air bubbles in system
   b. Ensure pressure bag is inflated to 300mmHg.

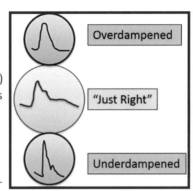

## PLACEMENT

1. There are markings on the PA catheter itself.
   a. Typically, from a thin line (tic mark) to another thin line is 10cm.
   b. Thick line to thick line is 50 cm.
2. Like most assessments, it's a good idea to get a baseline and know at what depth the PA catheter is positioned so that it can be monitored throughout transport.
3. This (insertion point for depth) will be the first place you should check after noting a pressure change on the pressure monitor because it will indicate if the PA catheter tip has migrated.
4. Always document the PA catheter at the beginning, throughout, and at the end of a patient transport.

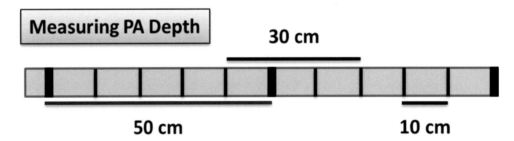

## PULMONARY ARTERY RUPTURE

1. Indicated when copious amounts of blood are coming from the patient's mouth or endotracheal tube.
2. Fluids and blood products needed to support the patient, and surgery is IMMEDIATELY REQUIRED.

## INTRA-AORTIC BALLON PUMP (IABP) MANAGEMENT

### INTRODUCTION

The Intra-Aortic Balloon Pump (IABP) is a circulatory assist device that is used to support the left ventricle. The IABP inflates a balloon to force blood backward into the aorta and coronary arteries and deflates just before the heart beat. This deflation reduces afterload the moment before ventricular contraction occurs, making it easier on the heart to pump blood.

Displaced blood during inflation pushes blood backward against the aortic valve. Some blood is pushed into the coronary arteries and increases coronary perfusion pressure, which increases myocardial oxygen supply. Basically, you're pushing oxygen into the myocardium.

Displaced blood during deflation occurs with essentially a cavity where the balloon used to be, and immediately upon deflation drastically reduces afterload. This reduction in afterload makes it easier for the heart to pump blood forward, and thus reduces afterload and myocardial oxygen demand.

The balloon is connected to a console that regulates the inflation or deflation of the balloon with the passage of helium. Helium is used as it is easily dissolved in blood and prevents the risk of air emboli if the catheter ruptures. Use CT or X-ray to confirm correct placement: between the subclavian artery and the renal arteries.

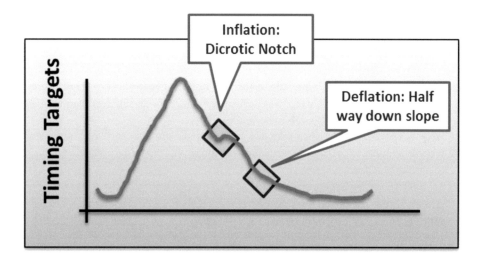

## INFLATION
1. Ideally, inflation occurs at the time of aortic closure. This is signified on the pressure waveform as the dicrotic notch.
2. If inflated correctly, a V shape should be shown on the balloon trace (see page 170 to review a normal tracing).
3. The effect of displacement of blood in the aorta causes an increase in diastolic arterial pressure and an increase in cardiac output.

4. IABP Rule #1: Inflate balloon directly prior to the dicrotic notch; this causes the augmented diastolic pressure to be greater than the patient's own systolic pressure (green arrow).

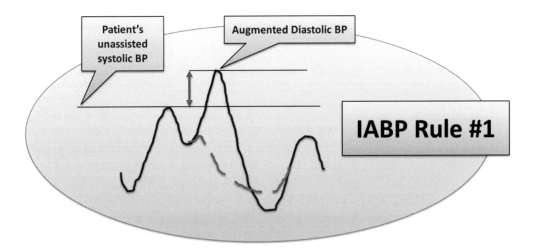

5. EARLY INFLATION: occurs when the balloon inflates prior to the aortic valve closure, and then there will be insufficient blood in the aorta, resulting in a ↓ in supply to coronary arteries, premature closure of aortic valve and ↑ afterload.
6. LATE INFLATION: occurs when the balloon inflates too late after the closure of the aortic valve. Blood is allowed to escape down the aorta to the rest of the body, instead of being directed toward the coronary arteries.
7. For inflation timing issues, on the console, move the timing closer to match the aortic valve closure. It can be one augmentation for every systole (1:1), or one augmentation for every other systole (1:2). These are the common timings.

## DEFLATION
1. Deflation is the depression of the balloon and the transfer of helium back into the console, which occurs in systole.
2. The effect is a decrease in aortic end diastolic pressure (afterload) by the balloon deflating and creating space in the aorta. This causes less impedance to the blood being expelled from the left ventricle once the balloon is deflated.
3. This results in a decreased ventricle wall tension, increased stroke volume and complete emptying of the ventricle.
4. Cardiac workload is reduced due to a decrease in left ventricular end systolic volume and preload, which reduces the cardiac workload, and myocardial oxygen demand.
5. IABP Rule #2: Augmented end– diastolic pressure should be LOWER or EQUAL TO the patient's unassisted end-diastolic pressure (orange arrow). Therefore, the augmented end– diastolic pressure should NEVER be higher than the patient's own inherent (unassisted) diastolic pressure.

6. IABP Rule #3: The augmented systolic pressure should be LOWER to the patient's inherent (unassisted) systolic BP (black arrow). Therefore, augmentation with IABP should reduce the patient's systolic BP (afterload).

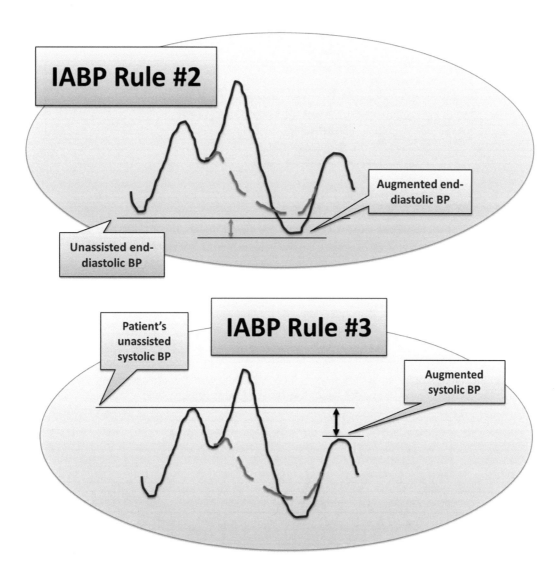

7. EARLY DEFLATION: This causes retrograde blood flow out of the coronary arteries and effecting forward blood flow to other vessels and ↑ afterload.
8. LATE DEFLATION: This has the effect of impeding the left ventricular ejection. The balloon acts as a roadblock in this scenario. It MUST be deflated once the heart begins to contract. This increases SVR DRAMATICALLY.
9. REMEMBER: the 'Double V' pattern = Late Deflation

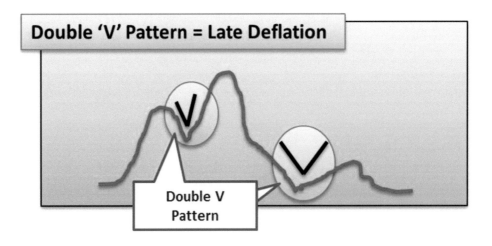

## INFLATION & DEFLATION ERROR SUMMARY

1. Early Inflation: Balloon inflates way before the dicrotic notch. This violates IABP Rule #1. Result: this forces the aortic valve closed, ⁻ stroke volume, and ↑ left ventricle workload.

2. Late inflation: the balloon inflates after the dicrotic notch and exposes the dicrotic notch for viewing. This also violates IABP Rule #1. Result: ⁻ coronary perfusion pressure.

3. Early Deflation: Swiftly dropping diastolic pressure which causes a U– shaped diastolic curvature. Also, the augmented systolic BP is not lower, but the same as the patient's unassisted systolic BP. This violates IABP Rule #3. Result: no ⁻ in afterload = no real IABP benefit.

4. Late Deflation: there is a widened diastolic pressure. Also, the augmented end– diastolic pressure is not lower, but the same or higher than the patient's unassisted end– diastolic pressure. This violates IABP Rule #2. Result: ↑ left ventricle workload.

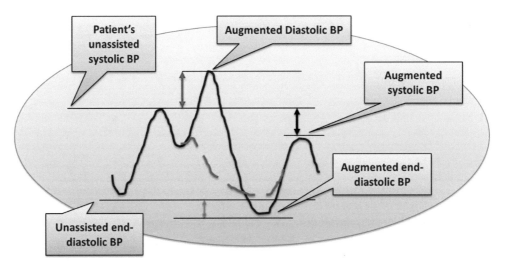

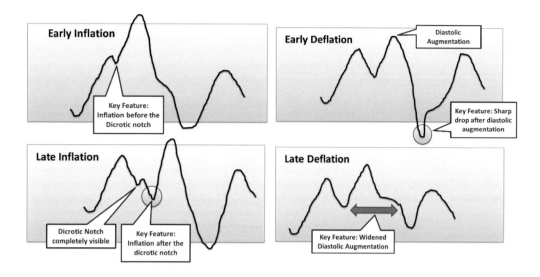

## BALLOON RUPTURE
1. The hallmark sign of a ruptured balloon is blood in the connecting tubing.
2. IMMEDIATELY stop counterpulsation to prevent cerebral embolization.
3. Never let the patient sit up more than 30 degrees and consider a knee immobilizer for the leg of insertion to prevent dislodgement.

## IABP TIMING
You can control how often the IABP balloon inflates by telling the machine to inflate the balloon after every systole (1:1 timing), after every other systole (1:2 timing), or after 2 normal systoles (1:3 timing). Sometimes patients may need more coronary perfusion pressure to maintain myocardial oxygen supply (from the balloon inflating and forcing blood retrograde from the aorta and into the coronary arteries), so the timing frequency is increased. Sometimes patients need more of a reduced afterload (deflation), so the timing frequency [meaning going from a slower timing (1:3) to a more frequent timing (1:1)] may be increased.

### 1:1 Timing
1. One counterpulsation per heartbeat
2. This can be tough because there is never a normal systole to compare inflation timing with the dicrotic notch– better explained below.
3. Most IABP will allow you to pause balloon inflations to see the underlying dicrotic notch so that you can best time the inflation
4. In 1:1 timing, there are ONLY assisted systoles with augmented diastoles– NO NORMAL or UNASSISTED heart beats.

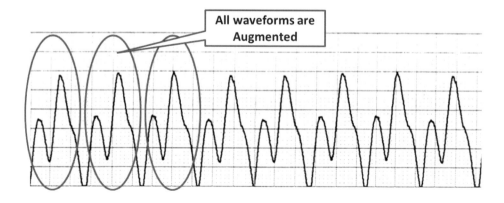

**1:2 Timing**

1. One counterpulsation every other heartbeat.
2. Ideally, the IABP inflation should match the height of the dicrotic notch, meaning the IABP inflation and the physiologic dicrotic notch should be at the same height on the waveform.
3. Notice below that the IABP balloon inflation point is HIGHER than the dicrotic notch.
4. This is the key to identifying correct inflation– is the height of the inflation the same height as the dicrotic notch in a non-assisted systole? If the answer is no, there is an inflation timing problem.
5. The higher than the dicrotic notch = EARLY inflation; the lower than the dicrotic notch = LATE inflation.

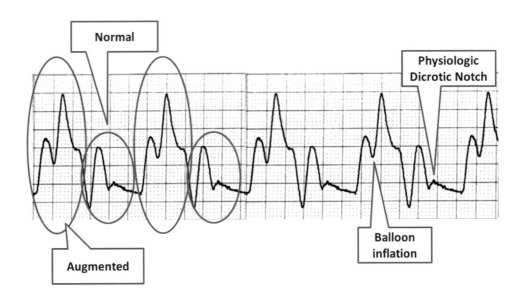

**1:3 Timing**

1. One counterpulsation every second heartbeat.
2. This is for when you need only a little augmentation.

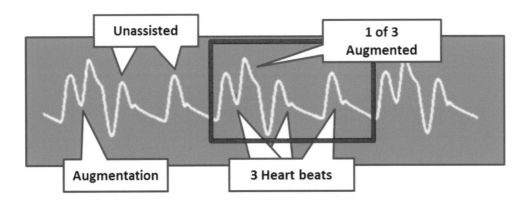

144

## CARDIAC PACING

Pacing is a procedure that is utilized when the heart's intrinsic pacemaker system fails. A slowing of the heart (< 60 beats per minute) leads to reduced cardiac output. There are four different routes for pacing that will be discussed in this text: epicardial, transvenous, transcutaneous, and transesophageal.

### *PACING TYPES*

#### Transcutaneous
1. This is a temporary method of pacing to stabilize a patient until a more definitive pacemaker can be implanted.
2. This mode is characteristic of adhesive skin pads (skin leads) that are positioned on the patients chest, or on the chest and back.
3. A set rate and output current are programmed, and the patient is assessed for mechanical capture.

#### Epicardial:
1. During cardiac surgery, electrodes (epicardial wires) are attached directly to the epicardial surface of the atrium and/or ventricle.
2. Leads are placed on the epicardial surface of either the right atrium, right ventricle, or both.
3. The wires then exit through the patient's sternum where they are then connected to a pulse generator.
4. Epicardial pacing is often used following cardiac surgery for the management of surgically related bradydysrhythmias.

#### Transvenous:
1. Leads can be placed by a PA catheter, or by an interventional radiologist or a cardiothoracic surgeon.
2. This type of pacing is usually utilized right after cardiac surgery.
3. Leads are placed on the endocardial surface of either the right atrium, right ventricle, or both.

#### Transesophageal
1. In transesophageal pacing is an electrode attached to an esophageal probe inserted into the esophagus just behind the left atrium to permit temporary atrial pacing.
2. The patient is to remain sedated for the duration of this type of pacing. Also, esophageal injury can be caused by long-term transesophageal pacing.

### *TEMPORARY PACING*

1. Temporary pacing is used in a variety of elective and emergent procedures. When the SA node fails to produce regular impulses between 60-100 beats per minute, cardiac output can be compromised. This can lead to poor tissue perfusion and arrhythmias.
2. Indications for Temporary Pacemakers:
   a. Bradydysrhythmias
   b. Heart blocks
   c. Sick sinus syndrome
   d. Cardiovascular surgery
   e. Drugs and medications that can suppress electrical conduction

## POLAR VS. CHAMBER

### POLAR

1. A pole is a conducting wire, and an electrode. Remember the defibrillation paddles from back in the day? The cord to the paddle is the conducting wire and the paddle itself is the electrode.
2. Unipolar Pacing: this is a method that is characteristic of one conducting wire and one electrode and is typically used in permanent (implanted) pacing systems. Not typically used with transcutaneous pacing.
3. Bipolar Pacing: this is the method of choice for transcutaneous pacing. There are two conducting wires and two electrodes. The impulse passes through one wire and the electrode, passes through the cardiac tissue and causes the depolarization and then completes the circuit by flowing through the second electrode and wire back to the pulse generator.
4. Remember, the term "polar" indicates how many sets of wires and electrodes you have.

### CHAMBER

1. Chamber, of course, refers to either the right atria or the right ventricle.
2. Single Chamber Pacing: typically, atrial pacing is preferable to ventricular pacing because this allows for atrioventricular synchrony.
   a. However, for atrial pacing to work, the AV nodal pathway must be intact and functioning normally. Otherwise, the electrical impulse generated by the pacemaker is not correctly distributed to the ventricle, and therefore, no benefit is gained.
   b. Even though atrial pacing is preferable, either the right atria or the right ventricle can be selected for single chamber use.
3. Dual Chamber Pacing: as you may have guessed, this type of pacing includes both the right atria and the right ventricle.
   a. Increasing the heart rate is not the only function of the pacemaker, in the dual pacing feature allows for another important function: AV synchrony.
   b. Remember the importance of atrial kick? It helps to increase the stretch of the ventricle which leads to higher stroke volume (blood pumped out of the heart). Using dual chamber pacing, you can ensure AV synchrony, therefore making sure that atrial kick and a maximal stretch of the ventricle occurs.

## DEMAND VS. ASYNCHRONOUS PACING

1. This essentially describes the modes of pacing. You can think of mode as WHEN the pacer initiates.
2. Demand Pacing: demand is the mode where the pacer discharges only when the patient's rhythm falls below a set rate. The pacer measures the QRS to QRS distance, and if they are too far apart (meaning the rate is too slow) then the pacer initiates.
3. Asynchronous Pacing: this mode of pacing doesn't discriminate as to what the patient is doing. It provides impulses at a set rate regardless of the patient's underlying rhythm.
4. Safety in choosing a mode of pacing (demand vs. asynchronous) is determined by the patient's underlying rhythm.
   a. Asynchronous pacing is only safe when the patient's underlying rhythm is asystole or if there is very little electrical activity produced by their heart.
   b. Demand pacing is safer because it provides pacing only when needed, therefore protecting the patient against electrical impulses firing during vulnerable periods of the cardiac cycle.

c. Remember R on T phenomenon?  If an electrical discharge causes depolarization of the ventricle (QRS, or R wave) at the height of the T wave, then lethal rhythms like V fib or ventricular tachycardia can occur.  Therefore, demand pacing is safer.

## GENERIC PACING MODE WITH NASPE CODES

1. NAPSE : N. American Society for Pacing and Electrophysiology
2. I know what you're thinking and stop rolling your eyes at this topic.  This is very simple, so we'll discuss it and move on.
3. We have already discussed most of the items and this chart.  This chart describes the various knobs you'll see on the control box of the pacer itself.  Now, you'll still have to be aware of the specific equipment at your hospital or transport service, but this will be an overview of the functions that can be dialed into a pacemaker.  The first three positions are the most common utilized by critical care clinicians.
4. Chamber Paced: Just because pacing wires are in place does not mean the pacer has to be on all the time.  You can set the pacer to not pace (O), to pace atrial only (A), to only pace ventricle (V), or to pace both (D; atria and ventricle) .
5. Chamber Sensed: Not all pacemakers are designed to sense the patient's intrinsic (natural) heart rhythm.  Additionally, even the ones that are designed to sense can be turned off.  The pacer can be set to sense none of the time (O), to sense only the atrial impulses (A), to sense only the ventricular impulses (V), or to sense both (D for dual).
6. Response to Sensing: This setting instructs the pacer what to do once impulses are detected.
   a. Inhibited: Delivery of an impulse is inhibited if a beat is detected from that chamber.  If no intrinsic beat is detected within a predetermined time period, the pacemaker goes ahead and paces.  So basically, this is the backup plan. If the heart fails to generate an impulse, the machine fires.
   b. Triggered:
      i. This is another method of backup, and is specific to ensure a AV synchrony.
      ii. This is specific to dual chamber pacing and cannot be used unless both chambers are being sensed AND the ventricle is being paced.
      iii. If an impulse (generated by the patient or the machine) is not transmitted through the AV node efficiently, then the ventricular sensing wire will tell the ventricular pacing wire to fire.
      iv. Again, this is a backup plan in the case that poor conduction through the AV node occurs.  If it does, the ventricle will detect it and send an impulse to ensure AV synchrony, thus maintaining a solid cardiac output.

## SETTING THE PACEMAKER

1. Again, be sure to know your equipment at the hospital  and transport facility where you practice.
2. Identify the atrial and ventricular (if available) wires on your patient's chest.  Atrial wires exit from the right side of the chest, and ventricle wires exit from the left side of the patient's chest.
3. Attach the appropriate wires to the appropriate leads: positive to positive and negative to negative.
4. Set the rate to approximately 70 to 90 beats per minute.
5. Set Output:
   a. Set the milliamperage for the atrial leads: 10 to 20 mA.
   b. Set the milliamperage for the ventricular leads: 10 to 20 mA
6. Set Sensitivity
   a. Atria: Start at 0.5 mV
   b. Ventricle: Start at 2– 5 mV

# COMPLICATIONS MANAGEMENT

### Failure to Capture:
1. This describes the situation where the electrical pulse results in no pacer spike on the ECG.
2. Cause: output too low– increase the mA.
3. Cause: anti-arrhythmic drugs on board
4. Cause: lead migration or dislodgment

### Failure to Sense (Undersensing):
1. This describes the situation where the pacer cannot "see" the ECG waveforms. If you cannot "see" the ECG waveforms, then it cannot produce an impulse at the right time. It's like being blind and trying to walk across the street.
2. Cause: the device is set to an asynchronous mode- change to demand mode.
3. Cause: sensitivity is set too low- turn the sensitivity (mV) to a lower mV setting.

### Oversensing
1. This occurs when the pacer is too sensitive, picking up artifact (motor movements and shivering) and creating an impulse from them.
2. Cause: sensitivity set too high- turn the sensitivity (mV) to a higher mV setting.
3. Cause: shivering, seizures, skeletal muscle movements

### Failure to Pace:
1. This occurs when the pacemaker is set, but it is not creating impulses.
2. Cause: output turned off- turn on and set the output.
3. Cause: pacemaker turned off or low battery– ensure adequate power supply.
4. Cause: loose connection or disconnected lead- make sure all connections are snug.

# 12 LEAD ECG PACER MORPHOLOGIES
1. The key indicator is the pacer spiked itself, which is a very skinny vertical black line imbedded in the ECG tracing.
2. The best place to look is before the P-waves and before the QRS waves.
3. Examples:
   i. Paced Atrial Rhythm:

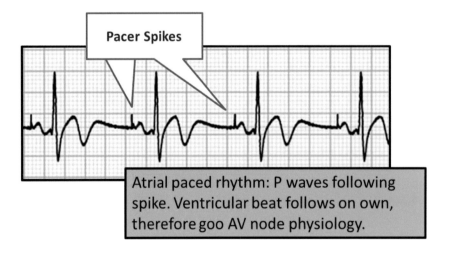

**Pacer Spikes**

Atrial paced rhythm: P waves following spike. Ventricular beat follows on own, therefore goo AV node physiology.

ii. Paved Ventricular Rhythm

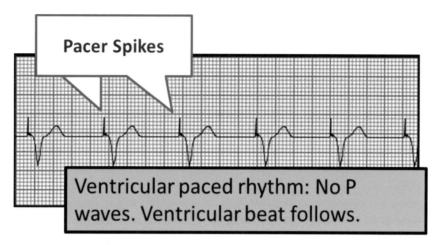

iii. Dual Paced Chamber

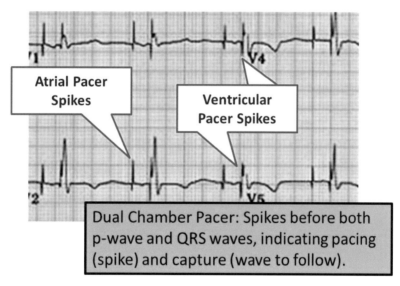

iv. Failure to Capture

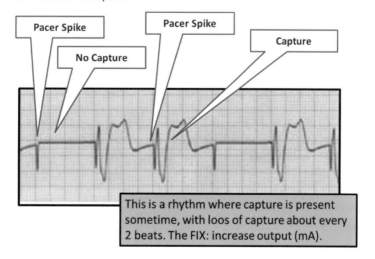

# VENTRICULAR ASSIST DEVICES

A VAD is essentially a device that takes over the pumping of blood from the heart when the heart gets too sick to do it alone. Ventricular assist devices (VADs) and the technology that drives them are improving every year, therefore it is quite possible you could see an increasing number of patients with these devices. It typically consists of a pumping device, a controlling device (control panel), battery packs and backup batteries, and tubes going to various portions of the heart.

## TYPES

1. Left ventricular assist device (LVAD): in this particular configuration, blood leaves the left ventricle through a tube, is propelled forward by the pump, and is deposited in the ascending aorta.
2. Right ventricular assist device (RVAD): in this configuration, blood leaves the right atrium or the right ventricle through a tube, is propelled forward, and is deposited in the pulmonary artery.
3. Bilateral ventricular assist device (BiVAD): this configuration utilizes both of the above flow paths. It includes the two from the left ventricle to the aorta as well as a two from either the right atrium or right ventricle to the pulmonary artery.

## INDICATIONS

1. Bridge to Recovery: the VAD will act as a temporary solution to improve ventricular function in cardiac output until the heart is healed enough to generate the appropriate cardiac output on its own.
2. Bridge to Heart Transplantation– to buy time to find a suitable donor heart.
3. Bridge to Decision-Making Moment: the VAD will act as a temporary solution until a decision can be made between allowing the heart to heal or transplantation.
4. Destination Therapy: this means that the VAD is the last treatment option and will require continued use until the end of life.

## TYPES OF PUMPS

1. There are two basic types of VAD pumps: pulsatile and continuous flow.
2. As you imagine, the pulsatile pumps produce a palpable pulse; however, the continuous flow does not produce a palpable pulse. This creates confusion from a treatment perspective to a clinician who has never treated a VAD before.
3. Pulsatile
   a. The first-generation type devices utilized ventricular sack- like bladders that would fill with blood then be ejected into systemic circulation.
   b. Electric motors or pneumatic pressures collapse the chamber and force blood into systemic circulation.
   c. These devices can be used for left ventricular support (LVAD), right ventricular support (RVAD), or bilateral ventricular support (BiVAD).
   d. These patients will have a palpable pulse and a measurable blood pressure, both generated by the device.
4. Continuous Flow (Non -Pulsatile)
   a. These devices are designed to produce flow throughout the cardiac cycle.
   b. Therefore, if the patient is completely dependent upon the device for cardiac output, there will be no pulse and no blood pressure.
   c. Conversely, if the patient has some ventricular function, and the device simply supports their circulatory effort, and then you might feel a weak pulse and be able to detect a weak, or lower, blood pressure.
   d. There are a few different designs, which therapeutically speaking is not that important, and they make up the second and third generation of this technology.

## FOCUSED ASSESSMENT

1. Assess for signs of bleeding:
   - a. Assess for: hypotension, neuro impairment, nosebleed, GI bleed
   - b. Any overt bleeding can lead to a drop in preload. Patients with left ventricular assist devices are dependent on adequate preload in order to maintain proper function.
2. Assess for signs of infection:
   - a. Assess for: fever, hypertension, hemorrhage from the exit point of implanted tubes/ wires, and history of infection
   - b. Fever can indicate sepsis which can lead to a lowering blood pressure (which means the preload is also reduced). Protect preload. VADs love them some preload.
3. Assess for Right Ventricular Dysfunction:
   - a. Assess for: edema, jaundice, and ascites.
   - b. Preload is important because it helps to establish the atrial kick as well as Starling's Law, which both increase ventricular stroke volume.
   - c. Right ventricular dysfunction means we may need to add more preload, meaning isotonic fluids.
4. Assess for Suckdown:
   - a. Assess for: hypotension, PVCs, ventricular tachycardia, or knocking sounds heard when the device is auscultated.
   - b. Because the device is pulling blood from the left ventricle to push into the aorta, it can collapse the left ventricle if hypovolemia is present or if the VAD is in overdrive: when the left ventricle collapses, it is known as suckdown.
5. Assess for Device Failure or Malfunction:
   - a. Determine if the device is operating properly (no alarms).
   - b. If alarming, read control panel for instructions.
   - c. Assess for signs of hypotension and hypoperfusion.
6. Assess for Arrhythmias:
   - a. Determine the patient's cardiac rhythm.
   - b. Determine if the patient's hemodynamics are stable or unstable.
     - i. Stable: even with a lethal arrhythmia, the patient is awake and alert and not showing signs of hypoperfusion or hypotension.
     - ii. Unstable: with a lethal arrhythmia, the patient has mental status changes, signs of hypoperfusion, and or signs of hypotension.
   - c. It is very important to consider the stability/ instability of a patient with an arrhythmia, or even a lethal arrhythmia because delivering electricity to a stable patient can damage the machine and hurt the patient.

## FIELD MANAGEMENT

1. Manage airway and breathing as appropriate.
2. Remember that all VADs need adequate preload in order to pump efficiently.
3. IV access should be initiated on every VAD patient.
4. Volume with isotonic crystalloid in an unstable VAD patient is the first line therapy.
5. Do not administer nitrates unless instructed by the sending physician, or unless ordered to do so by the implanting center's VAD coordinator.
6. Assess for other non- VAD related injuries and illnesses.
7. UNSTABLE: Cardiovert or defibrillate the patient only if they are UNSTABLE. VAD patients may have a lethal arrhythmia but be completely stable. Allow signs of hypoperfusion and patient's mentation to guide your definition of "stable". If they are awake with warm/ pink skin, capillary refill < 2 seconds, you're likely fine.
8. Identify the patient's resources:

a. Locate the phone number for the implanting centers VAD coordinator.
b. Listen to family members, because they are likely also trained on how to manage the device.
c. Look for manuals and quick guides in the patient's equipment bag to bring with you.

9. Consider allowing the patient's caregiver to remain with the patient if possible. They could be a great service, as well as calm the patient if the patient is awake.

10. Transport all VAD equipment with the patient, including equipment, cords, and manuals. Package them as securely as possible to prevent dislodgement.

11. Transport to a VAD implanting center when possible, because they are trained and equipped to handle VAD patients.

12. DO NOT INITIATE CPR, unless instructed by the implanting centers VAD Coordinator or physician.

# PART 10: CARDIAC MANAGEMENT QUESTIONS

1. When assessing your cardiac patient, you assess heart tones. You recall the "lub " sound is equivalent to which of the following:
   a. Closure of the AV valve
   b. The P wave on the ECG
   c. The aortic valve opening
   d. Isovolumetric relaxation

2. As blood flow though the heart continues, pressure changes occur. Once there is greater pressure in the aorta and pulmonary artery, the semilunar valves close. Which of the following sounds does this closure represent?
   a. S2
   b. S1
   c. S4
   d. S3

3. Preload, afterload and contractility are all components that can influence which of the following?
   a. PA pressures
   b. Cardiac output
   c. Stroke volume
   d. Systolic pressure

4. Your adult cardiac patient has a pulmonary artery (PA) cath in place. You receive the following information: BP 92/52 mmHg, CO 3 L/min, and the PA temperature is 98 degrees F. Which of the following is dangerous?
   a. All are normal
   b. Blood pressure
   c. PA temperature
   d. Cardiac output

5.  Which of the following patients appear  hemodynamically compromised?
    a.  57 y/o cardiac patient who has a CO 4.2 L/min
    b.  22 y/o trauma patient who has a CO 3.1 L/min
    c.  3 m/o infant with a cardiac output of 0.9L/min
    d.  4 y/o asthmatic patient who has a  CO 2.5 L/min

6.  Your patient suddenly becomes bradycardic. You understand that this lower heart rate will result in which of the following?
    a.  CO is reduced
    b.  CO is elevated
    c.  SV is reduced
    d.  SV is elevated

7.  Upon looking at your patient's hemodynamic parameters, you notice a very high afterload which you suspect is preventing adequate ventricular emptying. Which of the following is the best general treatment plan?
    a.  Administer a vasopressor
    b.  Administer a vasodilator
    c.  Administer isotonic fluids
    d.  Administer beta blockers

8.  You are transporting a patient who is complaining of chest pain. Currently, the patient has the following ECG findings: lead I and aVL are positive; lead II is isoelectric; and lead III, aVF, and aVR are negative. Which of the following conditions is the patient most likely suffering from?
    a.  Coronary artery block
    b.  Anteroseptal AMI
    c.  Aortic dissection
    d.  Left axis deviation

9.  Your patient has an upright deflection in aVF and a downward deflection in Lead I. With this information, you know that there is also most likely which if the following?
    a.  Myocardial ischemia
    b.  First-degree heart block
    c.  Posterior hemiblock
    d.  Anterior hemiblock

10. While assessing your adult chest pain patient, you note the morphology of the QRS waveform in V1. Which of the following indicates a bundle branch block?
    a.  QRS complex spanning 4 small boxes
    b.  ST depression with a positive QRS
    c.  A short and flat hyper acute T wave
    d.  Presence of a U-wave after the T wave

11. You have a patient with a wide QRS waveform (150ms). A retrograde (reverse direction) upward deflection from the J point in V1 on a 12 lead ECG. Which of the following is present?
    a. Right bundle branch block
    b. Left bundle branch block
    c. Present left axis deviation
    d. Present right axis deviation

12. Your patient exhibits the following ECG findings: ST segment elevation in lead I, II, III, aVL, and aVF, as well as a PR segment that is below the isoelectric line. Which of the following is the patient most likely experiencing?
    a. Aortic dissection
    b. An anterior AMI
    c. Acute pericarditis
    d. Cardiomyopathy

13. While assessing your cardiac patient, you notice a morphology that exhibits the "ladle effect". Because of this, your patient is most likely suffering which of the following?
    a. Hyperkalemia
    b. Digitalis toxicity
    c. Hypokalemia
    d. Mag toxicity

14. Your patient has tall peaked T- waves. With this 12- lead feature, what would you most likely expect to find with this patient?
    a. Hypocalcemia
    b. Potassium of 7 mEq/L.
    c. Digitalis toxicity
    d. Chloride of 99 mmol/L

15. When assessing a patient for WPW, which of the following findings would indicate WPW is present?
    a. Shortened PR and lengthened QRS
    b. Shortened QRS and lengthened PR
    c. Depressed ST segment and short PR
    d. Long PR and elevated ST segment

16. On a 12 lead ECG, you identify the following features: QRS notching and ST elevation. Which of the following assessments is most likely correct?
    a. STEMI
    b. Endocarditis
    c. Cardiac contusion
    d. Pericarditis

17. You are assessing a 12 lead ECG. You identify the following: PR interval of 90 milliseconds, QRS < 120 milliseconds, a Q wave that is 2/3 the height of the R wave, and no notching. Which of the following assessments is most likely correct?
    a.  Pericarditis is currently present
    b.  Acute MI is in progression
    c.  Pathological Q wave present
    d.  Osborne wave present currently

18. You are assessing a 12 lead ECG, and you notice a narrow QRS (< 120 milliseconds), an M-shaped P wave in lead II, Q wave < 1/3 the R wave height, and no ST elevation. Which of the following is most likely the current condition?
    a.  Right atrial enlargement
    b.  Silent AMI is occurring
    c.  P mitrale is present
    d.  Diseased tricuspid valve

19. You observe tall peaked P waves on your ECG tracing. This is caused by which of the following:
    a.  Massive hyperkalemia
    b.  Increased cardiac output
    c.  Reduced SVR and CVP
    d.  High right atrial pressures

20. Which of the following are criteria indicating biatrial enlargement?
    a.  Evidence of P pulmonale and biphasic P wave in V1
    b.  Evidence of P mitrale and biphasic T waves in V3
    c.  Biphasic T waves in V3 with profound QRS notching
    d.  Monophonic T waves in V1 and a delta wave in lead I

21. You are assessing a QRS complex for left ventricular hypertrophy. Which of the following would indicate LVH is present?
    a.  V2 S wave and V6 R wave together is 37 mm
    b.  V4 S wave and V5 R wave together is 41 mm
    c.  V5 S wave and V2 R wave together is 25 mm
    d.  V1 S wave and V5 R wave together is 30 mm

22. You are assessing a QRS complex for left ventricular hypertrophy. Which of the following would indicate LVH is present?
    a.  aVR R wave is 10 mm
    b.  aVL R wave is 12 mm
    c.  aVR S wave is 11 mm
    d.  aVL S wave is 15 mm

23. Your 24 y/o patient is experiencing sudden onset of shortness of breath. You observe the following findings: HR 22, BP102/70, SpO2 88%, an S wave in V1 of 10mm and R wave in V1 of 20 mm. Which of the following condition is most likely present?
    a. Congestive heart failure
    b. Status asthmaticus
    c. Myocardial infarction
    d. Pulmonary contusion

24. While assessing your AMI patient you notice ST segment elevation without hyperacute T waves and without pathological Q waves. Which phase of AMI progression is the patient currently in?
    a. Acute phase I
    b. Acute phase II
    c. Hyperacute T waves
    d. Age indeterminate

25. As you assess a patient with sudden onset chest pain, you do not observe any ST elevation. Instead you see a large, deep Q wave. There is evidence of elevated cardiac enzymes. Which phase of AMI progression is the patient currently in?
    a. Hyperacute T waves
    b. Acute phase I
    c. Acute phase II
    d. Age indeterminate

26. Your chest pain patient has the following 12 lead findings: ST depression in I and aVL, with ST elevation in leads II, III, and aVF. Which coronary artery is most likely occluded?
    a. Left circumflex artery
    b. Left coronary artery
    c. Right coronary artery
    d. Right circumflex artery

27. Your chest pain patient has the following 12 lead findings: ST depression in V8 and V9, with ST elevation in V3 and V4. Which coronary artery is the one most likely occluded?
    a. Right circumflex artery
    b. Right coronary artery
    c. Left circumflex artery
    d. Left anterior descending

28. Your chest pain patient has the following 12 lead findings: ST elevation in V5 and V6. Which coronary artery is most likely occluded?
    a. Right coronary artery
    b. Left anterior descending
    c. Left coronary artery
    d. The circumflex artery

29. Your chest pain patient has the following 12 lead findings: ST elevation in V5, V6, and lead I. Which coronary artery is most likely occluded?
    a.   Left circumflex artery
    b.   Left anterior descending
    c.   Right coronary artery
    d.   Right circumflex artery

30. If you assess a patient for chest pain and the 12 lead ECG reflects a left bundle branch block, which of the following diagnostic tools could be used to confirm an acute myocardial infarction?
    a.   Sgarbossa criteria
    b.   S to R wave ratio
    c.   Hyperacute T waves
    d.   Osborne waves in V1

31. You are assessing for an AMI in your patient. You notice in V6 ST elevation of 1 mm in height with a positive QRS, and ST depression in V3 of 2 mm with a negative QRS complex. How many points does this earn when the Sgarbossa criteria is applied?
    a.   4 points
    b.   6 points
    c.   8 points
    d.   2 points

32. Which of the following hemodynamic values are within their normal limits?
    a.   SVR of 33
    b.   CVP of 5
    c.   PCWP 22
    d.   CO of 18

33. Which of the following hemodynamic values are within their normal limits?
    a.   CO of 10
    b.   CVP of 15
    c.   SVR of 8
    d.   PCWP 5

34. Which of the following hemodynamic values are within their normal limits?
    a.   Systolic PAP 60
    b.   Diastolic RVP 12
    c.   Systolic RVP 27
    d.   Diastolic PAP 20

35. Which of the following hemodynamic values are within their normal limits?
    a. Systolic RVP 15
    b. Diastolic PAP 6
    c. Diastolic RVP 10
    d. Systolic PAP 10

36. Your patient presents with the following vitals and lab findings: BP 152/98, SpO2 96, CVP 5, PCWP 7, CO 7, and 1500 for SVR. Which of these parameters is MOST concerning?
    a. SVR 1500
    b. PCWP 7
    c. CVP of 5
    d. SpO2 96

37. Your patient currently presents with the following: HR 89, SpO2 88, BP 144/99, CVP 12, PCWP 10, CO 8, and 900 for SVR. Which of the following would you most likely assess in this patient?
    a. Wet lungs
    b. Wet system
    c. Dry PA
    d. Dry RVP

38. As you assess your medical patient, you observe the following: HR 118, SpO2 87, BP 78/50, CVP 2, PCWP 3, CO 4, and 1650 for SVR. What type of shock is this patient exhibiting?
    a. Cardiogenic
    b. Septic shock
    c. Distributive
    d. Hypovolemic

39. A patient presents to the ER after 3 days status post abdominal surgery he is diaphoretic, with malaise, and slightly short of breath. The patient has the following vitals and findings: HR 122, SpO2 96, BP 110/78, CVP 5, PCWP 5, CO 12, and 600 for SVR. What type of shock is this patient exhibiting?
    a. Cardiogenic
    b. Septic shock
    c. Hypovolemic
    d. Neurogenic

40. You note the following hemodynamic parameters on your patient's chart: CVP 10, PCWP 18, CO 3, and 1200 for SVR. What type of shock is this patient exhibiting?
    a. Anaphylactic
    b. Septic shock
    c. Cardiogenic
    d. Neurogenic

41. Your patient has been in a car crash and exhibits multi- system trauma, including crepitus to the back of the neck. Additionally, there is a line of demarcation at the level of the xyphoid (red skin below this level). Which of the following treatments should this patient likely receive?
    a. Provide NS, inotropes, and vasodilators
    b. Withhold fluids as well as vasopressors
    c. Administer volume and increase the SVR
    d. Deliver fluid boluses only- no vasopressor

42. Upon reviewing your IABP patient's AP chest X-ray, you notice the tip of the IABP balloon is observed at the 5th intercostal space. The critical care transport clinician understands that:
    a. This positioning is too low
    b. This positioning is too high
    c. The position is close enough
    d. The position doesn't matter

43. Examine the following IABP tracing, then choose the appropriate assessment of this tracing.

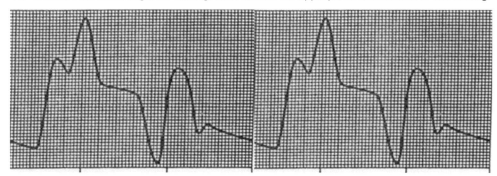

    a. Late deflation
    b. Late inflation
    c. Early deflation
    d. Early inflation

44. Examine the following IABP tracing, then choose the appropriate assessment of this tracing.

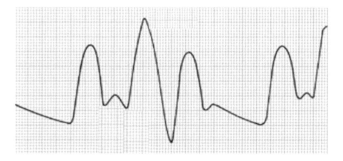

    a. Early deflation
    b. Late inflation
    c. Late deflation
    d. Early inflation

45. Examine the following IABP tracing, then choose the appropriate assessment of this tracing.

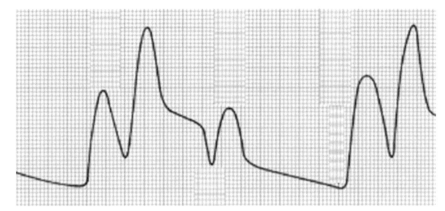

   a.  Late deflation
   b.  Early inflation
   c.  Late inflation
   d.  Early deflation

46. Examine the following IABP tracing, then choose the appropriate assessment of this tracing.

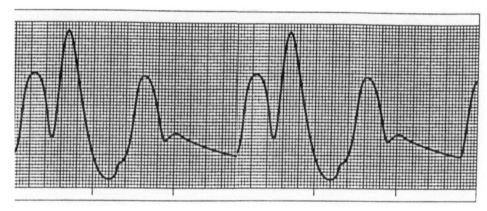

   a.  Early inflation
   b.  Late deflation
   c.  Early deflation
   d.  Late inflation

47. Examine the following hemodynamic pressure monitor tracing, and then choose the appropriate assessment of this tracing.

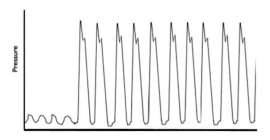

a. A superwedge is currently progressing
b. LV is throwing runs of ventricular tach
c. PA catheter has migrated to the RV
d. A retrograde PA cath movement

48. While reading up on cardiac pathophysiology, you recall that an infarction affecting the lateral wall of the heart means there was a blockage to which coronary artery?
    a. Right coronary artery
    b. Left coronary artery
    c. Left circumflex
    d. Posterior coronary artery

49. While discussing pathophysiology with a colleague, you recall that an infarction affecting the septal wall of the heart means there was a blockage to which coronary artery?
    a. RAD
    b. RCA
    c. LCA
    d. LCx

50. You are orientating a new employee, and they ask about a specific condition characterized by serum being forced into the alveoli from back pressure and produces a foamy liquid which prevents adequate ventilation. Which of the following best identifies this pathophysiology?
    a. Congestive heart failure
    b. Right-sided heart failure
    c. Left-sided heart failure
    d. Chronic heart failure

51. An internet blog site is discussing a cardiac condition caused by injury to the heart resulting in fluid accumulation under the pericardium which results in increasingly worsening cardiac output. What condition is this blog describing?
    a. Cardiogenic shock
    b. Congestive heart failure
    c. Cardiac tamponade
    d. Cardiomyopathy

52. A student asks you to summarize what happens in cardiogenic shock. Which of the following would best answer the student's question?
    a. Weakened pump, poor tissue perfusion, global acidosis
    b. Weakened pump, cardiac tamponade, global acidosis
    c. Weakened arterial walls, poor tissue perfusion, dysrhythmias
    d. Weakened arterial walls, cardiac tamponade, global edema

53. You are transporting a patient having an anterior myocardial infarction. Which of the following constitute the best pharmacological choices?
    a. Aspirin, nitro, heparin, warfarin
    b. Aspirin, nitro, heparin, beta blockers
    c. Nitro, heparin, beta blockers, AV shunt
    d. Nitro, high molecular weight heparin

54. The sending MD lets you know that you have a patient with an aortic dissection. You recall the treatment for this includes:
    a. Keep BP >120mmHg systolic, vasodilators first THEN negative inotropes if needed
    b. Keep BP >120mmHg systolic, negative inotropes first THEN vasodilators if needed
    c. Keep BP <120mmHg systolic, vasodilators first THEN negative inotropes if needed
    d. Keep BP <120mmHg systolic, negative inotropes first THEN vasodilators if needed

55. On your way to a dilated cardiomyopathy patient, you recall the treatment for this condition is which of the following?
    a. Copious fluid resuscitation
    b. Palliative care only
    c. Same as with heart failure
    d. Vasopressors are a must

56. Your partner brings up cardiac tamponade. You recall that the two common causes of this include which of the following?
    a. Pericarditis and chest trauma
    b. Chest trauma and pneumonia
    c. Pneumonia and cardiogenic shock
    d. Pericarditis and cardiogenic shock

57. Examine these fishbone labs and identify the value that is out of range:

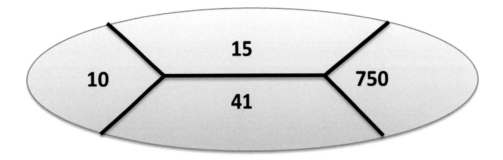

    a. Platelets
    b. The WBCs
    c. Hematocrit
    d. Hemoglobin

58. Examine these fishbone labs and identify the value that is out of range:

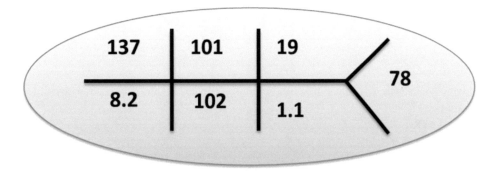

    a.    Serum BUN
    b.    Creatinine
    c.    Serum K+
    d.    Bicarbonate

59. Examine these fishbone labs and identify the value that is most out of range.

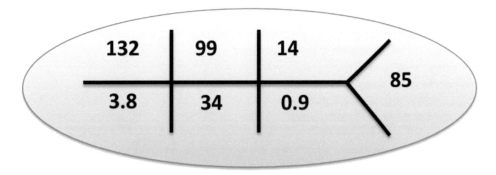

    a.    The chloride
    b.    Bicarbonate
    c.    Potassium
    d.    The glucose

60. You administer a medication that you know stimulates the alpha 1 and beta 1 receptors. What physiological changes would you anticipate following the administration of such a medication?
    a.    Increased BP and slower AV conduction
    b.    Bronchoconstriction with bradycardia
    c.    Lowering blood pressure and tachycardia
    d.    Vasoconstriction and increasing HR

61. Hemodynamically, what do you expect middle dose dopamine to do to your patient's hemodynamic parameters?
    a.  ↑ HR
    b.  ↓ PVR
    c.  ↑ SVR
    d.  ↓ CO


62. Hemodynamically, what do you expect dobutamine to do to your patient's hemodynamic parameters?
    a.  ↓ SVR
    b.  ↑ PCWP
    c.  ↑CVP
    d.  ↓ CO


63. Your elderly patient currently has the following hemodynamic profile: CVP 12, PCWP 15, CO 4, and 1175 for SVR. Which of the following medications would best treat this patient?
    a.  LMW Heparin
    b.  Nitroglycerin
    c.  Metoprolol
    d.  Integrillin


64. You administer levophed to a critical patient. What are the expected physiologic changes following the administration of this medication?
    a.  Reduced BP and increased HR
    b.  Reduced vasoconstriction and HR
    c.  Elevated HR and vasodilation
    d.  Slightly ↑ HR and blood pressure


65. A patient's vital signs are pulse 80, respirations 24, and BP of 124/60 mm Hg and cardiac output is 4.8 L/min. What is the patient's stroke volume?
    a.  80 mL
    b.  40 mL
    c.  120 mL
    d.  60 mL


66. The critical care transport clinician is caring for a patient receiving a continuous norepinephrine (Levophed) IV infusion. Which patient assessment information indicates that the infusion rate may be too high and that a second pressor may be warranted?
    a.  SVR
    b.  CO
    c.  PCWP
    d.  CVP

67. An intraaortic balloon pump (IABP) is being used for a patient who is in cardiogenic shock. An assessment finding indicating to the critical care transport clinician that the goals of treatment with the IABP are being met is a:
    a. SVR 550
    b. CO of 5
    c. PCWP 6
    d. CVP 15


68. When monitoring for the effectiveness of treatment for a patient with left ventricular failure, the most important information for the critical care transport clinician to obtain is which of the following:
    a. SV waveform
    b. CVP tracing
    c. PA waveform
    d. PCWP tracing


69. Following surgery, a patient's central venous pressure (CVP) monitor indicates low pressures. Which action will the critical care transport clinician anticipate taking?
    a. Increase the IV fluid infusion rate
    b. Administer the pressor levophed
    c. Begin a nitroglycerine infusion
    d. Start the vasopressor dobutamine


70. When evaluating an IABP waveform strip, you notice a characteristic 'double V' pattern. You quickly recognize this timing pattern as which of the following?
    a. Early deflation
    b. Late deflation
    c. Early inflation
    d. Late inflation


71. Your patient began having shortness of breath and chest pain over the last 2 hours. The patient reports that he is a CHF patient for 10 years with multiple stents placed in his heart, he has a pacer and has been hospitalized twice in the last decade for his cardiac conditions. Examine the ECG tracing below. Which of the following is the patient most likely experiencing?

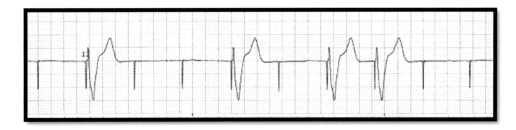

    a. The pointy P waves indicate p- pulmonale
    b. Hypoxia is present and will soon exacerbate

    c.    Failure of the ventricular pole to capture

    d.    There is a left bundle branch block present

72. Your LVAD patient doesn't have a pulse at any pulse site. The patient is calm, awake, and answering all questions. What kind of VAD does the patient have?
    a.    Pulsatile Flow
    b.    Continuous Flow
    c.    Pneumatic Flow
    d.    Asynchronous Flow

73. You are treating a patient involved in a MVC with massive external damage. The patient is a VAD patient and currently presents with the following: awake and alert, in pain, open clear airway, with a HR of 0, BP of 0, RR 22/min, SpO2 91%, EtCO2 44, skin cool and pink, with good capillary refill (< 2 seconds), however ventricular fibrillation is on the monitor. What is the next most appropriate action?
    a.    Supportive care
    b.    Defibrillation
    c.    Cardioversion
    d.    Precordial Thump

74. Look at the 12- lead below and identify which wall of the myocardium is affected.

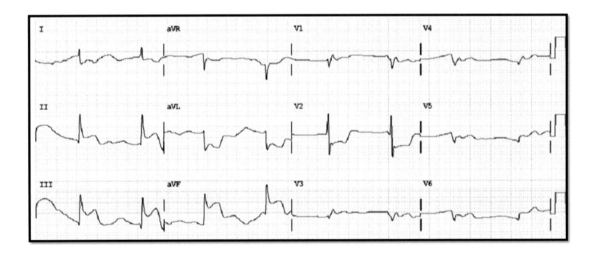

    a.    Septal wall AMI
    b.    Lateral wall AMI
    c.    Anterior wall AMI
    d.    Inferior wall AMI

75. Look at the 12- lead below and identify which wall of the myocardium is affected.

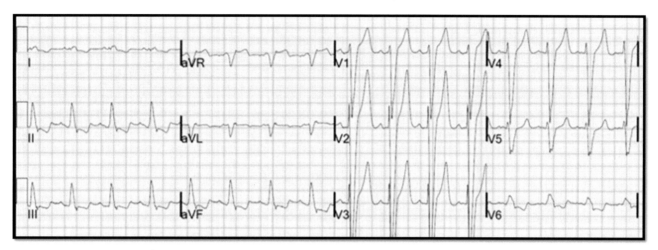

    a.   Inferolateral wall AMI
    b.   High lateral wall AMI
    c.   Anteroseptal wall AMI
    d.   Inferioseptal wall AMI

76. Look at the 12- lead below and identify which wall of the myocardium is affected.

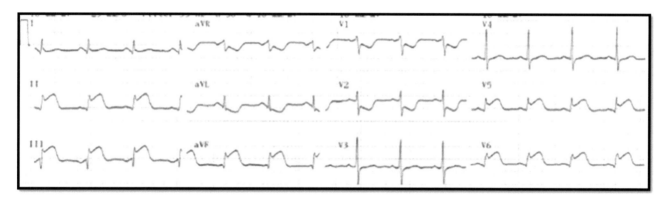

    a.   Inferior wall AMI
    b.   Inferolateral wall AMI
    c.   Anteroseptal wall AMI
    d.   Posterior wall AMI

# PART 11: CARDIAC MANAGEMENT RATIONALES

1. **(A)** Understanding the components of the cardiac cycle is imperative for these certification exams. When the AV valve closes, it makes a dull 'thump' sound that we recognize as the "lub" sound, also known as the S1 heart tone. "Lub-Dub" is equivalent to the S1 and S2 respectively.

2. **(A)** Understanding the components of the cardiac cycle is imperative for these certification exams. When the AV valve closes, it makes a dull 'thump' sound that we recognize as the "lub" sound, also known as the S1 heart tone. When the semilunar valves close (the pulmonic and aortic valves), then the "dub" sound is generated. Lub-Dub is equivalent to the S1 and S2 respectively. S3 and S4 are extra sounds caused by various conditions. S3 occurs with S1 and S2, but the way that it is generated it presents with an S1, followed by S2 and S3 that are very close together. This makes the KEN----tuck-y sound that is mentioned in this literature. This indicates heart failure or volume overload. The S4 sound is heard BEFORE S1 and progresses as follows: S4 and S1 very close together, a short pause, and then the S2 sound. This gives the characteristic pattern like saying the word: TEN-NES----ee. This occurs from forcing blood into a failing or hypertrophic left heart.

3. **(B)** Cardiac output is defined by the equation CO = HR x SV, where stroke volume (SV) is determined by the preload, afterload, and contractility.

4. **(D)** It is important to know ALL the value ranges for the various cardiac parameters. In this case, you are asked to know the ranges for core body temperature (which is 98.6 degrees), cardiac output (which is 4-8 L/min), and blood pressure (which is typically perfusing when above 90 systolic, or above 60 mmHg of MAP- which is 65 mmHg in this case). The only one that seems dangerous is the low cardiac output because 3 L/min for an adult is low- that patient is dry as can be. Fluid, fluid, fluid. The temperature is 0.6°F low, but that isn't enough to call it 'dangerous'.

5. **(B)** It is important to know ALL the value ranges for the various cardiac parameters. In this case, you need to know not only the normal range of cardiac output, but you need to know the cardiac output for each of the major age ranges: adult, pediatric, and infant. Adult is 4-8 L/min, pediatric is 1-3 L/min, and an infant is 0.8-1 L/min. The only patient in the question that is exhibiting abnormal hemodynamics is the 22 y/o trauma patient. Trauma patients' mortality drastically increase with a single episode of hypotension- this 22 y/o has a low cardiac output, suggesting he needs lots of fluids and/or blood products.

6. **(A)** To answer this question, you need to understand how cardiac output is affected by heart rate and by stroke volume. CO= HR x SV, so any increase in HR or stroke volume will INCREASE cardiac output. Therefore, any decrease in HR or SV will DECREASE cardiac output. We know that bradycardia is a HR less than 60, therefore, the patient experienced a drop in cardiac output.

7. **(B)** To answer this question, you need to know what afterload is and what treatments affect it. Afterload represents the pressure the heart must pump against to eject blood into the aorta (left ventricle) and lungs (right ventricle). It is measured as the SVR (systemic vascular resistance). If SVR is normal, then there isn't excess pressure the heart has to pump against. If SVR is low, then it is very easy for the ventricles to pump blood out of the heart. If SVR is high, then there is an awful lot of excess pressure the ventricles must overcome in order to pump blood. Medications like **vasodilators** will dilate the arterial system, and thus reduce the SVR- which is the answer. Administering vasopressors will increase SVR- bad in this case. Adding fluid could also worsen this issue and ultimately will not fix the issue. Beta blockers would reduce cardiac output but won't directly affect the afterload. The best choice here is to

administer a vasodilator to reduce SVR and thus making it easier for the heart to pump (which also directly decreases myocardial oxygen demand).

8.  **(D)** This is testing your knowledge on axis deviation. You'll need to know how to identify axis deviation. Normal is lead I and aVF are positive. Left axis deviation (physiologic) is where lead I is positive, and aVF is negative, and pathologic left axis deviation is where lead I is positive, Lead II is negative, and aVF is negative. Right axis is where lead I is negative, and aVF is positive. Extreme axis deviation is where both lead I and aVF are both negative.

9.  **(C)** This patient has a right axis deviation (negative waveform in lead I and a negative waveform in aVF). A right axis deviation also means there is a conduction block of the left posterior hemifasicle, or also known as posterior hemiblock. To be able to answer this question, you'll have to be able to know the criteria for axis deviation. Normal is lead I and aVF are positive. Left axis deviation (physiologic) is where lead I is positive, and aVF is negative, and pathologic left axis deviation is where lead I is positive, Lead II is negative, and aVF is negative. Right axis is where lead I is negative and aVF is positive. Extreme axis deviation is where both lead I and aVF are both negative.

10. **(A)** To answer this question, you'll have to be able to identify the criteria of a bundle branch block. The main criteria taught in this text includes a prolonged QRS waveform. Prolonged QRS is defined as greater than 120ms, or longer than 3 small ECG boxes. In this case, the answer of 4 small QRS boxes is correct because that means that the impulse takes 160ms to get through the conductive tissue (40ms per small box). It is important to be able to describe the same concept in different ways, such as here, where 120ms equals 3 small boxes.

11. **(A)** To answer this question, you'll need to know how to identify left and right bundle branches. Left bundle branch blocks can be identified by a wide QRS complex (> 120ms) and a downward deflection from the J point (retrograde in direction) on a 12 lead ECG. Right bundle branch blocks can be identified by a wide QRS complex (> 120ms) and an upward deflection from the J point (retrograde in direction) on a 12 lead ECG.

12. **(C)** You need to be able to identify pericarditis to be able to answer this question. Pericarditis presents with global ST elevation (exhibited here with ST elevation in lead I, II, III, aVL, and aVF), PR depression (exhibited here as PR segment below the isoelectric line), notching of the QRS, and a scooping and upward concave ST segment.

13. **(B)** To answer this question, you'll need to know the morphology of digitalis toxicity. It presents with a "ladle effect" or mustache sign which looks like a concave ST segment to the right of the QRS complex. This is specific to digitalis toxicity.

14. **(B)** High and peaked T-waves occur clinically with a K+ of typically 5.5 or above. Digitalis toxicity presents with the ladle effect morphology. Hypocalcemia essentially has benign 12 lead morphology. The correct answer is a potassium of 5.5.

15. **(A)** WPW presents with a delta wave, which is identified by a shortened PR segment (from a re-entry pathway) which then creates a delta shape and a lengthy QRS. The two factors that identifies the delta wave is the short PR segment (< 120 milliseconds) and a long QRS (or at least not a short one) at < 100 milliseconds.

16. **(D)** Notching with ST elevation is most likely 100% NOT an acute MI, therefore, the 'AMI is absent' answer selection is the correct answer.

17. **(C)** A Q wave that is either greater than 1/3 the height of the R wave or > 0.03 of a second (or 30 milliseconds) is indicative of a pathological q wave, therefore, this is the correct answer.

18. **(C)** An M- shaped P wave indicates left atrial enlargement. This is commonly caused by a diseased mitral valve. Therefore, answer choices right atrial enlargement and diseased tricuspid valve is incorrect. This also doesn't meet the criteria for a silent AMI. P mitrale is also known as left atrial enlargement- therefore this is the correct answer.

19. **(D)** Tall peaked P waves are an indication of right atrial enlargement, which is typically caused by high right atrial pressures. Increased Q wouldn't cause RAE, and neither would reduce q, reduced CVP, nor hyperkalemia. If you choose hyperkalemia, remember that hyperkalemia causes peaked T-waves, not peaked P waves.

20. **(A)** To identify a biatrial enlargement, you need to identify a biphasic p wave in V1 as well as either p- mitrale (M- shaped P wave) or P- pulmonale (tall peaked P wave). This needs to be committed to memory.

21. **(A)** For LVH to be present, there are multiple criteria. This question presents answers referring to the Deep/ tall criteria. If the deepest S wave (V1 or V2) plus the tallest R wave (in V5 or V6) is 35 mm high it higher, then LVH is present. In this question only one answer matches this criteria is the answer: V2 S wave and V6 R wave together is 37 mm. Remember, it's S depth in V1 or V2 PLUS the R height in V5 or V6; if it's > 35 mm high then LVH is present.

22. **(B)** For LVH to be present, there are multiple criteria. This question presents answers referring to the aVL criteria. Under these criteria, if the aVL R wave must be larger than 11mm then LVH is present. In this question the correct answer is the only one meeting these criteria: aVL R wave is 12 mm.

23. **(D)** To answer this question, you need to understand what information the question is offering you. SUDDEN onset of shortness of should put PE on your radar. The S/ R wave data should prompt you to investigate for LVH or RVH. Any time R and S wave heights are provided, apply your hypertrophy criteria to identify if hypertrophy is present. Then recall what common causes of these hypertrophies are. In this case, RVH is present (because in V1 the R wave is bigger than the S wave). RVH is caused by anything that prevents blood flow through the lungs- resulting in back pressure. Contused lungs would swell and reduce blood flow through them, thus increasing the pressures in the right side of the heart, and boom- RVH. Congestive heart failure is close, but the onset probably wouldn't be sudden-it would probably be gradual. Asthmaticus is more an airway issue, instead of vascular.

24. **(A)** The typical ST elevation MI (or STEMI) involves ST elevation changes. These changes occur in a pattern as the MI runs its course. In the acute phase I progression phase, the key feature is an elevated ST segment. The key feature of hyperacute T-waves is: hyperacute T waves (shocker). With possible ST depression. The key feature in the acute phase II progression phase is the introduction of pathological Q waves and residual ST segment elevation (residual ST segment elevation from acute phase I). The Age Indeterminate phase of MI progression, the key feature is a pathological Q wave WITHOUT any ST elevation. Therefore, the correct answer selection for this question is acute phase I- because there is no mentioning of a pathological Q wave.

25. **(D)** This question is illustrating an age indeterminate phase of an AMI. Pathological Q waves indicate a previous AMI (meaning the patient is predisposed to it). In the acute phase I progression phase, the key feature is an elevated ST segment. The key feature of hyperacute T waves is: hyperacute T waves (shocker) with possible ST depression. The key feature of the acute phase II progression phase is the introduction of pathological Q waves and residual ST segment elevation (residual ST segment elevation from acute phase I). The Age indeterminate phase of MI progression, the key feature is a pathological Q wave WITHOUT any ST elevation. Therefore, the correct answer selection for this question is age indeterminate- since there is only a pathologic Q waves observed in the presence of chest pain and elevated cardiac enzymes.

26. **(C)** The ECG ST elevation pattern (elevation in leads II, III, and aVF with possible ST depression in leads I and aVL) in this question is specific to an inferior wall AMI. These AMIs occur mostly from a blockage of the right coronary artery.

27. **(D)** The ECG ST elevation pattern (elevation in V3 and V4 with possible ST depression in V8 and V9) in this question is specific to an anterior wall AMI. These AMIs occur mostly from a blockage of the left anterior descending artery.

28. **(B)** The ECG ST elevation pattern (elevation in V1 and V2) in this question is specific to a septal wall AMI. These AMIs occur mostly from a blockage of the left anterior descending artery.

29. **(A)** The ECG ST elevation pattern (V5, V6, aVL and lead I) in this question is specific to a lateral/ high lateral wall AMI. These AMIs occur mostly from a blockage of the left anterior descending artery and left circumflex arteries.

30. **(A)** The Sgarbossa criteria is a method of assessing chest pain patients with left bundle branch blocks (LBBBs) for an active AMI.

31. **(C)** Earning 5 points from criteria 1 (upright QRS and 1 mm ST segment elevation in V6-concordance) and 3 points from criteria 2 (negative QRS in V3 with ST segment depression- also concordance) yields 8 points.

32. **(B)** Normally, CVP is 2-8 mmHg, SVR is 800-1300 dynes/sec/cm^3, PCWP is 4-12 mmHg, and CO is normally 4-8 L/min. Therefore, the only one in its normal range, in this case, is the CVP of 5.

33. **(D)** Normally, CVP is 2-8 mmHg, SVR is 800-1300 dynes/sec/cm^3, PCWP is 4-12 mmHg, and CO is normally 4-8 L/min. Therefore, the only one in its normal range, in this case, is the PCWP of 5.

34. **(C)** Normally, systolic RVP is 25-30 mmHg, diastolic RVP is 0-5 mmHg, systolic PAP is 15-30 mmHg, and diastolic PAP is 5-10 mmHg. Therefore, the only answer selection here that is within normal limits is the systolic RVP of 27.

35. **(B)** Normally, systolic RVP is 25-30 mmHg, diastolic RVP is 0-5 mmHg, systolic PAP is 15-30 mmHg, and diastolic PAP is 5-10 mmHg. Therefore, the only answer selection here that is within normal limits is the diastolic PAP of 6.

36. **(A)** The BP is out of normal limits but is not an answer selection. The only other number out of range, and concerning, is the SVR. Normal SVR is 800- 1200 dynes/sec/cm^3. At 1500, there is some serious AFTERLOAD happening (very high). This means the heart must work extra hard to push blood out of the left ventricle against the high pressures (from afterload). While there isn't much context in this question, this gets me thinking of a heart failure patient of some kind. We'd need to consider a vasodilator to reduce SVR and make it easier for the heart to pump blood into the aorta.

37. **(B)** In this patient, there is a high CVP, which directly indicates a WET SYSTEM. Heart failure (right side issues in this case) prevents easy, forward flow, thus, a back pressure occurs from the right side of the heart. The left heart is not affected (normal PCWP), therefore, the lungs are dry in this case. High CVP means wet system and a high PCWP means wet lungs.

38. **(D)** Hypovolemic shock presents with low CVP and PCWP, normal or low CO, but for sure presents with high SVR- so most everything is low, or low side of normal, and SVR is high. Here CVP, PCWP are both low with the CO on the low side of normal, while the SVR is extremely high, representing HYPOVOLEMIC shock.

39. **(B)** High CO and low SVR with the other hemodynamic parameters mostly normal, is difficult to diagnose confidently. However, if there is evidence of fever/ shock, then the diagnosis becomes clear. Here, the patient returns 3 days after surgery diaphoretic (probably because they are warm/hot with fever), which suggests sepsis by itself, but add it to the high cardiac output with a low SVR, it's a dead giveaway for septic shock. Remember, high temp and CO with low SVR are strongly suggestive of septic shock.

40. **(C)** All the hemodynamic parameters are all high except one: **cardiac output**. This is very telling for cardiogenic shock. It makes sense too, right? The heart is damaged, so it cannot push

blood forward. This causes a backup which leads to building pressure. High pressures and not a lot being pushed forward = cardiogenic shock.

41. (C) This patient is suffering from neurogenic shock (fractured neck with a demarcation line on the skin illustrating massive vasodilation). Fluids are needed, but a pressor is also needed to take control of the vasoconstriction because the cut nerves below the injury no longer can stimulate vasoconstriction– we must give medicine to make vasoconstriction occur. If you only administer fluids, then the patient most likely would remain hypotension due to lack of neurologic control of the peripheral blood vessels. Here the SVR is extremely low- we can fix it with a pressor.

42. (A) This is TOO LOW of a positioning. The AP chest should show the IABP balloon at about the 2nd or 3rd intercostal space, which places it 1-2 cm under the subclavian artery and also above the renal arteries. If placed too low (like at the 5th intercostal space) then it occludes the renal arteries, and if placed too high it will occlude the subclavian, brachiocephalic, and carotid arteries.

43. (D) Note a VERY high inflation point. First remember where the dicrotic notch should be. Now, look at this one. It is very high to the peak of the systole, most likely way before the dicrotic notch. This causes a lot of pressure against the compressing ventricles. This is the MOST DANGEROUS timing error.

44. (B) Look at the very noticeable dicrotic notch following the systolic peak. The dicrotic notch begins, ends, and then the balloon is inflated. The dicrotic notch is COMPLETELY visible. This is clear late inflation.

45. (A) First off, the dicrotic notch looks in the appropriate location. Second, there is incredibly wide diastolic augmentation (balloon inflation). The elongated distance between systolic peak and the next systolic peak indicate this is late deflation. Late inflation results in increased effort the left ventricle has to push against the balloon.

46. (C) First, the dicrotic notch looks to be in the right spot. Secondly, there is a very severe drop after the balloon inflation. This indicates early deflation.

47. (C) Look at the CVP pressures, or otherwise recognize the CVP waveform- it goes from low to MUCH higher. This occurs when the PA catheter that is sitting in the right atrium accidentally migrates into the right ventricle. The right ventricle HATES this and can start throwing PVCs or runs of V-tach. Therefore, this is the PA cath migrating from the right atrium (RA) to the right ventricle (RV).

48. (B) The lateral wall (V5-V6, Lead I, & aVL) is fed mostly by the left circumflex artery. Memorize these.

49. (D) The septal wall (V1-V2) is fed mostly by the left anterior descending coronary artery. Memorize these. This isn't a typo.

50. (C) The condition described is pulmonary edema, which is found MOST SPECIFICALLY with left sided heart failure. Congestive heart failure might be a tempting answer selection, but it is not the best answer in this case because congestive heart failure consists of BOTH left and right heart failure findings (thus congestive = both sides in failure).

51. (C) The condition being discussed is cardiac tamponade: fluid accumulating between the pericardium and the pericardial sac.

52. (A) In cardiogenic shock, some pathophysiology damages the heart or prevents it from functioning normally. This weakens the pump. With a weak pump the heart cannot produce enough pressure to perfuse the distal tissues (skin, brain, liver, lungs, etc). This poor perfusion leads to widespread acidosis and, if uncorrected, death.

53. (B) In treating AMI, or any active MI for that matter, ASA will prevent further sticking of platelets, nitro with act as a vasodilator (especially on the coronary arteries), heparin thins out

the blood so the heart doesn't have to pump as hard to propel the blood forward, and beta blockers slow the hearts efforts to reduce myocardial oxygen demand. Warfarin and AV shunt (really?) aren't indicated.

54. **(D)** Before you treat an aortic dissection with vasodilators, you need to treat with a medication that reduces the force of the velocity of the blood being ejected out of the heart. High ejection pressures further tear the dissection. Therefore, slowdown that velocity with a negative inotrope (like a beta blocker- which is common) before adding a vasodilator.

55. **(C)** Dilated cardiomyopathy patients are treated just like heart failure patients: heart failure management with CPAP, nitrates, loop diuretics, morphine, ACE inhibitors, inotropes.

56. **(A)** The two most common etiologies of cardiac tamponade is pericarditis and chest trauma. Therefore, if you come across a pericarditis patient, routinely rule out signs/ symptoms of tamponade. If you are looking for this stuff, you'll catch things earlier.

57. **(A)** Here the only value that is not within its normal limits is the PLATELETS of 750. Platelets should be in the ballpark of 150 -400 [x 103/mL]. All the other values are within normal limits.

58. **(C)** Here the only value that is not within its normal limits is the POTASSIUM of 8.2. Potassium (K+) should be in the ballpark of 3.4-4.5 [mEq/L]. All the other values are within normal limits. Any potential causes of hyperkalemia (high K+) or evidence of actual hyperkalemia (a high serum potassium) would be an indication NOT to use SUCCINYLCHOLINE if you were to intubate.

59. **(B)** Here the only values that are out of range is BICARBONATE of 34 and SODIUM of 132. Bicarbonate should be in the ballpark of 22-26 [mEq/L] and sodium should be between 135-145 mEq/L. There isn't an answer option for sodium, but there is an option for bicarbonate, therefore, it is the correct selection. All the other values are within normal limits.

60. **(D)** By stimulating the alpha 1 receptor, you will increase vasoconstriction (which raises blood pressure). By stimulating the beta 1 receptor, you increase HR via increasing SA node firing (chronotropy) and increasing the speed through which electrical impulses travel through the conductive system (dromotropy). Additionally, beta 1 stimulation increases cardiac contractility, but that isn't a factor in this question since there isn't any mention of contractility in the answer selections.

61. **(A)** Dopamine administered in the middle dosing range (5-10 mcg/kg/min will elicit a mixed adrenergic effect (meaning it will stimulate more than one receptor). At this dose, it will primarily stimulate beta 1, but can stimulate a little alpha 1 as pharmacology is never black and white- just shades of grey. Stick to the tenets for these exams. In this case, the middle dose of dopamine will stimulate beta 1 which will increase HR.

62. **(A)** Dobutamine will improve contractility and stimulate a vasodilation effect, making it an ideal CHF medication. This medication makes the heartbeat more efficiently (↑ contractility) in addition to making it easier for the heart to pump out to the aorta (↓ SVR). This action would indirectly reduce PVR and PCWP thus making these answer selections incorrect. Dobutamine also increases CO (by increasing contractility); therefore, this answer selection is also incorrect. The correct answer then is increasing HR. The big difference between dopamine and dobutamine is dopamine causes vasoconstriction while dobutamine causes vasodilation.

63. **(B)** There is only one medication in the answer selections that act as a vasodilator, and that's nitroglycerin. Please note that the CVP and PCWP are both high- meaning there is fluid backing up on both sides of the heart and thus requiring a relief in this pressure. To relieve this pressure and correct the hemodynamics in this situation, nitro can be administered to act as a vasodilator. This would help relieve the increased intracardiac pressure.

64. **(D)** Levophed is a medication that is a catecholamine, or a chemical that mimics epinephrine to varying degrees. Levophed highly stimulates alpha 1 and *slightly* stimulates beta 1;

therefore, BP will go up primarily (from increased SVR) and with it, the HR will increase (which increases CO and BP, but only a little). Here, the "Slightly ↑ HR and blood pressure" is the correct answer.

65. **(D)** Cardiac Output = HR x SV. So, if you know both HR and CO, then you can calculate the SV. This has been asked on critical care certification exams, even though it doesn't change our care. I included it to make sure you have seen it.

66. **(A)** Levophed increases alpha 1 stimulation (therefore increases SVR), which increases blood pressure. If you monitored SVR and it got very high without correcting blood pressure, then a new pressor may need to be added.

67. **(B)** A CO of 5 L/min is normal and indicates that the IABP has been successful in treating the shock.

68. **(D)** PCWP reflects left ventricular end diastolic pressure (or left ventricular preload). Because the patient in left ventricular failure will have a high PCWP, a decrease in this value will be the best indicator of patient improvement. The other values would also provide useful information, but the most definitive measurement of improvement is a drop in PCWP.

69. **(A)** A low CVP indicates hypovolemia and a need for an increase in the infusion rate. The diuretic administration will contribute to hypovolemia and elevation of the head may decrease cerebral perfusion. Documentation and continued monitoring are an inadequate response to the low CVP. The goal is to increase the CVP to normal levels and to ensure an adequate urinary output (~ 0.5 - 1.0 cc/kg/hr).

70. **(B)** This is a characteristic finding in the LATE DEFLATION.

71. **(C)** If the patient has a ventricular pacer, then where is the pacer spike on the ventricular beat? In this case, there is no ventricular pacer spike, so we have a failure to capture. We don't have the information to identify if hypoxia is occurring, nor do we have enough information to identify if a left bundle branch block is present. Finally, these are no p- waves.

72. **(B)** There are two main types of VADs with regards to flow- pulsatile (produces pulse) and continuous flow (doesn't create a pulse). The best approach with VADs and cardiovascular pathophysiologies is to allow their mental status and perfusion status guide your concerns. If the patient is calm and following commands without a pulse or in v-tach, then just apply supportive treatment as opposed to drastic ACLS protocols.

73. **(A)** In this case, supportive care (fluid bolus and monitoring) is all that is warranted. Remember, this patient has his blood being pumped by the machine essentially, so protect with supportive care (oxygen/ fluid) as long as their mental state and perfusion state are adequate. Here perfusion is adequate as measured by being alert awake patient with good capillary refill.

74. **(D)** Notice the pattern of ST elevation in leads II, III, and aVF. This is typical of inferior wall AMI.

75. **(C)** Notice the pattern of ST elevation in leads V1 –V4. This is typical of anteroseptal wall AMI.

76. **(B)** Notice the pattern of ST elevation in leads II, III, and aVF as well as V5 and V6. This is typical of inferolateral wall AMI.

# CHAPTER 4: TRAUMA MANAGMENT

## PART 1: TRAUMA TRIAGE

### INTRODUCTION

Trauma triage is the use of specific assessment tools to prioritize trauma patients according to their injuries, or the response to their injuries. There are primary and secondary triage. Primary triage is done at the site of injury, and secondary triage is done at a casualty clearing station in between the scene and the hospital. The big picture is to assess for the presence of either SHOCK or DEATH.

### TRIAGE

1. The big picture is that we will be answering questions concerning:
   a. Respirations
   b. Perfusion
   c. Mental Status
2. What we are really doing is assessing for DEATH or SHOCK. Everything else can wait for later reassessment.
3. There are 4 Classifications:
   a. GREEN- walking wounded
   b. YELLOW- delayed treatment
   c. RED- immediate treatment
   d. BLACK- dead
4. There are adult and pediatric versions:
   a. START- method of triaging adults
   b. JumpSTART- method of triaging pediatrics
      i. < 8 years old
      ii. < 100 lbs.
5. Keep It Simple:
   a. Walking Wounded- GREEN.
   b. Persistent Apnea– DEAD.
      i. Reposition and give a single breath in adults.
      ii. Give five breaths in pediatrics.
   c. Breathing too fast or slow- IMMEDIATE.
   d. Weak pulse and/or delayed cap refill- IMMEDIATE.
   e. Follows simple commands- DELAYED.
   f. Does not follow commands/ painful stimuli- IMMEDIATE.

# PART 2: TRAUMA CENTER CRITERIA

## INTRODUCTION

In 2011, American College of Surgeons Committee on Trauma established guidelines for the triage and transport of patients based on physiological and anatomical criteria. To be successful on critical care transport exams, you will need to be able to read information on a patient and determine if they need to go to a Level I trauma center.

## FIELD TRIAGE GUIDELINES

### Step 1: Assesses physiology (vital signs)—> GO TO LEVEL 1
1. GCS < 13
2. Systolic BP < 90
3. RR < 10 or > 30

### Step 2: Assesses anatomy of injury—> GO TO LEVEL 1
1. All penetrating trauma (above elbow and knee)
2. Chest wall instability/ deformity
3. Two or more proximal long bone fractures
4. Crushed, degloved, mangled, or pulseless extremity
5. Amputation (proximal to wrist/ ankle)
6. Pelvic Fx
7. Paralysis
8. Open or depressed skull Fx

### Step 3: Assesses mechanism of injury—> GO TO APPROPRIATE TRAUMA CENTER (not necessarily a Level 1)
1. Falls
   a. Adults: >20 feet (one story = 10 feet)
   b. Children: >10 feet or two to three times the height of the child
2. High-risk auto crash
   a. Intrusion, including roof: >12 inches occupant site; >18 inches any site
   b. Ejection (partial or complete) from automobile
   c. Death in the same passenger compartment
   d. Vehicle telemetry data consistent with a high risk for injury
3. Automobile versus pedestrian/bicyclist thrown, run over, or with significant (>20 mph) impact; or
4. Motorcycle crash >20 mph

### Step 4: Assesses for special patient and system types—> transport to a trauma center or hospital capable of timely and thorough evaluation and initial management.
1. Older adults
   a. Risk for injury/death increases after age 55 years
   b. SBP <110 might represent shock after age 65 years
   c. Low impact mechanisms (e.g., ground-level falls) might result in severe injury
2. Children: Should be triaged preferentially to pediatric capable trauma centers

3. Anticoagulants and bleeding disorders: Patients with head injury are at high risk for rapid deterioration
4. Burns
    a. Without other trauma mechanism: triage to burn facility
    b. With trauma mechanism: triage to trauma center
5. Pregnancy >20 weeks
6. EMS provider judgment– meaning if a reasonable rationale for transporting a patient to a trauma center exists, then proceed. Medical control here is suggested.


# PART 3: INJURY PATTERNS

## INTRODUCTION

Injuries are most categorized by either mechanism, place of injury, or intent. Mechanisms refer to a specific object or way the injury occurred, such as a stab wound, fall, or blunt injury. Intent is the classification that illuminates whether the injury happened by accident or if it was intentional.

## BASICS
1. Kinematics- The process of predicting injury patterns based on certain mechanisms
2. Big Players:
    a. Mechanism of Injury: Specific chain of events in trauma leading to injury.
    b. Force of Energy Applied: Relates the mass and acceleration of an object at impact .
    c. Anatomy: Relates the organ or organ system involved in an impact.
    d. Type of Energy: Mechanical, thermal, electrical, or chemical.

## BLUNT INJURY PATTERNS
### *Down and Under Pathway*
1. Frontal Impact
2. Occurs when the patient slides under the steering wheel
3. Injuries:
4. Knee, Hip, and Ankle fracture/ dislocation
5. Thoracic Trauma
6. Abdominal Trauma
7. Facial Trauma

### *Up and Over Pathway*
1. Frontal Impact
2. Occurs when the patient flies over the steering wheel
3. Injuries:
4. Knee, Hip, and Ankle Fx/dislocation Bilateral Femur Fxs
5. Thoracic Trauma
6. Abdominal Trauma
7. Facial Trauma

### *Lateral Impacts*
1. Side impact/ T–bone impact

2.  Injuries:
3.  Head: coup-contrecoup, shear of brain vessels (brain hemorrhage)
4.  Neck: Odontoid fx
5.  Thorax: Flail chest, pneumothorax, aortic arch shear
6.  Abdomen: Liver or spleen (side impact dependent), shear of renal vessels
7.  Extremities: Unilateral injury patterns

### Rear Impacts
1.  Struck from rear
2.  Injuries:
3.  Head: coup-contrecoup, whiplash, shear of brain vessels
4.  Neck: Hyperextension with stretched ligaments/ tendons
5.  Torso: Usually minimal
6.  Extremities: Usually minimal

### Rotational Impacts
1.  A strike causing vehicle and occupants to spin/rotate, along with objects in the vehicle.
2.  Injuries:
    a.  Head: coup-contrecoup, shear of brain vessels (brain hemorrhage), contusions
    b.  Neck: Compression Fx, Odontoid Fx
    c.  Thorax: Fx ribs, hemo/pneumothorax, flail segment, myocardial rupture or contusion, aortic arch shear/ rupture
    d.  Abdomen: Liver or spleen (side impact dependent), shear of renal vessels
    e.  Extremities: Pelvic Fx, clavicle Fx, humeral compression fx

### Rollovers
1.  Very difficult to predict
2.  Typically, is a mixture of multiple injury patterns mentioned above.

### Motorcycle: Up and Over Pathway
1.  Bilateral Femur Fractures
2.  Head/ Neck Trauma: Direct (skull Fx, cerebral contusion)/ Axial loading
3.  Thoracic/ abdominal: Lung or heart contusion or rupture, hemo/pneumothorax/ Sheared aorta, sheared liver/ Intestine or diaphragm rupture
4.  Pelvis/ Extremities: Pelvic Fxs, groin trauma
5.  Road rash on skin

### Motorcycle: Laying the Bike Down
1.  Massive Road Rash
2.  Unilateral extremity fracture/ amputations
3.  This mechanism is less likely to be severe when compared to the motorcycle up and over pathway.

### Pedestrian vs. Motor Vehicle
1.  Adults:
    a.  Turn to their side: Unilateral injuries/ Severe lower extremity injuries
    b.  Hood Impact: Face, thoracic and abdominal injuries
    c.  Ground Impact: Head strikes ground/ Hip and shoulder injuries/ Patient can be run over
2.  Pediatrics:
    a.  Turn and face the vehicle: Frontal injuries/ Severe femur and/or pelvic Fxs
    b.  Hood Impact: Face, thoracic and abdominal injuries
    c.  Ground Impact: Head strikes the ground/ Patient can be run over

    d.  Waddell's Triad:
        i.  Femur Fracture
        ii.  Intratorso Injury
        iii.  Head Injury

## *Critical Fall*

1. Fall 15-20 feet, or 3 times a person's height
2. Injuries:
   a. Calcaneus Fx/ Tib/fib; femur, pelvic Fxs;  Spinal Fxs
   b. Bilateral Colles' Fx (from outstretched hand)
   c. Classic deceleration injures (all the compressions and shearing injuries)
   d. Lethal dose 50 (LD 50) describes a mechanism that kills 50% of the people that experience it. LD 90 kills 90% of the people experiencing it. For falls, LD 50 is 4 stories (48 ft) and LD 90 is 7 stories (84 ft).

## *Blast Injury Patterns*

There are 4 phases of a blast injuries: primary, secondary, tertiary, and quaternary

### Primary

1. Occurs from the blast pressure wave
2. Burns, Confusion, Tinnitus, rupture/ bleeding: lungs, GI tract, thoracic and abdominal organs
3. A ruptured tympanic membrane should raise suspicion of other hollow organ injury.

### Secondary

1. Occurs from the debris thrown from the blast
2. Abrasions/ Lacerations, Penetrating chest and abdominal injuries

### Tertiary

1. Occurs as the blast turns the patient into a missile
2. Flail chest, compression of spine, extremity fxs

### Quaternary

1. Occurs from structural collapse or building fire
2. Smoke inhalation, crush injuries, burns from structural fires, traumatic amputations

## PENETRATING INJURY PATTERNS

### *Low Energy Projectiles/ Weapons*

1. Ex: Knives, tree branches, fence posts
2. Tissue crush is usually small- unless a fence post
3. The more blunt a penetrating object, the more force is needed to cause penetration
4. Greater wound effect can be caused by rotating the handle or exterior portion of the object

### *Mid to High Energy Projectiles/ Weapons*

1. Handguns to high power rifles
2. Injury patterns caused by several factors
3. Cavitation
   a. Temporary cavitation: temporal cavity caused as a projectile passes through the body and stretches the tissue from the sonic pressure wave.
   b. Permanent: residual cavity formed after tissue has been disrupted by a penetrating object

4. Deformation: Some bullets, like hollow points, deform at impact making a larger striking surface
5. Tumble: Some mid energy bullets spin in mid air, thus creating more damage if it strikes a victim at full profile
6. Fragmentation: Some bullets are designed to break apart completely causing more damage (shatter)
7. Range: The closer you are to a firearm at the time of discharge, the more damage can occur.
8. Burns: The skin can be burned when a muzzle is held close to the skin and the hot gasses from discharge burn the skin.

## Specific GSW Injury Patterns

### Skull GSW (mid-energy)
1. Usually not enough energy to leave the skull
2. Bullet follows the curvature of the skull

### Skull GSW (high-energy)
1. Massive destruction to brain and skull
2. At closer ranges, heated gas training behind the projectile will enter the skull just behind the bullet and create an explosive effect

### Thoracic GSW
1. Pulmonary and vascular disruption
2. Hemo/pnumothorax- can lead to tension pneumothorax
3. Massive internal hemorrhage

### Abdominal GSW
1. Multiple air-filled structures
2. Assume a major injury- requires surgery to identify all damage

### Neck GSW
1. Vascular and nervous tissue at risk
2. Can lead to disabling injuries

# PART 4: TRAUMA ASSESSMENT

## INTRODUCTION

The ultimate goal in the trauma assessment is to identify and then immediately manage any life threats. Examples would include apnea or tension pneumothorax because they would need to be fixed RIGH AWAY or the patient could die.

## THE TRAUMA ASSESSMENT

### Airway:
1. Open using trauma (modified) jaw thrust
2. Assess for patency
   a. Clear any objects or material in the airway

b. Noises like snoring, gurgling or silence indicate a threat and should be treated right away (positioning, suction, BVM ventilation).

c. Treat with the simplest methods because advanced methods take too much time.

## Breathing

1. Usually performed with the assessment of the airway
2. Provide ventilation if respirations are inadequate
   a. Inadequate: < 10/min, >30/min, shallow (Adults)
   b. Treat with supplemental oxygen and assist ventilations if SpO2 are < 95% generally.
3. Expose and inspect chest (back too)
   a. Redness to chest wall- injury
   b. Asymmetric chest movement- flail chest or tension pneumothorax
   c. Retractions- inadequate respirations
   d. Sucking chest wound- occlusive dressing taped on 3 sides
4. Auscultate
   a. Make sure air is going in and out on each side equally
   b. This isn't the time to diagnose underlying physiology- just assess for adequate respirations.

## Circulation

1. Assess skin color, temperature, and condition
   a. Pale, mottled, blue skin= poor perfusion
   b. Cool skin= hypothermia or poor perfusion
   c. Diaphoretic skin= sympathetic response (sick)
2. Assess pulses (radial and carotid)
   a. BP not confirmed w/ or w/o a radial pulse, but perfusion is.
   b. (+) carotid, (-) radial= poor perfusion
3. Assess Capillary Refill
   a. >2 seconds= poor perfusion
4. Rule out significant hemorrhage (quick full body sweep)

## Disability

1. Assess mental status
   a. Pt looking at you= good
   b. Calculate baseline GCS (practice this)
2. Assess for pulses x 4 extremities
3. Assess for sensation that is "normal" or "numb/ pins and needles"
   a. Relate numbness to dermatomes
4. Assess movement
   a. If pt can move/lift/hold all extremities equally= good
   b. Note if one side is weaker than the other
5. Assess for spinal step-off or crepitus
6. Apply spinal precautions

## Exposure

1. Identify any other injuries hidden by clothing
2. KEEP PT WARM IN THIS PROCESS

## Secondary Assessment

1. Head-to-Toe
   a. Looking for DCAP-BTLS-TIC for all regions of the body
   b. Obtaining quantitative vital signs
   c. Obtain SAMPLE history

2. Reassess. Reassess. Reassess.
3. Obtain the FULL Clinical Picture:
   a. Clinical Assessment: what we have been doing
   b. History: patient, situation, prior treatment (meds/fluids)
   c. Labs/ Studies: CBC, BMP, H/H, Lactate (obtain from sending facility or utilize iStat– DO NOT DELAY transport to obtain).
   d. Images: X-rays, CTs, FAST/ Ultrasound
4. Specific Findings and Management
   a. Gurgling-- Suction
   b. Snoring-- Reposition
   c. Apnea--Assist ventilations
   d. Hemorrhage--Pressure and tourniquet
   e. Tension Pneumothorax-- Needle decompression
   f. Flail segment--PPV or intubation/ mech vent
   g. Tamponade-- Fluid Bolus/ Pericardiocentesis
   h. Diaphragmatic Rupture-- Assist ventilations
   i. Pelvic/ Open Book Fx-- Bind pelvis
   j. Pulmonary Contusion--SIMV w/ PEEP @ 10-15/ Or CPAP at 10-15/ Fluids

# PART 5: THORACIC TRAUMA

## INTRODUCTION

You will be exposed, repeatedly, to moderately complex traumatic conditions, and at times, you will be forced to contend with a highly complex traumatic situations. Fix what you can fix and treat what you can treat. Use medical control if needed. Consider PAM = Pathophysiology, Assessment (S/S), and Management (MGT).

## THORACIC TRAUMA CONDITIONS

### Open Pneumothorax
1. Patho: penetrating chest trauma--> air able to enter chest through wound--> sucking chest wound
2. S/S: sucking chest wound, dyspnea, hypoxia
3. MGT: ABCDE, O2, occlusive dressing, be ready to needle decompress, consider chest tube

### Tension Pneumothorax
1. Patho: injured lung--> continuously allows air into pleural cavity--> building pressure--> mediastinal shift away from injured side--> lung/ heart compromised--> cardiac arrest
2. S/S: dyspnea, concurrent drop in BOTH BP and pulse oximetry, JVD, tracheal deviation/ tugging (LATE), worsening compliance with bagging or PIP alarms if on vent, hyper-resonant chest
3. MGT: Support ABCs, needle decompression or chest tube

### Hemothorax
1. Patho: trauma--> disruption of thoracic vasculature--> hemorrhage occurs spilling into the chest--> reducing lung volumes and circulating blood volume--> hypoxia--> cardiac arrest
2. S/S: hypoxia, hypotension, decreased BS to affected side, 'dull' chest percussion, worsening shock, low hematocrit and hemoglobin
3. MGT: support ABCs, IV fluids to target 90 systolic or 65 MAP, consider a chest tube

## Flail Segment
1. Patho: Blunt trauma--> 2 or more ribs broken in 2 or more places--> altered chest wall mechanics--> reduced lung volumes/pressures--> hypoxia
2. S/S: dyspnea, hypoxia, crepitus to chest, possible paradoxical movement, tenderness/ bruising over area
3. MGT: support ABCs, oxygenate, consider mechanical ventilation to splint the flail segment, be suspicious of tension pneumo and shock

## Pericardial Tamponade
1. Patho: penetrating trauma to heart--> excess blood accumulates in the pericardial sac--> compresses the heart inward at large pressures--> pump failure--> cardiogenic shock--> death
2. S/S: Beck's triad (muffled heart tones, JVD, pulsus alterans), hypoxia syndrome, rising CVP (>15cm H2O), hypotension
3. MGT: ABCs, IV fluids, pericardiocentesis

## Aortic rupture
1. Patho: traumatic dissection/ transection--> massive bleeding into chest cavity--> shock--> death
2. S/S: 15-20mmHg difference form one arm to another, hypotension, AMS, fractures to 1st and 2nd ribs, chest contusions
3. MGT: ABCs, O2, IV fluids, trauma surgeon

## Myocardial Contusion
1. Patho: blunt trauma--> bruised heart muscle--> damaged vessels at bruise not perfusing the downstream muscle--> mimics MI--> cardiogenic shock
2. S/S: trauma with arrhythmias, STEMI in right side leads, bundle branch blocks (especially right side), hypotension
3. MGT: ABCs, arrhythmia specific treatments, be suspicious for tamponade

## Tracheobronchial Disruption
1. Patho: trauma the trachea and /or either bronchus--> massive air leakage--> reduced lung volumes, pneumothorax, pneumomediastinum, and/or tension pneumothorax--> severe hypoxia syndrome
2. S/S: severe dyspnea, hypoxia, subcutaneous air, JVD or tracheal deviation
3. MGT: ABCs, oxygen, PPV unless it worsens the pt condition, consider needle decompression if indicated, consider chest tube

## Pulmonary Contusion
1. Patho: blunt trauma--> damages smaller lung vessels--> disrupts oxygen transfer to the RBC--> severe hypoxia
2. S/S: increasing hypoxia with chest trauma, worsening ABGs over time, opacity on chest x ray
3. MGT: ABCs, Mechanical vent/ CPAP with 10-15 PEEP, fluids and pain meds

## Esophageal Perforation
1. Patho: ruptured esophagus--> free air into thorax/ gastric contents into thorax--> subcutaneous air, bacteria, acids in thorax
2. S/S: pain, fever, subcutaneous air/ stiff neck, widening mediastinum, pleuritic type pain
3. MGT: ABCs, antibiotics, surgeon

## Traumatic Asphyxia
1. Patho: compressive force to chest--> blood forced backward out of right side of heart--> engorging veins of the neck/head/face--> cyanotic appearance from deoxygenated blood

2. S/S: cyanotic chest/ neck/ head, JVD, conjunctival bleeding, sharp line of demarcation with normal skin color below
3. MGT: ABCs, tx associated injuries of compressive forces, if pt is trapped- IV and fluids before removing the weight to ensure hemodynamics; consider bicarbonate infusion.

### Laryngotracheal Injuries
1. Patho: blunt trauma to throat (clothesline, steering wheel, etc)--> disrupts the integrity of the neck structures--> open air to trachea and larynx
2. S/S: bubbling neck wound, subcutaneous air, dysphonia, stridor, dyspnea, edema
3. MGT: ABCs, intubation carefully, occlusive dressing to open wounds, spinal precautions, surgeon; be ready to perform cricothyrotomy.

# PART 6: ABDOMINAL TRAUMA

## INTRODUCTION
You will be exposed, repeatedly, to moderately complex traumatic conditions, and at times, you will be forced to contend with a highly complex traumatic situation. Fix what you can fix and treat what you can treat. Use medical control if needed. Consider PAM = Pathophysiology, Assessment (S/S), and Management (MGT).

## ABDOMINAL TRAUMA CONDITIONS

### Abdominal Injury
1. Patho: blunt trauma--> disrupts structures and vessels in the abdominal compartment--> hypotension--> hypoxia syndrome--> shock
2. S/S: AMS, hypoxia syndromes, hypotension, loss of palpable pulses, pale/cool/moist skin
3. MGT: ABCs, O2, IV fluids/ pressors- target 90mmHg systolic or 65mmHg MAP, keep warm, dress open abdominal wounds, Foley- unless contraindicated

### Spleen Injury
1. Patho: Blunt/ penetrating trauma--> direct rupture of very vascular spleen (lots of bleeding)
2. S/S: Pain in LUQ, Kehr's Sign (left shoulder pain)
3. MGT: ABCs, O2, IV fluids/ pressors- target 90mmHg systolic or 65mmHg MAP, keep warm, dress open abd wounds, Foley- unless contraindicated

### Liver Injury
1. Patho: Blunt/ penetrating trauma--> damages the liver itself, which is a very vascular organ (lots of bleeding)
2. S/S: Pain in RUQ, right shoulder pain as blood accumulates in the diaphragm
3. MGT: ABCs, O2, IV fluids/ pressors- target 90mmHg systolic or 65mmHg MAP, keep warm, dress open abd wounds, Foley- unless contraindicated

### Intestinal Injury
1. Patho: Blunt/ penetrating trauma--> damages the intestine itself, which is a very vascular organ (lots of bleeding), also intestinal contents spill out into abdominal cavity

2. S/S: Abdominal pain, seatbelt sign, guarding, abdominal distension, rebound tenderness, vomiting, fever
3. MGT: ABCs, O2, IV fluids/ pressors- target 90mmHg systolic or 65mmHg MAP, keep warm, dress open abdominal wounds, Foley- unless contraindicated

### Abdominal Vascular Injury
1. Patho: Blunt/ penetrating trauma--> damages the abdominal vessels (lots of bleeding)
2. S/S: Potentially none other than abdominal pain, AMS, hypotension in the absence of external bleeding
3. MGT: ABCs, O2, IV fluids/ pressors- target 90mmHg systolic or 65mmHg MAP, keep warm, dress open abdominal wounds, Foley- unless contraindicated

### Abruptio Placenta
1. Patho: blunt/ penetrating trauma--> disrupts the connections of the placenta with the uterine wall--> bleeding--> fetal demise--> mother hypotension and shock--> death
2. S/S: vaginal bleeding, abdominal/ back pain, shock, loss of fetal heart tones or slowing fetal heart tones
3. MGT: ABCs, O2, tilt left lateral 15 degrees if > 20 weeks gestation, aggressive fluid resuscitation, rapid transport

# PART 7: ORTHOPEDIC TRAUMA

## INTRODUCTION
You will be exposed, repeatedly, to moderately complex traumatic conditions, and at times, you will be forced to contend with a highly complex traumatic situation. Fix what you can fix and treat what you can treat. Use medical control if needed. Consider PAM = Pathophysiology, Assessment (S/S), and Management (MGT).

## ORTHOPEDIC TRAUMA CONDITIONS
### Pelvic Fracture
1. Patho: blunt trauma--> breaks bones of the pelvis--> massive internal hemorrhage--> shock
2. S/S: rotation or uneven pelvic crests, uneven leg lengths, pain, crepitus to inward or lateral compression, perineal bruising
3. MGT: ABCs, Splint fx, proactive for shock

### Femur Fracture
1. Patho: blunt trauma--> breaks femur bone--> significant hemorrhage (1-2 L in cavity)--> shock
2. S/S: Pain, swelling, deformity, open wound (compound fracture), crepitus
3. MGT: Control bleeding, assess PMS, IV fluids, pain meds, traction splint, reassess PMS

### Dislocation
1. Patho: blunt trauma--> bones come out of their joints--> nervous and vascular damage as well as tendon and ligament damage
2. S/S: Pain, swelling, deformity, crepitus

3. MGT: Assess PMS, pain meds, reduce the dislocation if no pulses are present distal the injury, reassess PMS

### Compartment Syndrome
1. Patho: blunt trauma to extremities--> muscle bundles within a fascia swell--> pressure within the bundle increases--> once the compartment pressure gets within 30mmHg of diastolic BP, blood flow stops--> muscle cell death
2. S/S: pain, pallor, pulselessness, paresthesia, paralysis, pressure,
3. MGT: ABCs, O2, PMS reassessments, ice pack extremities affected, IV fluids to improve perfusion, pain meds, proactive for rhabdomyolysis/ hyperkalemia/ myglobinemia

### Rhabdomyolysis
1. Patho: blunt trauma/exercise/ seizures--> damage to the muscle cell wall--> influx of calcium, sodium, and water--> cell wall ruptures--> K and myoglobin spills into circulation--> hyperK--> myoglobin and hypovolemia--> renal tubal blockage--> acute renal failure
2. S/S: dark colored urine, weakness/ dehydration, creatine kinase elevation (5 times normal), hyper K (>5.5mEq/L) with tall T waves on ECG, HypoCalcemia (<4.3mEq/L)
3. MGT: ABCs, IV fluids- at least 2 L, 1mEq/kg bicarb, 1-2g calcium q 4 minutes if ECG signs of hyperK, consider mannitol and adding bicarb to NS to alkalinize the urine (keep urine pH over 6.5)

# PART 8: TRAUMA PHARMACOLOGY

## INTRODUCTION
These medication or fluids are very important in the management of traumatic conditions. Permissive hypotension is encouraged to prevent hemodilution. Consider withholding fluid unless the mean arterial pressure (MAP) is 60 mmHg or less. Remember, MAP is calculated by doubling the systolic, adding it to the systolic value and then divide by the number three (3).

## MEDICATIONS USED IN TRAUMA
### Packed Red Blood Cells (PRBCs)
1. Action: Increases the number of RBCs
2. Side Effects: Hypersensitivity/ hemolytic reactions
3. Used to evaluate PRBC therapy and for ongoing bleeding.
4. 1 unit of PRBCs = 250cc
   a. Raises hemoglobin by 1g/dL
   b. Raises hematocrit by 3%

### Opiates
1. Mechanism: Pain control
2. Action: Reduces the sensation of pain
3. Side effects: Respiratory depression, hypotension
4. Noteworthy: Fentanyl: minimal effect on hemodynamics

### Sedatives
1. Mechanism: Reduces anxiety and agitation
2. Side effects: Hypotension

3. Cautions: Use in hemodynamically stable patients
4. Potentiates opiates
5. Noteworthy: Ativan, Versed are examples

## Antibiotics
1. Mechanism: Prevents bacterial infection
2. Side effects: Hypotension (vancomycin/ Levaquin)/ Allergic reaction/ Cautions
3. On intubated patients, use waveform capnography to detect bronchoconstriction from allergic reaction
4. Vancomycin, Penicillin or Gentamycin or Ampicillin

## Anticoagulants
1. Mechanism: Prevents clots (from PE or DVTs)
2. Side effects: Bleeding
3. Cautions: Delicate balance in trauma- need clotting, but prevent DIC in the severely bleeding patient
4. Examples: Heparin, Warfarin, ASA, LMWH
5. Protamine Sulfate is heparin's antidote
6. Vitamin K is Warfarin's (Coumadin) antidote

## Tranexamic Acid
1. Mechanism: Slows bleeding (antifibrinolytic)
2. Indication: significant bleeding from trauma
3. Dose: 1 g in 100 cc NS over 10 minutes; then followed by 1 g in 500cc NS over 8 hours.


# PART 9: TRAUMA LABS

## INTRODUCTION
These are lab values that can help in trauma cases. As is in more any lab , image, or study, the entire clinical picture should be considered and never a single value.


## TRAUMA LABS
### Hemoglobin (HGB)
1. HGB indicates oxygen carrying capacity
2. Norm: ~ 13-18 g/dL
3. Critical Value:
   a. < 5 g/dL indicates bleeding, iron deficiency, and anemia
   b. 20 g/dL indicates dehydration/ hemochromotosis

### Hematocrit (HCT)
1. Crit indicates oxygen carrying capacity
2. It is the percentage of RBCs in a sample of blood.
3. Norm: 35-45% in women/ 40-50% in men
4. Critical Value:
   a. < 15% indicates bleeding, iron deficiency, anemia
   b. 60% indicates dehydration

## Lactate

1. Produced in large amounts during anaerobic metabolism
2. Norm: 4-20 mg/dL (SI units = 0.5-2 mmol/L)
3. Critical Value:
   a. 45 mg/dL this indicates that there is ischemic disease or hypoperfusion, or both
   b. (SI >4.5 mmol/L) this indicates that there is ischemic disease or hypoperfusion, or both

## Oxygen Saturation of Venous Blood (SvO2) aka Mixed Venous Gas

1. Physiology
   a. Oxygen is released in the arterial/ capillary system
   b. When hypoperfusion is present, the cells on the venous side are so O2 starved, they steal O2 from the venous blood. Measured from a central line.
   c. A reduction in SvO2 indicates hypoperfusion or ischemic disease.
2. Norm: 70-75%
3. Critical Value: < 60%

# PART 10: TRAUMA MANAGEMENT QUESTIONS

1. You are responding to a mass casualty at an industrial facility where an explosion has occurred. The authorities have deemed the scene safe and you proceed inside. You find 2 patients on the ground. You call out to the victims to stand and move toward your voice, and none stand. There is no reply or action after you call out to them. Patient #1 is a an obese male lying on his back with 70% 2nd degree burns and a traumatic amputation of both upper extremities. He doesn't answer you when you ask his name. There are no respirations. What is the most appropriate first action for patient #1?
   a. Tag Red
   b. Reposition airway
   c. Tag Black
   d. Move to next patient

2. Patient #2: You find this patient on the ground also with 70%+ burns and their clothes have also been burned off. They moan incomprehensibly when you ask for their name. They are currently breathing twice in a 6 second period. What is the first most appropriate action for patient #2?
   a. Tag this patient with the green tag
   b. Move to respiration assessment
   c. Move this patient to walking wounded
   d. Tag this patient with the black tag

3. Categorize the respiratory rate of patient #2.
   a. 2-4 bpm
   b. 5-10 bpm
   c. 12-20 bpm
   d. 30 bpm

4. A patient presents with bilateral femur fractures, muffled heart tones, and a large facial laceration status post MVC where they were driving. What injury patterns are they displaying?
   a. Lateral Impact
   b. Down and Under
   c. Laying the bike down
   d. Up and Over Pathway

5. A patient presents with a patellar fracture, open book pelvis, pulmonary contusions, and a large facial laceration after a frontal impact MVC. What injury patterns are they displaying?
   a. Lateral Impact
   b. Down and Under Pathway
   c. Up and Over Pathway
   d. Laying the bike down

6. Which would cause greater tissue crush?
   a. Sledgehammer
   b. Samurai sword
   c. Tomahawk axe
   d. Ice pick

7. Your trauma patient is dead. Their entire cranial vault looks to have exploded. From this injury pattern what could you infer about the firearm that killed them?
   a. It was high velocity a long distance away
   b. It was low velocity a long distance away
   c. It was low velocity at a nearby distance
   d. It was high velocity and at closer range.

8. A patient is struck by cement from a building wall moments after an explosion in the building. The resulting pattern is due to what?
   a. Primary blast
   b. Secondary blast
   c. Tertiary blast
   d. Quaternary blast

9. A patient has been stabbed with a steak knife through the hand. There is no significant bleeding and the patient can still feel and move hand. With this information you know that the patient meets criteria for which hospital?
   a. Teaching hospital
   b. Closest appropriate
   c. Level 1 Trauma
   d. County hospital

10. Your patient is exhibiting deep respirations and doesn't answer when you call out to him. He has dry, rattling breath sounds. What is the most appropriate management strategy?

a. Suction
b. Reposition
c. Intubation
d. Ventilation

11. Your patient was the victim of a frontal impact MVC. They present with asymmetrical chest wall with each inspiration. There is no paradoxical motion. What is the most appropriate management for this patient?
    a. Splint with bulky pad
    b. Immediate ventilation
    c. Reposition the airway
    d. Needle decompression

12. You identify faint heart tones and (+) JVD in your rollover MVC patient. What immediate treatment is warranted?
    a. Remove air from the pleura
    b. Drain the pericardial space
    c. Increase the tidal volume
    d. Reduce PEEP on the vent

13. Your patient presents with difficulty breathing. They were involved in a 2 car MVC. The patient is tachycardic, has borderline blood pressure, and percussion of the chest produces a dull chest sensation. What is the patient's current condition?
    a. Tamponade
    b. Pneumothorax
    c. Hemothorax
    d. Flail Segment

14. A patient was involved in a 1 car MVC with frontal impact. There is crepitus over the rib just inferior to the right clavicle with ecchymosis and there is a 12 mmHg difference between the right and left arm. What condition is the patient moat likely experiencing?
    a. Cardiac contusion
    b. Aortic rupture
    c. Pulmonary contusion
    d. Flail segment

15. Your 23 year old assault patient (baseball bat to the chest) is exhibiting ST elevation in leads II, III, and aVF with a wide QRS in V1. What condition is the patient most likely experiencing?
    a. Cardiac contusion
    b. Cardiac tamponade
    c. Pericardial effusion
    d. Pulmonary contusion

16. Your partner is recalling a patient who suffered intraperitoneal bleeding. Which of the following findings indicates a pathology where blood collecting at the diaphragm?
    a. Cullen's Sign
    b. Kehr's Sign
    c. Bruzinski's Sign
    d. Beck's Sign


17. Your patient has suffered a rollover MVC and is concerned that her unborn child is injured or in danger. Which of the following would most indicate danger to the fetus?
    a. Left shoulder pain
    b. Right shoulder pain
    c. Sharp back pain
    d. Intense nausea


18. You have a patient that presents with the following vital signs and findings: HR 120, BP 82/55, RR24, (+) seatbelt sign, rebound tenderness, and vomiting. Which of the following conditions does this most suggest?
    a. Cardiac Injury
    b. Kidney Injury
    c. Great Vessel Injury
    d. Intestinal Injury


19. Your patient fell off a roof and landed mostly on his right foot. The patient presents as follows: HR 98, BP 99/60, RR 14, (+) pulses with a shortened right leg, (+) crepitus with pressure to anterior superior iliac spine and is awake and alert. No other injuries are present. What treatment MUST occur?
    a. Quickly apply SAM sling
    b. Begin bilateral large IVs
    c. Administer pain meds
    d. Initiate fluid bolus


20. A colleague is explaining that a football player had been recently transported in rhabdomyolysis. You know that this condition is best treated by which of the following:
    a. Fluids, bicarb, calcium
    b. Normal saline, potassium
    c. Potassium, bicarb, fluids
    d. Fluids, analgesics, B- blocker


21. You administer 2 units of PRBCs to your hypotensive trauma patient. What should their HGB elevate to if the HGB was 12g/dL before being administered blood?
    a. 13 g/dL
    b. 9 g/dL
    c. 14 g/dL
    d. 18 g/dL

22. You recognize that your patients clotting times take way too long. Which of the following medications should you reach for?
    a. Warfarin
    b. Vitamin K
    c. Heparin
    d. Cryoglobin

23. A patient has a critical low hematocrit. What is the best treatment for this patient?
    a. Hypertonic Saline
    b. Isotonic Crystaloids
    c. Blood Products
    d. Lactated Ringers

24. Your patient has a critical low SvO2. What is the best treatment for this patient?
    a. Hypertonic Saline
    b. Isotonic Crystaloids
    c. Blood Plasma
    d. Lactated Ringers

# PART 11: TRAUMA MANAGEMENT RATIONALES

1. **(B)** If there is no evidence of respiratory effort, you should at least clear and position the airway.
2. **(B)** Systematically, you have ruled out the ability to walk and are moving to assess the respiratory rate.
3. **(C)** Two breaths in a six second period equates to 20 because there are 10 six second periods in a minute, and 10 times the number of breaths each six second period is a total of 20. This is the "Six Count" method where you observe your watch's second hand click 6 times and multiple the breath count by 10.
4. **(D)** Up and Over- the patient flies over the wheel/dashboard fracturing both femurs (driver); then the thorax/abd impacts the wheel/dashboard causing trauma; then the face impacts the wheel/dash/windshield.
5. **(B)** Down and Under- the patient slides under the steering wheel or towards dashboard impacting knees causing knee, hip, and femur fxs; the chest strikes the wheel/dash causing thoracic and abd trauma; finally the head hits the wheel/ dash causing face and head trauma.
6. **(A)** The blunter an object, the more difficult it is to cause penetration, therefore, more tissue crush is needed to result in penetration. Each of these items are sharp except one: the sledgehammer.
7. **(D)** High power weapons can bring with the projectile a pressure wave that can make the cranial vault explode. This is more likely to occur at closer ranges with high power firearms. However, this can occur with high power firearms at larger distances away, but in this case the

high velocity/ close range answer is better because the fact that you're closer would cause more of an explosive effect. Therefore, its the best answer.

8. **(B)** Secondary- Debris thrown from the blast; Primary- damage from the blast itself; Tertiary- patient becomes a missile; Quaternary- burning from building or collapsing wall of a building.

9. **(C)** A depressed skull fracture meets Step II criteria for a level 1 trauma center.

10. **(B)** Dry and rattling is describing sonorous respirations, thus the tongue is falling to the back of the throat. Reposition is necessary.

11. **(D)** With asymmetrical chest wall in the absence of a flail segment (paradoxical chest wall movement) then it is anticipated that there is a tension pneumothorax, thus needle decompression is immediately warranted. If you ventilate before decompressing, then you could worsen the tension.

12. **(B)** Faint heart tones and JVD indicate cardiac tamponade, so a pericardiocentesis is needed. This procedure, simply stated, is removing fluid from the pericardial space.

13. **(B)** The dull element in this question points to the way a chest feels when it is filled with fluid. You won't get that feeling, or sensation, with these other conditions.

14. **(B)** The information of broken 1st/ 2nd ribs (crepitus below the clavicle) and the difference in BP from the right or left arm, indicates an aortic rupture. Some of these other conditions can be present too, but this info REALLY points to aortic rupture.

15. **(A)** Myocardial contusion is characterized by ST elevation in leads II, III, and aVF with a wide QRS in V1 (BBB) especially in the face of direct chest trauma.

16. **(B)** Kehr's sign classically indicates a splenic injury but can also refer pain from an irritated diaphragm where the irritation is caused by blood.

17. **(C)** The sharp back pain indicates an abruption. The shoulder pains also indicate bleeding, but the back pain is specific to an abruption.

18. **(D)** Remember the s/s of intestinal injury: abd pain, seatbelt sign, guarding, abdominal distension, rebound tenderness, vomiting, and fever.

19. **(A)** In this case, there is evidence of a pelvic fracture (shortened leg) and pelvic crepitus and therefore the hip needs to be bound to prevent significant hemorrhage into the pelvic cavity.

20. **(A)** Remember, the management for rhabdo is IV fluids- at least 2 L, 1mEq/kg bicarb, calcium q 4 minutes with ECG signs of hyperK, consider mannitol and adding bicarb to NS to alkalinize the urine (keep urine pH over 6.5).

21. **(C)** 2 Units should elevate this HGB by a measure of 2 g/dL, so it should change from 12 to 14. Remember, 1 unit = increase hemoglobin by 1 and increases hematocrit by 3%.

22. **(B)** If the patient has a high PTT, then it takes too long for their blood to clot- potentially due to over-aggressive anticoagulant therapy. Vitamin K is the reversal for warfarin.

23. **(C)** This patient needs the oxygen carrying capacity of red blood cells.

24. **(B)** This patient needs to improve perfusion, so ensure to support blood pressure aggressively and maximize oxygenation. The low SvO2 indicates oxygen is being stolen from the venous system, and thus indicates a poorly perfused patient.

# CHAPTER 5: BURN MANAGMENT

## PART 1: BURN PATHOPHYSIOLOGY

### INTRODUCTION

Significant changes occur to in physiology when our tissues are burned. Therefore, it is important to be able to differentiate pathophysiologies and management for specific burn injuries.

### PATHOPHYSIOLOGIES SEEN IN BURNS

#### Vascular changes resulting from burn injuries:
1. Circulatory disruption occurs at the burn site immediately after a burn injury.
2. Blood flow decreases or ceases due to occluded blood vessels.
3. Damaged macrophages within the tissues release chemicals that cause constriction of vessel.
4. Blood vessel thrombosis may occur causing necrosis.

#### Fluid Shifts:
1. Occurs within the first 12 hours after the burn and can continue to up to 36 hours.
2. Fluid shifts occur after initial vasoconstriction, and then dilation.
3. Blood vessels dilate and leak fluid into the interstitial space.
4. This is known as third spacing or capillary leak syndrome.
5. It causes decreased blood volume and blood pressure.

#### Fluid Imbalances:
1. Occur as a result of fluid shift and cell damage.
2. Hypovolemia– occurs from 'weeping' fluid loss from the burn itself and the shifting of fluids.
3. Metabolic acidosis– occurs because of shock that can quickly follow a burn (from hypovolemia) causing poor perfusion and acidosis.
4. Hyperkalemia– due to cellular wall damage, allowing potassium to spill out into the extracellular spaces.
5. Hyponatremia– occurs as the shifting of fluid moves from the intravascular space to outside the vessels, and the fluid brings with it sodium. Therefore, there is less sodium in the vasculature, which is hyponatremia.
6. Hemoconcentration– fluid leaving the vessels causes an increase in hematocrit, thereby concentrating the blood. Risk for thrombosis.

#### Fluid Remobilization:
1. Occurs after 24 hours.
2. Capillary leak stops.
3. Diuretic stage progresses- fluid shifts from the interstitial spaces into the vascular space
4. Blood volume increases leading to increased renal blood flow and diuresis.
5. Body weight returns to normal.
6. Hypokalemia– occurs as the fluid shifts back into the cell from the interstitial spaces, thus diluting the electrolyte potassium.

## Jackson's Theory of Thermal Burns

1. This is a theory centered around 3 different zones of a thermal burn, each characterized by a specific set of pathophysiological phenomena.
2. **Zone of Coagulation** (a): this is the area of the burning characteristic of cell membrane rupture and destruction, blood coagulation, and structural proteins are destroyed. Center of burn.
3. **Zone of Stasis** (b): this zone has characterized an area of labile injured cells with decreased blood flow. Because of this poor blood flow, cells can become necrotic.
4. **Zone of Hyperemia** (c): in this outermost zone tissue, perfusion is increased. The tissue here will invariably recover unless there is severe sepsis or prolonged hypoperfusion.

# PHASES OF BURN INJURIES

## EMERGENT Phase:

1. This is the initial pathophysiologic phase of burn injury
2. Immediate problem is fluid loss, edema, reduced blood flow (fluid and electrolyte shifts)
3. Goals: secure airway/ support circulation by fluid replacement/ keep the client comfortable with analgesics/ prevent infection through wound care/ maintain body temperature/ provide emotional support
4. Clinical Manifestations:
   a. Clients with major burn injuries and with inhalation injury are at risk for respiratory problems (Inhalation injuries are present in 20% to 50% of the burn patients.
   b. Burns of the lips, face, ears, neck, eyelids, eyebrows, and eyelashes are strong indicators that an inhalation injury may be present.
   c. Change in the respiratory pattern may indicate a pulmonary injury.
   d. The patient may: become progressively hoarse, develop a brassy cough, drool or have difficulty swallowing, produce expiratory sounds that include audible wheezes, crowing, and stridor.
   e. Upper airway edema and inhalation injury are most common in the trachea and main stem bronchi.
   f. If wheezes disappear, this indicates impending airway obstruction and demands immediate intubation.
   g. Cardiovascular will begin immediately which can include shock (Shock is a common cause of death in the emergent phase in clients with severe burns).
   h. Changes in renal function are related to decreased renal blood flow: urine is usually highly concentrated and has a high specific gravity
   i. Urine output is decreased during the first 24 hours of the emergent phase
   j. Fluid resuscitation is provided at the rate needed to maintain a urine output 0.5-1 cc/kg/hr.
   k. Measure BUN, creatinine, and Na2+ levels
   l. Sympathetic stimulation during the emergent phase causes reduced GI motility and paralytic ileus
   m. Clients with burns of 25% TBSA or who are intubated generally require an NG tube inserted to prevent aspiration and removal of gastric secretions

## ACUTE Phase:

1. In this stage, the patient is hemodynamically stable, has restored capillary permeability and has been showing signs of diuresis.
2. During this time, the emphasis is placed on restoration of the patient's capillary permeability, and the phase continues until the wound is totally closed.
3. The main goal of the acute phase is focused on prevention of infection, wound care, optimum nutrition and physical therapy.

## REHABILITATIVE Phase:

1. The rehabilitative phase is the final phase of managing a burn injury. Most frequently, it overlaps the acute phase, and it continues after hospitalization.
2. The main goals during this phase are helping the patient to gain independence and achieve maximal function.

## CLASSIFICATION OF BURNS

### Superficial Burns

1. These are burns found on the outside perimeters of higher magnitude burns and also from sunburns.
2. Characteristics:
   a. Only epidermis is affected
   b. Red skin, pain at site

### Partial Thickness Burns

1. These are burns that affect both the dermis and the epidermis.
2. Characteristics:
   a. Epidermis & dermis are affected
   b. Blisters, intense pain, white to red skin, moist mottled skin

### Full Thickness Burns

1. These are burns that continue through all 3 layers of the skin; sometimes this classification can include tissue destruction in excess of skin– it can include muscle, fat, and bone.
2. Characteristics:
   a. Epidermis, dermis, muscle, fat affected
   b. Charring, dark brown or white, skin hard to the touch, little or no pain, pain at periphery of burn

# PART 2: BURN ASSESSMENT

## INTRODUCTION

The burn assessment has received quite a lot of scrutiny over the last 10-15 years as prehospital providers were thought to "over-fluid resuscitation" their patients. Over-fluid resuscitation can lead to changes in metabolism that reduces survivability and worsens mortality. It is therefore, important to be as accurate as possible with respect to the burn assessment to be able to make the best clinical decisions possible.

## BURN ASSESSMENT

### Assess Mental Status

1. AVPU:  Awake– eyes open spontaneously; Verbal- arouses to stimulation my voice; Painful- purpose for movements to painful stimuli; Unresponsive- no response to any stimuli
2. Assess GCS
   a. Eye Opening: Spontaneous (4); to speech (3); to painful stimuli (2); no opening at all (0)
   b. Verbal Effort: normal conversation (5);  confused (4); inappropriate words (3); incomprehensible sounds (2); no verbal effort (1)
   c. Motor Effort: follows commands (6); localizes pains (5); withdraws from pain (4); decorticate posturing (3); decerebrate posturing (2); no motor effort (1)

### Airway: Ensure a patent airway.

### Breathing and Respiratory Effort:

1. Note rate
2. quality (normal or labored), and
3. rhythm (normal or abnormal respiratory patterns).

### Circulation:

1. Ensure the patient has a pulse and note the rate, strength (normal, bounding, or weak), and quality (regular or irregular).
2. Obtain and assess heart rate, blood pressure, pulse oximetry, cardiac monitoring, and labs/ images if available.

### Disability:

1. Assess for the ability to move, lift, and hold all 4 extremities. Assess for equal grip and pedal strength. Assess for the ability to maintain a seated posture, standing and walking. Assess for cranial nerve deficits.
2. Identify deficits that existed prior to your assessment.

### Exposure: Expose patient and perform a full exam to rule out life threats.

### Assess for Burn Complications:

#### AIRWAY: Inhalation injury requiring intubation
1. Facial burns/ stridor/ hoarse voice/ carbon deposits around airway/ explosion/ circumferential neck burns/ soot around nose
2. Any of the above findings warrants IMMEDIATE INTUBATION in the burned patient suspected of having inhalation injury.

#### BREATHING:
1. ABG/ High flow O2
2. Circumferential Burns- escharotomy
3. Hypoxia without cyanosis- carbon monoxide poisoning
4. Extreme air hunger with metabolic acidosis- cyanide poisoning
5. Calculate the Anion Gap
6. (Na + K) – (CL + HCO3)
7. 11-16 confirms anion gap metabolic acidosis

#### CIRCULATION
1. HGB- > 10g/dL for flight (transfuse if lower)
2. Circumferential extremity burns- escharotomy

3. Edematous extremities- Tx compartment syndrome

**Rule of Nines**
1. Torso- all the same between the ages: 9% for one arm, 18% for front and 18% for back
2. Head
   a. Adult: 9%
   b. Peds (1-10 ish): 12%
   c. Infant (< 1 y/o): 18%
3. Legs
   a. Adult: 18% per leg
   b. Peds: 16.5% per leg
   c. Infant: 13.5% per leg

# PART 3: FLUID RESUSCITATION CALCULATIONS

## INTRODUCTION

Look. Seriously, this is madness and one of the most difficult topics to find in the literature, potentially because of the medical literature telephone games that happens. If one person reports a procedure incorrectly, then another reports the incorrect procedure in a different way than the previous author, the actual information gets very clouded. I am at risk here too, however at least I am admitting it and talking about the problem. What you want is guidance on how to treat your burned patients. Luckily, the American Burn Association (ABA) has done a lot of the work.

The ABA, however, has a clear picture of fluid resuscitation formulas. They offer clear guidance on most patients. This is a plus in clinical practice, but there is another problem looming for the to-be critical care certified provider- how the certification exams set up burn resuscitation questions. Everyone wants the burn resuscitation formula to use, and it is important to understand, that it isn't just the formula, but how the ABA suggests the formulas are used for clinical practice.

For the IBSC certifications, flight paramedic certification (FP-C) and/or the critical care paramedic certification (CCP-C), the burn formula you should use on these exams depends on how the question is set up. They will ask you to use a particular formula, such as the Modified Brooke or the Parkland formula. Then you simply take the provided patient information (burned percentage and the patient's weight) and make the calculation based on the burn resuscitation formula they provide. For this reason, we will provide the 3 formulas seen on the IBSC exams: Parkland, Modified Brooke, and Consensus formulas. For the Board of Certifications in Emergency Nursing (BCEN), it is a little simpler: they use the Consensus formula.

In 2008, the American Burn Association released a statement mentioning the board's *consensus* that an upper and lower limits of fluid resuscitation should be established. They agreed the 2-4 mL/kg/%BSA burned would be appropriate. These limits were derived from the 2 most common burn formulas at the time: the Parkland formula and the Modified Brooke formula. Originally, the Parkland formula was 4 mL/kg/%BSA burned and the Brooke formula was 1.5 mL/kg/%BSA burned, but the Brooke was later modified to 2 mL/kg/%BSA burned. I am leaving out some important elements of these formulas, but they really do not matter as of now and its best we keep things simple.

## CURRENT FORMULAS

### *CONSENSUS FORMULA*

2-4 mL/kg/%BSA burned

### *MODIFIED BROOKE FORMULA*

2 mL/kg/%BSA burned

### *PARKLAND FORMULA*

4 mL/kg/%BSA burned

## ABA GUIDELINES:

Now, we already said the Consensus formula is 2-4 mL/kg/%BSA burned, but the ABA goes a little further. There isn't just a formula, but an initial fluid rate for prehospital and early hospital care, as well as set conditions to help decide on milliliter value (2, 3, or 4 mL/kg/% BSA burned).

**ALSO- the patient's weight should be in IDEAL BODY WEIGHT, as per the ABA!**

### *INITIAL*

There are 3 initial fluid rate starting points, and they based on weight. The ABA offers this initial rate so you can get fluid resuscitation going while you get the patient prepped for transport. It allows time to prep the patient and to make the needed assessments and calculations. Instead of memorizing all 3, I argue to always memorize the middle set of information when there are ranges. In this case, the ABA calls for:

- 5 years and younger: 125 mL/hr of lactated ringers (LR)
- 6-13 years of age: 250 mL/hr of lactated ringers (LR)
- 14 years or older: 500 mL/hr of lactated ringers (LR)

So, my suggestion is to memorize 6-13 years of age: 250 mL/hr of lactated ringers (LR), and if you have a patient that is younger, you half the rate. If they are older than 14, then you double the rate. Be on the lookout for an update (after 2019) where the ABA provides a guideline based on weight instead of age, but as of now, the guideline is based on age.

### *CALCULATED*

**Adult Thermal and Chemical Burns**
2 mL/kg/%BSA burned

**Pediatric Patients**
3 mL/kg/%BSA burned

**Adults with High Voltage Burns w/ myoglobinuria**
4 mL/kg/%BSA burned

**Pediatrics with High Voltage Burns w/ myoglobinuria**
CALL BURN CENTER/ REIVING PHYSICIAN

## GOALS OF FLUID RESUSCIATION

Fluids should be increased of decreased based on urine output.

### ADULTS/ PEDIATRICS (>30kg)
0.5 mL/kg/hr

### YOUNG CHILDREN (≤ 30 kg)
1 mL/kg/hr

### ADULT-HIGH VOLTAGE w/ Myoglobinuria
75-100 mr/hr (which is between 0.5-1 mL/kg/hr usually)

## THE PROCEDURE

### STEP 1: INITIAL FLUID RATE
1. < 6 years old:125 mL/hr of LR
2. 6-13 years of age: 250 mL/hr of LR
3. > 13 years old: 500 mL/hr of LR

### STEP 2: CALCULATE BSA
1. Tabulate the total body surface area percentage (%TBSA)
2. Use Lund and Bauer or the Rule of Nines

### STEP 3: OBTAIN PATIENT WEIGHT
1. Estimate the weight of the patient.
2. USE IDEAL BODY WEIGHT!

### STEP 4: CALCULATE TOTAL FLUID IN 24 HOURS
1. 2 x KG x %TBSA for adults
2. 3 x KG x %TBSA for peds
3. 4 x KG x %TBSA for adults w/ myoglobinuria.

### STEP 5: DIVIDE BY 2
1. The result is the volume needed in both the FIRST 8 hours as well as the volume needed in the NEXT 16 hours.

### STEP 6: DIVIDE BY 8- this gets the 'per hour' rate
1. The result is the rate to needed to achieve the first 8 hours of fluid needed.
2. ADJUSTMENTS:
   a. This rate should be from the MOMENT of the burn. If there is a delay in fluid resuscitation, then do not divide by 8- divide by the remaining hours left in the first 8 hours.
   b. Example: if the patient was burned 2 hours ago, you'd divide the total volume needed in the first 8 hours by 6 hours, not 8 hours, because 2 hours have already passed.
   c. Also- any fluid administered prior to your fluid resuscitation rate should be accounted for- unless it was used to correct blood pressure.

### STEP 7: AMINISTER THE CALCULATED RATE

# PART 4: NON-THERMAL BURNS

## INTRODUCTION

Look. Seriously, this is madness and one of the most difficult topics to find in the literature, potentially

### *Electrical Burns*

1. Electrical burns are typically classified by their voltage. HIGH voltage is generally thought of as being > 1000 volts with LOW voltage being under 1000 volts.
2. Current is measured in amperes (A) and has 2 major categories: alternating current (AC) and direct current (DC).
3. Electrical Mechanisms:
   a. Current (AC or DC): this results in a direct flow of electricity. AC reverses the flow of electrons every half electrical cycle (absent entrance/ exit wounds). DC flows in only one direction and, therefore, produces entrance and exit wounds.
   b. Arching: this is the ionization of air particles that superheat to over 4000*F, resulting in ignition of clothing and an arching explosion.
   c. Lightning Strikes: a DC current.
4. Conditions to Monitor
   a. Cardiac Arrest– follow ACLS/ PALS.
   b. Muscle Compartment Syndrome– escharotomy or fasciotomy may be required should perfusion become compromised due to a hardening of the skin.
   c. Rhabdomyolysis– electrical burns cause significant cellular damage internally resulting in the massive cellular destruction which can clog the kidneys ( rhabdomyolysis). Continue fluid resuscitation to maintain a urine output of 0.5– 1 cc/kg/hr.

### *Chemical Burns*

1. Sources
   a. Acids: Drain cleaners
   b. Alkali: Rust removers, swimming pool cleaners
   c. Organic compounds (petroleum): Phenols and petroleum cleaners
2. Assessment for Chemical Burns
   a. Erythema
   b. Edema
   c. Blisters
   d. Tissue necrosis
   e. Pain
3. Specific Electrical Burn Management:
   a. Injuries to the Eyes
      i. Copious amounts of water because the chemical can bind with proteins.
      ii. Use of Morgan's lens for a directed irrigation effort.
4. Hydrofluoric Acid
   a. Copious amounts of water
   b. Calcium gluconate (1g) with petroleum jelly (100g)- use topically
5. Anhydrous Ammonia
   a. Copious amounts of water
   b. Irrigate with water until the ammonia smell is gone

### Radiation Burns

1.  You must determine if there has been a radiation exposure and then whether ongoing exposure continues to exist.
2.  Most ionizing radiation accidents involve gamma radiation or X-rays.
3.  Types:
    a.  Alpha: Little penetrating energy, easily stopped by the skin
    b.  Beta: Greater penetrating power, but blocked by simple protective clothing
    c.  Gamma: Very penetrating, easily passes through the body and solid materials
4.  Management:
    a.  Patients with a radioactive source on their body must be initially cared for by a HazMat responder.
    b.  Irrigate open wounds.
    c.  Notify the emergency department.
    d.  Identify the radioactive source and the length of the patient's exposure to it.
    e.  Limit your duration of exposure.
    f.  Increase your distance from the source.
    g.  Attempt to place shielding between yourself and the sources of gamma radiation.

# PART 5: BURN PHARMACOLOGY

## INTRODUCTION

While the medications of burn management are very similar to general trauma pharmacology, there are some specific items that have been added for discussion. On your way to every burn call, not only direct burn management, but also airway management medications should be refreshed in your mind. If airway isn't paramount with a patient, then pain medications and sedatives can help soothe their suffering.

## MEDICATIONS

### Fentanyl

1.  Class: Narcotic/ Analgesic
2.  Mechanism: Competitively binds with narcotic receptors and prevents the sensation of pain.
3.  Indications: pain control
4.  Contraindications: Allergy/ History of rigid chest syndrome
5.  Hemodynamics: (~CVP/ ~PCWP/~CO/~SVR).
6.  Adult Dose: 1-2 mg/kg IV. Peds Dose: 1-2 mg/kg IV.
7.  Very safe hemodynamic profile (does not drop blood pressure much at all).
8.  Can be used in the hypotensive setting when a benzodiazepine would be unsafe for perfusion.

### Morphine

1.  Class: Narcotic/ Analgesic
2.  Mechanism: Competitively binds with narcotic receptors and prevents the sensation of pain.
3.  Indications: pain control
4.  Contraindications: Allergy/ History of rigid chest syndrome
5.  Hemodynamics: (~CVP/ ~PCWP/~CO/↓SVR).
6.  Adult Dose: 2-5 mg IV; Peds Dose: 0.1 –.02 mg/kg
7.  Can precipitously drop blood pressure.

### Ketamine
1. Class: Hypnotic
2. Dose: 1-2 mg/kg IV
3. Indications: sedation; pain control, bronchodilation
4. Contraindications: Allergy/ increased ICP
5. Used as both analgesia and sedation.
6. Ketamine will help to increase BP– ideal in trauma, but not in increased ICP conditions.
7. Ketamine also will reduce bronchospasm

### Versed
1. Class: Benzodiazepine
2. Mechanism: binds to the benzodiazepine receptor and enhances the effects of central nervous system depression.
3. Indications: sedation, anxiety, skeletal muscle relaxation
4. Contraindications: Allergy/ acute angle glaucoma
5. Hemodynamics: ($\downarrow$CVP/ $\downarrow$PCWP/$\downarrow$CO/$\downarrow$SVR).
6. Adult Dose: 1-5 mg IV. Peds Dose: 0.05-0.1 mg/kg IV.

### Ativan
1. Class: Benzodiazepine
2. Mechanism: binds to the benzodiazepine receptor and enhances the effects of central nervous system depression.
3. Indications: sedation, anxiety, skeletal muscle relaxation
4. Contraindications: Allergy/ acute angle glaucoma
5. Hemodynamics: ($\downarrow$CVP/ $\downarrow$PCWP/$\downarrow$CO/$\downarrow$SVR).
6. Adult Dose: 2-4 mg IV. Peds Dose: 0.1 mg/kg IV.

### Silvadene
1. Class: Antimicrobial
2. Mechanism: Silver sulfadiazine has broad antimicrobial activity. It is bactericidal for many gram-negative and gram-positive bacteria as well as being effective against yeast.
3. Indications: Silvadene Cream 1% (silver sulfadiazine) is a topical antimicrobial drug indicated as an adjunct for the prevention and treatment of wound sepsis in patients with second- and third-degree burns.
4. Contraindications: Allergy
5. Dose: The cream should be applied once to twice daily to a thickness of approximately 1/16 inch.

# PART 6: GENERAL BURN MANAGEMENT

## INTRODUCTION
Since burns can manifest in multiple ways, it is important to not just think of burns as a single management strategy, but one that is dynamic and can change. Study and practice through visualization or scenarios to keep up your skills.

## THE GENERAL APPROACH

1. Remove the patient from the burning source.
2. Irrigate: do not irrigate longer than 20 to 30 minutes.
3. Administer high flow oxygen.
4. Remove all wet clothing and linen.
5. Obtain vascular access with multiple large bore IVs.
6. Calculate affected body surface area involving partial and full thickness burns.
   a. This skill must be practiced to mastery.
   b. Once mastered, the skill must be maintained by routine practice probably at least once a month, although there are no studies to corroborate this suggestion.
7. Once body surface area for partial and full thickness burns has been calculated, calculate the fluid resuscitation volumes and rates.
   a. Calculate the fluid required per hour for your patient
      i. Use the formula (2cc)(KG)(% BSA) to obtain the total amount of fluid to be replaced in 24 hours.
      ii. Divide this total by 2 to obtain the amount of fluid to be replaced over the first 8 hours.
      iii. Divide this new total by 8 to identify the expected hourly rate of fluid resuscitation.
   b. Augment any fluid resuscitation based on fluid resuscitation incorrectly administered
      i. Use the above formula to calculate total fluid needed in 8 hours.
      ii. Subtract fluid administered prior to your arrival from this total fluid required in 8 hours.
      iii. Divide this new total by 8 to arrive at the per hour corrected low rate.
   c. Be sure to use warm fluids for fluid resuscitation.
8. Monitor perfusion status (blood pressure and oxygenation) as well as urine output (target 0.5-1 cc/kg/hr).
9. Leave all blisters intact.
10. Administer pain medication and reassess every 10 minutes, or as often as the patient requires.
11. Reassess the infusion, your output, the condition of linens (keep dry), and keep the patient warm.

# PART 8: BURN MANAGEMEMNT QUESTIONS

1. A burned patient presents with the following: patent airway, tachycardia and tachypnea, 22% BSA to the majority of the front half of his body, stridor and hoarse voice, and stable blood pressure. What condition are you most concerned about?
   a. Severe thermal burn
   b. Circumferential burn
   c. Compartment syndrome
   d. Inhalation injury

2. Your patient has experienced a thermal burn from an explosion and presents with the following: awake and alert with a patent airway, 35% BSA affected with full and partial thickness burns, and a BP of 102/64. What condition should be suspected?
   a. Inhalation injury

b.   Circumferential burn

c.   Compartment syndrome

d.   Tension pneumothorax


3.   You arrive on the scene where your patient has suffered a thermal burn. This patient presents with patent airway, (+) radial and carotid pulses- strong, absent pedal pulses, 42% BSA affected with partial thickness burns to the entire surface to both lower extremities. What should immediately be done?

a.   BVM ventilation

b.   Intubation

c.   Escharotomy

d.   Apply dry sheets


4.   You have a severely burned patient (> 90% BSA) on the mechanical ventilator, and the high-pressure alarm sounds after 20 minutes of silence. Which intervention may be indicated?

a.   BVM bagging

b.   Escharotomy

c.   Increase PEEP

d.   Needle chest


5.   You are transporting a patient who was the victim of a house fire. The patient currently has the following vitals: HR 122, RR 26, BP 122/70, SpO2 99%, and the skin is pink/ warm/ dry. Which of the following is the patient most likely experiencing?

a.   CO poisoning

b.   Stagnant hypoxia

c.   Inhalation Injury

d.   Hypovolemia


6.   Your patient is incredibly tachypneic and recently rescued from a house fire. Upon looking into the lab report, you discover these values: Na 144, Ca 10, K 3.9, Glu 102, Cl 100, HCO3 27, BUN 15, H/H 14 and 42. Does this patient exhibit signs of cyanide toxicity?

a.   Yes- metabolic acidosis is present

b.   Yes- the tachypnea alone indicates it

c.   No- the calcium is too low here

d.   No- cyanide isn't produced in fires


7.   A patient was involved in a vehicle fire and inhaled hot gasses. Upon assessment you discover: patent airway, (+) breath sounds with wheezes in the distal airways, calm respiratory effort, and symmetrical chest wall movement. What is the most appropriate next action?

a.   Prepare for CPAP

b.   Cricothyrotomy

c.   BVM ventilations

d.   Bronchodilator

8. The patient you are responding to was involved in an explosion and has suffered burns and bilateral hemothoraces. You discover the following lab values: Na 140, Ca 9, K 4.5, Glu 85, Cl 102, HCO3 22, BUN 11, H/H 9 and 31. What is the most appropriate action?
   a. Needle decompresses
   b. Prepare to intubate
   c. Transfuse PRBCs
   d. Place a central line

9. Fluid resuscitation has begun for a 75kg patient with 23% partial thickness burns. The burn was 2 hours ago, and the sending facility has infused 350cc LR. What does the astute critical care clinician recognize in reference to fluid resuscitation?
   a. Not enough information
   b. Adequate and appropriate
   c. Inadequate- 200cc low
   d. Inadequate- 81cc low

10. Fluid resuscitation has begun for a 92kg patient with 31% partial thickness burns. The burn was 4 hours ago, and the sending facility has infused 1500cc LR. What does the astute critical care clinician recognize in reference to fluid resuscitation?
    a. Inadequate- 81cc low
    b. Adequate and appropriate
c. Inadequate- 200cc low
    d. Not enough information

11. As you are reviewing the chart of the 85kg burn patient you are about to transport to a larger hospital, the RN reports the following: HR 99, RR 18, BP 118/72, SpO2 99%, EtCO2 41, temp 37C, Na 141, K 3.9, Cl 101, HCO3 22, BUN 15, Glu 94, Cr 0.9, UO 35cc/h, H/H 15 and 45. What is the next most appropriate action?
    a. Prepare mag infusion
    b. Prepare to intubate pt
    c. No changes are needed
    d. Increase isotonic fluids

12. As you are reviewing the chart of the 85kg burn patient you are about to transport to a larger hospital, the RN reports the following: HR 87, RR 15, BP 141/82, SpO2 97%, EtCO2 44, temp 37C, Na 144, K 4.1, Cl 104, HCO3 24, BUN 13, Glu 97, Cr 0.8, UO 33cc/h, H/H 17 and 47. What is the next most appropriate action?
    a. Increase isotonic fluids
    b. Prepare to intubate pt
    c. No changes are needed
    d. Prepare mag infusion

# PART 9: BURN MANAGEMENT RATIONALES

1. **(D)** The key here is the stridor and hoarse voice in a patient who was burned. This indicates an inhalation injury, and the patient should be intubated right away.

2. **(A)** The key here is the explosion. This indicates an inhalation injury is potentially present, and the continued assessment should be looking for those tell-tale findings indicating inhalation injury: facial burns/ stridor/ hoarse voice/ carbon deposits around airway circumferential neck burns/ soot around the nose.

3. **(C)** The loss of pedal pulses is key in this case and indicates the arterial blood supply to the feet are compromised by the circumferential burn.

4. **(B)** The patient is 90% burned, so circumferential burns are likely. The critical care clinician needs to be prepared for poor chest expansion due to these circumferential burns. This would cause peak inspiratory pressure to rise and alarm. If the high pressure is due to the hardening skin from the circumferential burn, then an escharotomy is indicated. BVM/ needle chest/increase PEEP- wrong because it would not fix the rigidity of the chest. The chest needs to be cut to allow for chest wall expansion .

5. **(A)** The HR and RR indicate the body is increasing efforts to push oxygen forward (a sign of hypoxia), but the skin is warm and pink (non- cyanotic). If you take these two pieces of information with the history of a house fire, then you have a situation consistent with CO poisoning. Stagnant hypoxia is when blood isn't moving forward as it should, there is nothing here to suggest an inhalation injury, and BP is normal, so hypovolemia is unlikely.

6. **(A)** Remember, air hunger (tachypnea) with metabolic acidosis indicates cyanide poisoning/ toxicity, so when given the components of the anion gap, be sure to calculate it. In this case, (144 + 3.9) - (100 + 27) = 21. Since the anion gap is > 16, then metabolic acidosis is evident. This information considered with the history of a house fire and air hunger confirms the diagnosis of cyanide toxicity.

7. **(D)** Wheezes indicate bronchoconstriction, so use bronchodilators to open them up. Don't rush to cut the neck here- try a less invasive therapy. BVM ventilations seems overkill here too because they are breathing calmly, indicating they are not acutely hypoxic. CPAP could worsen bronchoconstriction.

8. **(C)** The H/H is your indicator and specifically the hemoglobin (it's 9 here), therefore a transfusion is necessary. We have no information here to indicate intubation because we don't know mental or hemodynamic status. Needle decompression won't correct a hemothorax- chest tubes are needed. A central line is not an absolute in this case, sure it would help, but the correct answer is to transfuse some RBCs.

9. **(D)** The consensus formula is (2cc x %BSA x KG), so in this case we get (2cc x 23 x 75) = 3450cc to be given in 24 hours. Half this total volume is 1725 cc and is to be given in the first 8 hours. (1725cc/8h  = 215cc/h, so in 2 hours the patient should have received 430cc, but they only received 350 cc (430- 350 = deficit of 80cc), therefore, the answer is 81cc low .

10. **(B)** The consensus formula is (2cc x %BSA x KG), so in this case we get (2cc x 31 x 92) = 5704cc to be given in 24 hours. Half this total volume is 2852 cc and is to be given in the first 8 hours. (2852cc/8h  = 356cc/h, so in 4 hours the patient should have received 1426cc. They received 1500cc; thus, the fluid resuscitation is adequate.

11. **(D)** The key here is the low urine output (UO) of 35cc/hr. Adequate fluid resuscitation in a burn patient would be indicated by a UO of 0.5-1cc/kg/min. In this case, 85kg x 0.5cc/hr = 42.5cc/h. It is reported that the patient has a UO of 35cc/hr or a deficit of 7cc/hr. Therefore, we need to increase the fluids to meet this minimum UO.

12. **(C)** The key here is the low urine output (UO) of 33cc/hr. Adequate fluid resuscitation in a burn patient would be indicated by a UO of 0.5-1cc/kg/min. In this case, 65kg x 0.5cc/hr = 32.5cc/h. It is reported that the patient has a UO of 33cc/hr. Additionally, all other values are normal; therefore, no changes are needed.

# CHAPTER 6: ENVIRONMENTAL EMERGENCIES

## PART 1: THE ENVIRONMENTAL ASSESSMENT

### INTRODUCTION

The environment poses several different conditions that affect the human body. You will face these calls and need to be able to quickly differentiate these conditions so you can treat them efficiently and effectively. The critical care transport professional can significantly impact patient outcomes positively by quickly recognizing when an environmental emergency is present and by executing the correct management strategies early.

### THE INITIAL ASSESSMENT

#### *GENERAL IMPRESSION*

1.  As you approach the patient, look at their body position, work of breathing and skin condition and color.
2.  Their body position provides important information: tripod means they are short of breath/ hypoxic, laying on the ground with weak muscles mean they are extremely hypoxic or intoxicated.
3.  Normal respiratory effort indicates they are receiving adequate oxygen, but labored respirations indicates they are hypoxic.
4.  Normal skin color indicates adequate perfusion, but pale or mottled skin can indicate poor perfusion.

#### *Assess Mental Status*

1.  AVPU:  Awake– eyes open spontaneously; Verbal- arouses to stimulation by voice; Painful- purpose for movements to painful stimuli; Unresponsive- no response to any stimuli
2.  Assess GCS
    a.  Eye Opening: Spontaneous (4); to speech (3); to painful stimuli (2); no opening at all (0)
    b.  Verbal Effort: normal conversation (5);  confused (4); inappropriate words (3); incomprehensible sounds (2); no verbal effort (1)
    c.  Motor Effort: follows commands (6); localizes pains (5); withdraws from pain (4); decorticate posturing (3); decerebrate posturing (2); no motor effort (1)
    d.  Max score is 15. Coma is 8 or less. Dead is 3.

#### *Airway: Ensure a patent airway.*

#### *Breathing and Respiratory Effort:*

1.  Note rate
2.  Quality (normal or labored)
3.  Rhythm (normal or abnormal respiratory patterns).

#### *Circulation:*

1.  Ensure the patient has a pulse and note the rate, strength (normal, bounding, or weak), and quality (regular or irregular).

2.  Obtain and assess heart rate, blood pressure, pulse oximetry, cardiac monitoring, and labs/ images if available.

### Disability:
1.  Assess for the ability to move, lift, and hold all 4 extremities. Assess for equal grip and pedal strength. Assess for the ability to maintain a seated posture, standing and walking. Assess for cranial nerve deficits.
2.  Identify deficits that existed prior to your assessment.

### Exposure: Expose patient and perform a head to toe r/o life threats.
1.  Expose that patient and rule out life threats
2.  Remove them from a hot or cold environment

# PART 2: ENVIRONMENTAL EMRGENCIES

## INTRODUCTION

The ultimate goal in the focused environmental assessment is to identify and then immediately manage any life threats and to remove them from a harmful environment. Examples would include apnea or tension pneumothorax because they would need to be fixed RIGH AWAY or the patient could die. Continue considering using the PAM method of assessment.

## HEAT-RELATED CONDITIONS

### Heat Cramps
1.  Patho: exertion--> profuse sweating--> sodium loss--> abdomen/ lower extremity cramping
2.  S/S: cramping (in abd and lower ext); profuse sweating; poor sodium replacement; prolonged time exerting self in hot environment
3.  MGT: remove from hot environment; replace sodium PO (if no aspiration risk); consider 1-2 L NS (if no hyponatremia present)

### Heat Syncope
1.  Patho: prolonged standing or lying in the heat--> upon movement from this position peripheral vasodilation occurs--> vertigo/ dizziness/ syncope
2.  S/S: hx of being in heat (standing or lying); syncopal episode/ fainting spell; (+) volume depletion (sweating/ dehydration thought to be an etiology)
3.  MGT: Remove from heat; recovery position prn; provide PO fluids (if no aspiration risk); manage ABCs as appropriate. Consider IV fluids.

### Heat Exhaustion
1.  Patho: heat exposure and exertion--> causes sodium loss and vasodilation (from dehydration)--> cramping and syncope together
2.  S/S: Profuse sweating; pale, cool clammy skin; dark brown urine; HA; Dizziness; cramping; low EtCO2 with carpopedal spasm (from hyperventilation); Temp 100.4-104°F
3.  MGT: remove from heat and excess clothing; elevate legs; rehydrate w/ sports drinks (if no aspiration risk); IV/ O2/ monitor; obtain blood samples and consider IV fluids; AVOID: antipyretics, active cooling; consider benzos for uncontrolled muscle movements

210

## Heat Stroke

1. Patho Types
2. Types
   a. Classic: high ambient temp--> elderly/ peds/ chronically ill very susceptible--> physiologic thermolysis occurs (body turns off heat production)--> chronic illness/ medications/ age extremes prevent heat loss--> temp continues to rise--> hyperthermia--> damage to hypothalamus with AMS--> coma--> death
   b. Exertional: an active person exerting himself in high ambient temp with humidity--> ambient temp reaches that of the body--> convection/ radiation are no longer effective--> humidity (>75%) slows down evaporative cooling (from sweating) heat continues to rise unchecked--> hyperthermia--> damage to hypothalamus with AMS--> coma--> death
3. S/S: red, dry skin; AMS (irritable, confused, or coma); temp > 104°F; constricted pupils; Sz; posturing
4. MGT: remove from heat/ excessive clothing; IV/ O2/ Monitor; fan pt/ sponge water on the pt (improves evaporation/ convection); active cooling (ice packs to neck, axilla, groin); consider fluids- lactated ringers; prepare for Sz management; prepare to protect airway as needed; stop the cooling process once your patient reaches 102° F- further: could result in rebound hypothermia.

# COLD EMERGENCIES

## Frostbite

1. Superficial: cold temps (>32°F)--> prolonged exposure--> develops slowly--> slows blood flow and nervous response--> capillaries can leak--> local edema--> burning sensation can occur for weeks after event
2. Deep: cold temps (< 32°F)--> prolonged exposure--> fluid in cells form ice crystals--> damages cell walls--> sludging effect of blood (high viscosity, thrombus, ischemia)--> upon warming, skin becomes purple and very painful--> gangrene--> digit/ extremity loss
3. S/S: history of cold exposure; extremity/ digit is hard, cold, and waxy; white- yellow colored skin; mottled blue- white skin also a variant
4. MGT: remove from cold; minimize patient movements; AVOID massaging frostbitten tissue; transport time < 1 hour– leave the part frozen; If > 1 hour transport time consider active rewarming (submerge part in 95-104°F water; establish IV and administer pain meds, dry once thawed, dress part).

## Hypothermia

1. Patho: exposure to cold temps--> alcohol/ malnutrition/ thyroid dz exacerbates--> mild hypothermia (increased HR/ BP, "umbles")--> glycogen stores run out and things slow down--> severe hypothermia (HR/ BP lowers, vasoconstriction, cold diuresis, fluids shift from vasculature to extracellular spaces)--> repeated defib and medications are not effective at 30°C--> arrhythmia/ poor conduction at 28°C--> coma--> death
2. S/S: temp < 95°F; shivering (or absent at 91°F); "umbles" (stumbles, mumbles, fumbles, grumbles); increased HR/BP/cardiac output (above 90°F); decreased HR/BP/cardiac output (below 90°F); cardiac arrhythmias; Osborne waves (notching between Q wave and T wave)
3. MGT: Remove pt from environment and remove wet clothing; dry pt; warm pt; IV/O2/Monitor; consider warmed IV fluids, warmed humidified O2, and/or peritoneal lavage of a KCL-free solution; Avoid repeated defib until their temp is >86°F; give ACLS meds more frequently if temp between 86-93.2°F; hold ACLS meds until temp >86°F.

| Umble: | Core Temp | Type of Hypothermia | Description |
|---|---|---|---|
| Fumbles | 98.6-95°F | Mild | One of the first signs of hypothermia is an inability to perform complex tasks with your hands. Blood is shunted away from your extremities and your hands become numb as you lose dexterity in fine motor control. |
| Stumbles | 95-90°F | Moderate | Below 95°F it becomes increasingly difficult to walk. Movements become slow and labored. |
| Mumbles | 95-90°F | Moderate | Speaking also requires focus and extra effort. Speaking is difficult and slurred. Sluggish thinking and confusion become apparent. |
| Crumbles | $\leq$ 90°F | Severe | You lose the ability to walk. Your body stops shivering in a last-ditch effort to conserve energy. Your behavior becomes extremely confused and increasingly incoherent. |

## WATER EMERGENCIES

### Drowning

1. Patho: water into lungs or stopped at spasmodic larynx--> significantly reduces gaseous O2--> anaerobic metabolism--> acid production--> failing physiology/ chemistry from acid/ waste build up--> AMS--> coma--> death
2. Freshwater: water moves from alveoli to the vascular space (osmotic pull)—> this movement destroys surfactant—> atelectasis—> shunting—> ventilation-perfusion (VQ) mismatch
3. Saltwater: Immediate washout of surfactant—> exudate—> blocks small airways—> shunt—> VQ mismatch
4. S/S: spinal stabilization (you never know if they dove in and injured spine)--> IV/O2/Monitor--> consider ETT placement--> set increased PEEP on vent (pushes water from interstitial space into capillaries)-> consider beta-2 agonist to reduce bronchospasm
5. MGT: IV/O2/Monitor; rapid transport to a facility with HBOT (hyperbaric O2 therapy)
6. Drowning vs. Near-Drowning
   a. Drowning: death from being submerged in a liquid within 24 hours of submersion.
   b. Near– drowning: surviving submersion 24 hours after the incident

### Diving Problems

**Decent Problems:**
1. As a diver descends, pressure is applied to his body in greater and greater amounts.
2. Increased pressure can rupture the tympanic membrane (ear drum) as well as the inner ear.
3. Sinus Squeeze: descending to depth—> pressure applied to body (sinuses)—> shrinking sinus space is replaced by fluid (tissue fluid or blood)—> leads to infections after resurfacing
4. Prevent these issues by purging (breathing against closed nostrils which forces air out of your Eustachian tube and equalizes pressure) on descent. Also, avoid diving while ill with a cold.

**Ascent Problems: Decompression illness (DCI)**
1. As a diver ascends, compressed gasses begin expanding.
2. Since the air that divers breathe is mostly nitrogen (N), if they come up too fast nitrogen can come out from being dissolved in body fluids and collects in different anatomical locations. This leads to specific pathophysiologic conditions.

a. Bends: results from mild DCI; nitrogen collects in the joints and causes pain; aka "Diver's paralysis".
b. Creeps: nitrogen collects along nerve tracks giving the sensation of pins and needles.
c. Chokes: results from moderate DCI; nitrogen collects in airways causing micro–pulmonary emboli
d. Staggers: results from severe DCI; this is where nitrogen is coming out of the patient's body fluids in such amounts that it begins to cause mini– cerebral emboli (strokes)
e. The key here is a diver is trained to ascend from a depth slowly, and proportional to their length of dive and depth (among other variables, but those are the more important ones).

**S/S: S/S:**

Hypoxia; fatigue; weakness; AMS; HA; dyspnea; joint pain (bends); itchy skin or paresthesia (creeps), dyspnea and coughing (chokes); altered mentation & unstable gait (staggers); tachycardia

**MGT:**

Maintain ABCs, return to depth (if ascending) or deliver to a hyperbaric chamber (if already ascended).

# HIGH-ALTITUDE ILLNESS

## BACKGROUND

1. **HIGH** altitude is between 5,000 ft and 11,500 ft, and altitude illness can happen beginning at 8,000ft.
2. **VERY HIGH** altitude is between 11.5K and 18K ft, which can result in oxygen saturation less than 90% and PaO2 of less than 60 mmHg.
3. **EXTREME** altitude is above 18K feet where oxygen is required (mostly) and extreme hypoxias and hypocarbias will be seen.

## CONDITIONS

1. Patho Types: High altitude pulmonary edema (HAPE) vs. High altitude cerebral edema (HACE)
2. Types:
   a. HACE: low partial pressures of O2--> hypoxia--> reduced Na+ transport that normally drives the re-absorption of capillary ultra-filtrate --> EDEMA --> HA/AMS/ataxia/Sz
   b. HAPE: low partial pressures of O2--> hypoxia--> reduced Na+ transport that normally drives the re-absorption of capillary ultra-filtrate --> fluid not reabsorbed as well combined with increased vasculature pressure due to hypoxia--> pink, frothy sputum indicating pulmonary edema
3. S/S: Hypoxia; fatigue; weakness; AMS; HA; dyspnea; pulmonary edema; chest pain; tachycardia
4. MGT: IV/O2/Monitor; DESCEND; Dexamethasone 4-8 mg; Albuterol; Nifedipine 30 mg (↓ pulmonary vascular pressure); Lasix 20-40 mg; **RAPID** transport to a facility with HBOT (hyperbaric O2 therapy) in severe cases or use portable pressure chamber.

# PART 3: ENVIRONMENTAL CONDITION QUESTIONS

1. You are transporting your patient from a motor vehicle accident scene in January. As you are leaving the ground, you remind your orientee to be careful with the patient and to avoid jostling them. This is because the patient is susceptible to which of the following?
   1. Rewarming shock
   2. Status epilepticus
   3. Myocardial infarction
   4. Ventricular fibrillation

2. Your heat stroke patient has myoglobinuria. What is the best treatment for this condition?
   a. Monitor oxygen saturation
   b. Aggressive fluid therapy
   c. Administer glycogen
   d. Administer H2 blockers

3. Severe hypothermia is recognized as a body temperature below what temperature (in degrees Fahrenheit)?
   a. 93
   b. 86
   c. 82
   d. 90

4. Your patient is a hiker who got caught in a snow storm. They were discovered with frostbitten feet and hands. As you approach the patient in the ER, you note the patient is lying down on the bed, the family is rubbing his hands to keep them warm, and the patient has pushed off the blanket from covering him. Which of the following is the most appropriate response to this situation?
   a. Replace the blanket to cover patient
   b. Receive report and transport patient
   c. Ask family to stop rubbing hands
   d. Have the family sit up the patient

5. You arrive to help rescue a patient who has fallen from a ravine in February near Seattle. Once the patient has been accessed, you notice that they stop shivering. You immediately know their core temperature to be which of the following?
   a. 86° F
   b. 91° F
   c. 93° F
   d. 89° F

6. A 17-year old female drove off a cliff into a frozen lake. Thirty–five minutes later, the fire department extricated the patient and found her to be unconscious and pulseless. The patient's pupils were fixed and dilated, and the skin was cold to touch. The vehicle had been filled with water. Which of the following is the most appropriate action?

a. Support ventilations and withhold CPR
b. Call the time of death and the coroner
c. Begin CPR and attempt to re-warm patient
d. Begin CPR immediately and transport

7. You arrive to find your patient in a cold environment with an altered mental status. If the patient was only suffering from hypothermia, then you could assume the patient's temperature (in degrees Celsius) to be lower than which of the following?
a. 32
b. 34
c. 30
d. 28

8. Your patient is an unconscious homeless person who had been found outside in the cold. He responds to only painful stimuli and is very cold to the touch. The patient presents with the following: HR 50, BP 80/40, and RR 6. Which of the following is the most appropriate management for this patient?
a. Active rewarming
b. Assist ventilations
c. Apply ECG monitor
d. Intubate the patient

9. You confirm that your hypothermic patient is in cardiac arrest. At what temperature (in degrees F) can you begin administering medications?
a. 86
b. 82
c. 90
d. 93

10. A football player experiences heat stroke in the middle of two-a-day practices in August. What would be your most likely finding?
a. Hyponatremia
b. Hyperglycemia
c. Hypokalemia
d. Hypercalcemia

11. Your hypothermic patient is < 30 degrees Celsius. What characteristic finding would you expect to see on a 12-lead ECG?
a. Delta wave
b. Dicrotic notch
c. Osborne waves
d. Slurred R wave

12. You're transporting a 35-year old male found by a friend unconscious in a non- air conditioned house. The patient was presented to the ER unresponsive to verbal and painful stimuli; dry flushed and warm skin; and a history of alcoholism. The ambient temperature has reportedly been over 100° F for about a week. Which of the following is your primary goal with respect to treatment?
    a. Administer 100% O2
    b. Stimulate sweating
    c. Lower temp to 102
    d. Provide fluid bolus

13. Heat stroke is recognized as a body temperature above what temperature (in degrees Fahrenheit)?
    a. >103
    b. >106
    c. >105
    d. >104

14. A 69-year old female with a history of heart disease and type two diabetes was found unconscious in her backyard on a July afternoon. The temperature had been 104° F for about six days. Currently, the patient presents with hot, dry skin and rapid & labored respirations. A neighbor claims that she had been acting funny all day. Which of the following conditions is the patient most likely suffering from?
    a. Major heat syncope
    b. Exertional heat stroke
    c. Mild heat cramps
    d. Classic heat stroke

15. A flight request comes out to a local lake used as a SCUBA training site. The 37-year old was at depth and panicked when his mask filled up with water and he could not clear it. He rapidly surfaced and lost consciousness immediately. Which of the following is most likely to happen?
    a. massive electrical discharge
    b. severe brain herniation
    c. Immediate cerebral edema
    d. Cerebral vascular accident

# PART 4: ENVIRONMENTAL CONDITION RATIONALES

1. **(A)** Ultimately, myoglobinuria should be treated with lots of fluids to prevent blockage within the kidney itself.
2. **(C)** This is simply a memorization question. You'll need to know the various temperatures that relate to physiological changes in your environmental emergency patient.
3. **(C)** You should never rub frozen body parts. Ice crystals form in the frostbitten tissues. Rubbing a frostbitten area will move the ice crystals in the tissues, causing trauma and worsening the injury.

4. **(B)** As a patient's body temperature continues to drop, once they reach 91° F, shivering stops. Commit this temperature and concept to memory.

5. **(D)** You should begin CPR immediately and transport the patient. After a patient has been submerged in cold water, the effects of hypothermia and the mammalian diving reflex will increase the time during which the patient could be successfully resuscitated. Rewarming severely hypothermic patients must begin from the core and work outward to prevent lactic acid wash out. Once vasoconstriction in the periphery is relieved from rewarming, the periphery opens and dumps all of the previously sequestered lactic acid into systemic circulation causing near-immediate acidosis. Therefore, the answer to this question involves being giving CPR immediately WITHOUT rewarming the patient.

6. **(A)** This is simply a memorization question. You'll need to know the various temperatures that relate to physiological changes in your environmental emergency patient.

7. **(B)** The best answer, in this case, is to assist ventilations. Even though we do not know the exact temp, cold to touch with depressed vital signs indicates an advanced hypothermic state. Anytime all vitals drop because of hypothermia; it must be an advanced progression of the pathophysiology. When patients are this cold, then active re-warming is contraindicated until the patients are warmed passively. Rewarming too early will cause a reduction of peripheral vasoconstriction and the release of lots of lactic acid into central circulation.

8. **(A)** This is simply a memorization question. You'll need to know the various temperatures that relate to physiological changes in your environmental emergency patient.

9. **(A)** A key piece of information here is the fact that this is a football player practicing twice a day in August. Football players drink a lot of hypotonic fluids (water), which can stimulate hyponatremia. Additionally, player sweats a lot of sodium out. Sodium loss to sweat and drinking hypotonic fluids both suggest hyponatremia. The liver will usually release glucose in lower glucose states unless the liver is damaged. It is safe to assume that this patient most likely has a healthy liver. Hyperkalemia is not the same thing as heat stroke, however, the answer selection in this question is hypokalemia. Therefore, it is an incorrect answer selection. Hypocalcemia typically occurs because dense muscle will bind more calcium, however, in this case, the answer selection is "hypercalcemia", therefore it is an incorrect answer selection.

10. **(C)** An Osbourne wave is characterized by a notch found to the right of the QRS waveform in the last third of the QRS complex. It is a confirmation of severe hypothermia.

11. **(C)** The primary goal here is to reduce your patient's core body temperature to 102° F. This is where the cooling process should stop because it continues residually, even after you have stopped the cooling process. If you continue to cool lower than the 102° F benchmark, then you could potentially make the patient hypothermic.

12. **(D)** This is simply a memorization question. You'll need to know the various temperatures that relate to physiological changes in your environmental emergency patient.

13. **(B)** This patient seems to be suffering from classic heat stroke. Classic heat stroke tends to occur in patients with chronic health problems that interfere with the body's ability to move heat. Classic heat stroke is characterized by altered mental status and hot, dry skin.

14. **(D)** As you breathe gas under water (and thus under pressure), nitrogen bubbles are forced to dissolve into the blood. You are supposed to come up slowly so that nitrogen can slowly un-dissolve out of the blood. If you come out rapidly, then emboli can occur. This patient is experiencing a neurological event, therefore, with this mechanism, it's strongly suggestive that the patient is experiencing a CVA from a cerebral embolus.

# CHAPTER 7: GENERAL MEDICAL

## PART 1: THE MEDICAL ASSESSMENT

### INTRODUCTION

There are so many conditions that you will face as a critical care clinician, and most will not be isolated. We typically study conditions as if they manifest solely on their own, but your experience (even if you just started in this field) probably dictates that isolated conditions in critical care are more rare than complex and compounding clinical situations. This section will dive into some of the most common medical conditions seen in critical care.

### INITIAL ASSESSMENT

#### *GENERAL IMPRESSION*

1. As you approach the patient, look at their body position, work of breathing and skin condition and color.
2. Their body position tells you great information: tripod means they are short of breath/ hypoxic, laying on the ground with weak muscles means they are extremely hypoxic.
3. Normal respiratory effort indicates they are receiving adequate oxygen, but labored respirations indicates they are hypoxic.
4. Normal skin color indicates adequate perfusion, but pale or mottled skin can indicate poor perfusion.

#### *Assess Mental Status*

1. AVPU: Awake– eyes open spontaneously; Verbal- arouses to stimulation by voice; Painful- purpose for movements to painful stimuli; Unresponsive- no response to any stimuli
2. Assess GCS
   a. Eye Opening: Spontaneous (4); to speech (3); to painful stimuli (2); no opening at all (0)
   b. Verbal Effort: normal conversation (5); confused (4); inappropriate words (3); incomprehensible sounds (2); no verbal effort (1)
   c. Motor Effort: follows commands (6); localizes pains (5); withdraws from pain (4); decorticate posturing (3); decerebrate posturing (2); no motor effort (1)

#### *Airway*

1. Ensure a patent airway.
2. Utilize basic or advanced measured as needed.

#### *Breathing*

1. Note rate,
2. Quality (normal or labored)
3. Rhythm (normal or abnormal respiratory patterns).

#### *Circulation*

1. Ensure the patient has a pulse
2. Note Rate

      a. Strength (normal, bounding, or weak)

      b. Quality (regular or irregular).

      c. Obtain and assess heart rate, blood pressure, pulse oximetry, cardiac monitoring, and labs/ images if available.

## *Disability*

1. Assess for the ability to move, lift, and hold all 4 extremities. Assess for equal grip and pedal strength. Assess for the ability to maintain a seated posture, standing and walking. Assess for cranial nerve deficits.
2. Identify deficits that existed prior to your assessment.

## *Exposure*

1. Expose patient
2. Perform a full exam to rule out life threats.

# PART 2: COMMON MEDICAL CONDITIONS

## INTRODUCTION

You will be exposed, repeatedly, to moderately complex medical conditions, and at times, you will be forced to contend with a highly complex medical situation. Fix what you can fix and treat what you can treat. Use medical control if needed.

Consider using a system I use to study where I know the 3 domains of a medical condition: Pathophysiology, Assessment (S/S), and Management, or PAM for short. If you know the pathophysiology of a condition, you should be able to describe the signs and symptoms, as well as how to manage the condition. Similarly, if you are provided with a series of treatments, you should be able to backtrack (usually with a little history) what the pathophysiology is and therefore how to identify it. Finally, if someone gives you a set of signs and symptoms, then you should be able to identify the condition and the management. So, you see, from any of these domains are known, then you should be able to figure out the other two. Therefore, we will study the content in this way.

## MEDICAL CONDITIONS

### *Allergy*

1. Patho: An immunologic hypersensitivity reaction: allergen into system (medication/ substance)--> the immune system recognizes the drug molecule as dangerous--> activates the immune response--> immune system tries to neutralize it .
2. S/S: LOCAL: itching; hives; flushing. Systemic: bronchospasm; laryngeal edema; shock; LABS: increased IgE levels
3. MGT: LOCAL: Benadryl (combats histamine response); SYSTEMIC: Airway management (Albuterol 2.5 mg for bronchospasm); Epinephrine (raises BP, opens airway, reduces edema), Corticosteroids (decrease inflammation)

## Hemophilia

1. Patho: a genetic disorder--> low amounts of clotting factor--> prevents stabilization of a platelet plug--> excessive internal and external bleeding can occur.
2. Causes:
    a. Hemophilia A→ Factor VIII deficiency
    b. Hemophilia B→ Factor IX deficiency
3. S/S: tendency to bruise, excessive bleeding from minor cuts, bruises, and abrasions; labs show prolonged PTT but NORMAL PT and bleeding time
4. MGT: maximize oxygenation; avoid ASA/ antiplatelet meds; admin factor VIII or IX; if specific factors not available- admin cryoprecipitate

## Sickle Cell (vaso-occlusive) Crisis

1. Patho: genetic disorder--> sickling RBCs--> Logjam of sickled cells obstructs blood flow at entrance of capillary beds--> vasospasm occurs--> vascular occlusion causes ischemia--> ischemia causes distal hypoxia ( lactic acidosis)--> cellular injury--> organ infarction .
2. S/S: Finger swelling; pain in back/ extremities; priapism; elevated reticulocyte count (replacing sickled cells)
3. MGT: ABCs; Pain management; Fluids, fluids, fluids

## Acute Chest Syndrome

1. Patho: (mimics pneumonia): low hemoglobin--> clumping of cells in the lungs--> decreased gas exchange--> hypoxia--> further sickling .
2. S/S: fever, cough, chest pain, shortness of breath, and decreased oxygenation; Increased WBC; (+) pulmonary infiltrates on X-ray
3. MGT: ABCs; Pain management; bronchodilators; steroids; antibiotics; fluid resuscitation; transfusion

## Disseminated Intravascular Coagulation

1. Patho: (sepsis/ massive hemorrhage/ burns/ CA)--> endothelial lining of blood vessels damaged--> coagulation factors triggered--> coagulation factors used up--> more bleeding; microvascular clots also formed and cause ischemia .
2. S/S: Ecchymosis, prolonged bleeding, petechial hemorrhages, depleted clotting factors, mucous membrane hemorrhage, (+) increased PT/ PTT, fibrin split products, and D-dimer
3. MGT: Treat the underlying cause; maximize oxygenation; transfuse platelets, FFP; cryoprecipitate

## Potassium (Norm: 3.5– 4.5 mEq/L)

### Hyperkalemia (> 4.5 mEq/L)

1. Patho: excess potassium in the bloodstream; mostly excreted by kidney, so renal failure pts are at risk for hypoxia ( lactic acidosis)--> cellular injury--> organ infarction.
2. S/S: Numbness/ weakness, reduced reflexes, K+ >5.0mmol/L; ECG changes (tall, peaked T waves- widening QRS); BUN/Cr (to r/o RF)
3. MGT: Stabilize cardiac membrane with calcium; move K intracellularly (insulin, D50, beta agonists, HCO3); increase K excretion (K wasting diuretics, resin binders that pull K out with the stool, dialysis)

### Hypokalemia (< 3.5 mEq/L)

1. Patho: excess renal loss, decreased potassium intake.
2. S/S: Numbness/ weakness, ECG changes (flattened T waves, U waves present); (+) hypomagnesimia or hypophosphatemia helps confirm this electrolyte issue
3. MGT: replace K+ slowly; 10 mEq/L should ↑ serum K+ by 0.1 mEq/L.

## Calcium (Norm: 8.5– 10.5 mEq/L)

### Hypercalcemia (> 10.5 mEq/L)
1. Patho: Increased calcium in the blood due to a multitude of metabolic conditions
2. S/S: altered mental status, low blood pressure, hypotonia
3. MGT: ABCs; NS fluids; calcitonin; loop diuretics

### Hypocalcemia (< 8.5 mEq/L)
1. Patho: allows sodium to move into excitable cells; results in increased nerve excitability and sustained muscle contraction (tetany); this can occur in renal failure patients.
2. S/S: Trousseau's and Chvostek's sign; Decreased cardiac output, prolonged QT interval, and may develop ventricular tachycardia
3. MGT: Treat the cause; Oral or IV supplements

## Metabolic Acidosis
1. Patho: a condition characterized by a deficiency of bicarbonate ions in the body in relation to the amount of acid in the body, in which the pH falls to less than 7.35
2. S/S: Low pH with $HCO_3$ < 22; (+) anion gap >20; elevated lactate; (+) etiology from MUDPILES
3. MGT: ABCs; maintain hemodynamics with fluids and inotropes; specific txs: (methanol/ ethylene glycol OD- dialyze/ ethanol; uremia- dialysis, iron OD- dialyze)

## Metabolic Alkalosis
1. Patho: a condition characterized by an excess of bicarbonate ions in the body in relation to the amount of acid in the body; the pH rises to greater than 7.45
2. S/S: High pH and $HCO_3$ >26; Weakness, Muscle cramps; Hyperactive reflexes; Tetany; Confusion; Convulsions; Atrial tachycardia;
3. MGT: ABCs; Tx underlying cause; Normal Saline to replace volume; KCl if it needs to be replaced

## Respiratory Acidosis
1. Patho: A drop in blood pH due to hypoventilation (too little breathing) and a resulting accumulation of $CO_2$.
2. S/S: Low pH and $pCO_2$ >45; drowsiness, disorientation, dizziness, HA, coma, decreased BP, warm flushed skin, seizures hypoventilation with hypoxia
3. MGT: ABCs; increase minute ventilation, consider CPAP, treat underlying cause

## Respiratory Alkalosis
1. Patho: A rise in blood pH due to hyperventilation (excessive breathing) and a resulting decrease in $CO_2$.
2. S/S: High pH and $CO_2$ < 35; hyperventilation; dizziness, paresthesias, muscle spasms (carpopedal spasms), seizures, and coma.
3. MGT: ABCs; treat underlying cause; coach to slow down ventilations

## Diabetic Ketoacidosis
1. Patho: (T1 DM) Insulin deficiency--> hyperglycemia--> catecholamines/glucagon released--> proteins used for energy--> ketones released--> acidosis
2. S/S: Elevated glucose (>200); (+) anion gap; (+) meta acidosis on ABG; (+) ketones in urine; N/V and ABD pain; Kussmaul's respirations- attempting to normalize pH by getting rid of $CO_2$; lethargy or coma; hypotension.
3. MGT: Fluids, insulin, K+ monitoring (as acidosis is corrected, K+ flows into cell -> hypoK+), bicarb if severe DKA (pH < 7)

### Hyperosmolar Hyperglycemia Non-Ketotic Coma (HHNK)

1. Patho: (T2 DM); partial insulin deficiency (just present enough to prevent need for protein breakdown)--> massive hyperglycemia--> sugar 'spills' into urine--> osmotic diuresis--> profound dehydration; occurs over days to weeks
2. S/S: polydipsia, polyuria, AMS, dry/ viscous mucous membranes; sunken eyes; (+) flat neck veins, hypotension; elevated glucose (>1000); serum osmolality >320mOsm; Urine- no ketones
3. MGT: LOTS OF FLUIDS (usually the fluid deficit is > 10L); 1L replaced in 1st hour, correct half the deficit in 12 hours and then the correct the remaining deficit over the following 24 hours; IV insulin possible, but do not reduce blood sugar by more than 50- 80 mg/dL/hr.

### Hyperthyroidism

1. Patho: infection or trauma--> stimulates thyroid--> releases large amounts of thyroid hormone--> heat intolerance/ tachycardia/ weakness--> HTN/ lethargy/ seizure
2. S/S: heat intolerance; tachycardia; weakness; HTN; lethargy; seizure; mania; serum T4 and T3 are elevated
3. MGT: Propylthiouracil (inhibits TH release), iodine inhibits release of stored TH), B-blockers (counteracts symptoms), IV steroids (inhibits hormone releases), dialysis (clears T4/T3), thyroidectomy

### Hypothyroidism

1. Patho: condition of hyposecretion of the thyroid gland causing low thyroid levels in the blood that result in sluggishness, slow pulse, and often obesity
2. S/S: fatigue, bradycardia, cold intolerance, delayed DTRs, hypotension, constipated, Elevated TSH, low T4/ T3.
3. MGT: ABCs; Synthroid or Levothyroxine

### Syndrome of Inappropriate Anti-Diuretic Hormone (SIADH)

1. Patho: ↑ secretion or continued secretion of anti-diuretic hormone (ADH) → water not excreted from kidneys→ increased fluid volume→ dilution of serum→ hyponatremia and hypo-osmolality
2. S/S: hyponatremia, hypoosmolality, and a urine osmolality above 100 mOsmol/kg. Urine sodium concentration is usually above 40 mEq/L.
3. MGT: IVF, 4 to 6 mEq/L in a 24-hour period. In patients who require emergency therapy, this goal should be achieved quickly, over six hours or less. Keep the rise in serum sodium less than 9 mEq/L in any 24-hour period.

### Acute Renal Failure (pre-renal)

1. Patho: due to conditions that reduce renal blood flow--> failure to clear toxins/ wastes--> kidneys lose effectiveness--> kidney completely fails
2. S/S: metallic taste in mouth, n/v; abd pain, oliguria; Hx of poor oral intake, (+) volume overload (like CHF); Increasing BUN/ Cr, 100-400mL/d urine suggests pre-renal cause
3. MGT: ABCs; treat hypovolemia (fluids); Foley cath; consider renal dose dopamine

### Sepsis

1. This characterizes a condition in which pathogenic microorganisms, usually bacteria, enter the bloodstream, causing a systemic inflammatory response to the infections
2. Two Types: SIRS and MODS
3. S/S: AMS, temp changes (first hot/ warm then cool extremities), hyperventilation, hypotension and tachycardia
4. MGT: ABCs; hypotension- treat with IVF (4-6L), vasopressors for refractory hypotension; obtain cultures; prevent adrenal insufficiency; avoid Etomidate with RSI– can worsen adrenal insufficiency

## GI bleed

1. Patho (UPPER): Peptic ulcer dz-- most common cause; esophageal varices-- occurs with cirrhosis/ portal HTN; Mallory-Weiss tears-- from forceful vomiting
2. Patho (LOWER): diverticulitis- diverticular erosion; inflammatory bowel dz (crohn's, CA, angiodysplasia)
3. S/S: n/v/d; abd pain; hematochezia; melena; hematemesis; anemia
4. MGT: support ABCs; NPO; large bore IVs; fluid resuscitation; NG/OG

## Intestinal Obstruction

1. Patho: hernia- protrusion; volvulus- twisting of intestine on itself; intusseption- prolapsed intestine; mechanical blockage
2. S/S: pain/ tender abdomen; foul smelling vomit; fever (septic); hyperactive bowel sounds (initially)--> absent sounds; cool- clammy skin; hypotension
3. MGT: support ABCs; fluid resuscitation/blood/pressors if hypotensive; NPO; OG/NG tube; antibiotics

## Esophageal Varices

1. Patho: inflammation of liver--> bile drainage inhibited--> increased portal resistance--> high resistance to blow flow--> blood backs up into the portal vein system--> blood further backs up into esophageal veins
2. S/S: jaundice/ gray feces/ dark urine (increased bilirubin); ascites; esophageal bleeding; hypotension
3. MGT: support ABCs; fluid resuscitation/blood/pressors if hypotensive; NPO; OG/NG tube; antibiotics, corticosteroids; avoid meds metabolized in the liver

## Pancreatitis

1. Patho: inflammation to pancreas--> pancreatic enzymes (acids) activated before arriving in the GI tract--> enzymes begin digesting the surrounding tissue--> digestion of pancreatic tissue reaches pancreatic blood vessels--> hemorrhage--> infection and necrosis
2. S/S: upper abd pain; n/v; fever; Turner's sign or Cullen's sign; ⁻ BP
3. MGT: support ABCs; fluid resuscitation/blood/pressors if hypotensive; NG/OG tube; pain management

## Adrenal Insufficiency

1. Patho: The reduction in one or more of the hormones secreted by the adrenal cortex as the result of dysfunction of the hypothalamic-pituitary adrenal axis: PRIMARY: d/t destruction or dysfunction of adrenal cortex; SECONDARY: from lack of ACTH secretion from the anterior pituitary gland
2. S/S: weakness, emaciation, hypoglycemia, increased pigmentation, hypotension, hyponatremia, malaise, loss of appetite, reduced ability to respond to stress, hyperkalemia; serum cortisol <20; PRIMARY- high K+ and BUN with low Na; SECONDARY- high Na, low K+
3. MGT: IVF, dexamethasone/ hydrocortisone; fludrocortisone (primary AI for co-morbid mineralocorticoid deficiency); avoid etomidate with RSI– can worsen adrenal insufficiency

## Appendicitis

1. Patho: obstruction of appendix lumen (fecal matter)--> distention of appendix--> increased appendicular pressure--> venous engorgement--> reduced arterial blood supply--> bacterial infection--> necrosis and rupture
2. S/S: RLQ pain, rebound tenderness, low-grade fever, fatigue, N/V; elevated WBC, CT is >90% sensitive
3. MGT: IV fluids, narcotics (pain), antibiotics, SURGERY

### Diverticulitis

1. Patho: inflammation of a diverticulum in the digestive tract (especially the colon)--> bleeding/ infection--> sepsis
2. S/S: LLQ pain, fever, increased WBCs, cramping, N/V, chills, GIB; CT w/ contrast
3. MGT: Antibiotics, IV fluids, pain management, blood transfusion, r/o other GIB etiologies, surgery

### Hepatitis

1. Patho: inflammation of the liver caused by a virus or a toxin--> cirrhosis/ liver failure
2. S/S: Jaundice; Fatigue; Low-grade fever; Headache; Abd pain; N/V; Diarrhea; elevated ALT, AST, ALP
3. MGT: diet, rest, small meals, IV fluids; transplantation; viral meds (interferon, vaccines)

# PART 3: PAIN SCALES

## INTRODUCTION

Pain is a sensation produced by noxious stimulation of the terminal branches of nerve fibers. As critical care clinicians, we will need to be a patient advocate and to that end need to develop strong skills at assessing for the presence of pain- even in the unconscious patient. The goal of pain management is relief without jeopardizing hemodynamics.

## TYPES OF PAIN

1. Acute pain: this type of pain typically has an identifiable cause and remits as the cause is resolved
2. Chronic pain: this has no specific etiology and is generally difficult to vocalize, quantify, and treat
3. Somatic pain: this typically involves the skin, subcutaneous tissue, or bones, and usually is well localized and described
4. Visceral pain:
    a. This pain arises from internal organs that share nerve innervation with another somatic anatomy.
    b. This type of pain to be localized or referred.
    c. These visceral to some somatic nerve connections are what make referred pain possible.

## PAIN ASSESSMENT

### OPQRST Pneumonic

It is important to get an adequate history of the pain, and this can be accomplished by simply utilizing the pneumonic: OPQRST.

1. (O)nset: when did the pain begin?
2. (P)rovocation: does anything make the pain worse or better?
3. (R)adiation: does the pain radiate anywhere?

4. (S)everity: rate the pain on some descriptive scale so that efforts at pain management can be assessed.
5. (T)iming: is it constant or intermittent?

## *RATING SCALES*

There is a multitude of different rating scales. The scales differ in depth of information obtained, target audience, as well as the way the pain is described. In this text, we'll offer two very common pain rating scales.

1. Numeric Scale: this is the common pain scales rated 1 (for almost no pain) to 10 (which is the worst pain you have ever felt in your life).
2. Faces Scale: the faces scale is a visual representation of a character who transitions from very happy to very hurt. This is great for individuals who cannot read as well as children. It provides a visual representation of pain. What is important to remember is that no matter what scale you use, any time the patient is in pain it is inhumane to withhold pain medication if it is available.

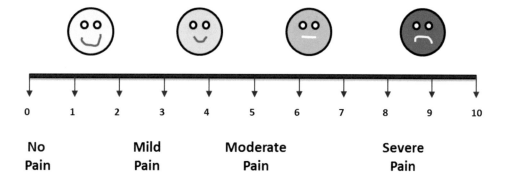

## *REASSESSMENT*

1. Reassess pain often and help keep your patient as comfortable as possible.
2. In the ventilated patient, heart rate should be utilized to assess for pain. Any increase in heart rate greater than 5 to 10 beats per minute from baseline is suggestive of pain and should be attenuated with the medications.

# PART 4: COMMON MEDICAL LABS

## INTRODUCTION

There are so many conditions and many have similar findings. Sometimes in the critical care transport environment having access to valuable laboratory data can help a clinician identify the correct diagnosis from a dense set of differential diagnoses. For this reason, lets investigate these lab studies.

PLEASE NOTE: Some labs that have already been discussed, may not be included in this chapter.

## MEDICAL LABS

### *URANALYSIS (positive or negative)*

1. pH: This is related to the acid-base balance maintained by the body. Therefore, consumption of acidic or basic foods, as well as the occurrence of any condition in the body that produces acids or bases, will directly affect the pH of the urine.
2. Protein: Proteins (Albumin is usually the first) excreted in the urine whenever there is a kidney problem. Conditions that usually produce high amounts of protein in the urine include preeclampsia, multiple myeloma, inflammation, urinary tract injuries, malignancies and other disorders that destroy red blood cells.
3. Glucose: Glucose should not be present in the urine. The conditions that can cause glycosuria are pregnancy, diabetes mellitus, liver diseases and hormonal disorders.
4. Ketones: Like glucose, ketones should not be present in the urine. Ketones are by-products of fat metabolism that form when there are not enough carbohydrate present for energy production. Other conditions that produce ketones in the urine are diabetes mellitus, frequent vomiting, strenuous exercise, and high protein diet.
5. Blood: The presence of blood in the urine is called hematuria, and this usually happens when there is an injury to the urinary tract. Other conditions that may induce hematuria include cigarette smoking, strenuous exercise, kidney problems, and trauma.
6. Nitrate: When a bacterial infection is present in the urinary tract, the bacterial flora can convert the urine's nitrate compound to nitrite.

### *ELECTROLYTES*

#### Phosphorus

1. Phosphorus is involved in the intracellular metabolism of proteins, fats, and carbohydrates. It also participates in the production of ATP, which is the chemical compound that supplies energy to the cell.
2. Phosphorus plays an important role in the acid-base balance of the body and glycolysis. It also helps in the release of the oxygen molecule from the hemoglobin of the blood.
3. Normal: 2.4 to 4.1 mg/dL
4. HIGH: Hypoparathyroidism, diabetic ketoacidosis, liver disease, kidney failure.
5. LOW: Poor nutrition, alcoholism, hyperparathyroidism, hypercalcemia.

#### Magnesium

1. Magnesium is important for muscle and nerve functions, blood pressure regulation and immune system. It also plays a role in blood sugar regulation. Although half of magnesium in the body is stored in bones, magnesium can also be found in cells of organs and body tissues.
2. Magnesium levels are determined whenever there are changes in motor functions or when patients are suspected of metabolic diseases.
3. Normal: 1.7 to 2.2 mg/dL
4. HIGH: Oliguria, dehydration, Addison's disease, chronic renal failure, diabetic acidosis.
5. LOW: Chronic diarrhea, alcoholism, hemodialysis, ulcerative colitis, delirium tremens, hypoparathyroidism, hyperaldosteronism, hepatic cirrhosis, pancreatitis, toxemia of pregnancy.

### *LIVER AND PANCREAS FUNCTION LABS*

#### Alanine Transaminase (ALT)

1. This is an enzyme that is found mainly in liver tissue, but also can be found in the kidneys, heart, and skeletal muscle. But when the liver is injured, it will release this enzyme.
2. Normal: 10-35 IU/L
3. HIGH: liver pathologies. When ALT > AST) then acute viral hepatitis is likely present.

4. LOW: Poor nutrition, vitamin D deficiency.

**Aspartate Transaminase (AST)**
1. This is an enzyme that is found inside tissues that have increased metabolic rates, such as heart, skeletal, brain, spleen, pancreas, kidney, lung, and liver.  When the stations are injured, AST is released.
2. Normal: 10-35 IU/L
3. HIGH: liver pathologies. When AST > ALT then alcoholic hepatitis is likely present.
4. LOW: Poor nutrition, vitamin D deficiency.

**Lipase**
1. An elevated level of serum lipase is an indicator of pancreatitis.  This is more specific to pancreas injury than the amylase test is.
2. Normal: < 160 IU/L
3. HIGH: pancreatitis or pancreatic injury, diabetes mellitus, Crohn's disease.
4. LOW: pancreatic dysfunction or insufficiency.

**Amylase**
1. This enzyme catalyzes the breakdown of starch into sugars and is found mainly in the pancreas. It is not as specific as lipase for pancreatic injury/ illness.
2. Normal: 30- 100 U/L
3. HIGH: pancreatitis or pancreatic injury, gallbladder injury/ illness.
4. LOW: pancreatic dysfunction or insufficiency.

# PART 5: MEDICAL PHARMACOLOGY

## INTRODUCTION

With all the different conditions, it is important to have a strong grasp on the pharmacology used in common conditions seen in the critical care transport environment.

## MEDICATIONS

### Albuterol
1. Class: Beta agonist
2. Mechanism: Stimulates the beta 2 receptor, which relaxes bronchiole smooth muscle which causes bronchodilation.
3. Indications: Acute bronchospasm (from COPD, asthma, allergic reaction or any other cause of bronchoconstriction.
4. Contraindications: tachycardia, hypertension, dysrhythmia
5. Hemodynamics: (~CVP/ ~PCWP/~CO/~SVR).
6. Adult Dose: 2.5 mg in 3 cc NS and nebulized
7. Peds Dose: 1.25 mg in 3 cc NS and nebulized

### Calcium Chloride
1. Class: Electrolyte

2. Mechanism: Essential in neurotransmission and muscle contractions; calcium competes with magnesium, so it's given in magnesium overdoses.
3. Indications: Hypermagnesemia, beta blocker OD, hypocalcemia
4. Contraindications: VFib during CPR, hypercalcemia, risk for digitalis toxicity, hypophosphatemia, renal calculi; pulseless ventricular tachycardia
5. Hemodynamics: (↑CVP/ ↑PCWP/↑CO/↑SVR)
6. Dose: 1-2 grams over 5 minutes.

## Dextrose

1. Class: Antihypoglycemic
2. Mechanism: increases blood glucose concentrations
3. Indications: hypoglycemia.
4. Contraindications: intracranial hemorrhage, delirium tremens
5. Hemodynamics: (~CVP/ ~PCWP/~CO/~SVR).
6. Adult Dose: 10- 25g of D50%
7. Peds:
    a. Over 2 years: 1g/ kg (D50% or D25%)
    b. Under 2 years: 0.5-1g/kg (D10%)
    c. D10: using a 30 CC syringe, remove 3 g of dextrose from an ampule of D50%. Then draw up 27 cc's of normal saline for a total of 30cc. So, 3 g in 30 cc's is a 10% solution; herefore, you have D10%.
    d. D25: using a 30 cc syringe, remove 7.5 g of dextrose from an amp D50%. Then draw up 22.5cc of normal saline for a total of 30cc. So, 7.5 g in 30 cc's is a 25% solution; therefore, you have D25%.

## Diphenhydramine

1. Class: Antihistamine
2. Mechanism: this medication binds and blocks H1 histamine receptors, reducing the effects of massive histamine release.
3. Indications: Anaphylactic reactions
4. Contraindications: allergies, acute asthma (this thickens secretions)
5. Hemodynamics: (~ CVP/ ~PCWP/~CO/~SVR)
6. Dose:
    a. Adult: 25-50 mg IV, IO, IM
    b. Peds: 1 mg/kg
7. This medication will cause drowsiness, dizziness, wheezing possible, hypotension

## Ethanol 10%

1. Class: Toxic alcohol antidote
2. Mechanism: Competes with methanol & ethylene glycol for alcohol dehydrogenase to inhibit production of toxic metabolites
3. Indications: Methanol Toxicity, Ethylene Glycol Poisoning.
4. Contraindications: hypersensitivity
5. Hemodynamics: (~CVP/ ~PCWP/~CO/~SVR).
6. Dose: Loading: 10 mL/kg of a 10 percent ethanol solution in D5W; Maintenance dose: 1 mL/kg of a 10% solution administered

## Fentanyl

1. Class: Narcotic/ Analgesic
2. Mechanism: Competitively binds with narcotic receptors and prevents the sensation of pain.
3. Indications: pain control
4. Contraindications: Allergy/ History of rigid chest syndrome

5. Hemodynamics: (~CVP/ ~PCWP/~CO/~SVR).
6. Adult Dose: 1-2 mg/kg IV. Peds Dose: 1-2 mg/kg IV.
7. Very safe hemodynamic profile (does not drop blood pressure much at all).
8. Can be used in the hypotensive setting when a benzodiazepine would be unsafe for perfusion.

## Ipratropium Bromide
1. Class: Anticholinergic Bronchodilator
2. Mechanism: blocks acetylcholine with results in bronchial smooth muscle relaxation
3. Indications: Acute bronchospasm (from COPD, asthma, allergic reaction or any other cause of bronchoconstriction.
4. Contraindications: tachycardia, hypersensitivity
5. Hemodynamics: (~CVP/ ~PCWP/~CO/~SVR).
   a. Adult Dose: 500mcg every 4-6 hours
   b. Peds Dose: 125– 250mcg nebulized

## Ketamine
1. Class: Hypnotic
2. Dose: 1-2 mg/kg IV
3. Indications: sedation; pain control, bronchodilation
4. Contraindications: Allergy/ increased ICP
5. Used as both analgesia and sedation.
6. Ketamine will help to increase BP– ideal in trauma, but not in increased ICP conditions; ketamine also will reduce bronchospasm.
7. Hemodynamics: (~CVP/ ~PCWP/↑CO/↑SVR)

## Magnesium Sulfate
1. Class: Electrolyte, Muscle relaxant
2. Mechanism: decreases the excitability of muscles, therefore, relaxes skeletal and smooth muscle: reduces BP, relaxes uterine contractions, bronchodilators, slows HR.
3. Indications: ventricular tachycardia refractory to other treatments, eclampsia, tocolytics for pregnancy
4. Contraindications: Bradycardia, hypotension, heart block
5. Hemodynamics: (↓CVP/ ↓PCWP/↓CO/↓SVR).
6. Dose:
   a. Adults: 1-2 g administered IV over 10-20 minutes
   b. Peds: 25-50 mg/kg IV or IM

## Morphine
1. Class: Narcotic/ Analgesic
2. Mechanism: Competitively binds with narcotic receptors and prevents the sensation of pain.
3. Indications: pain control
4. Contraindications: Allergy/ History of rigid chest syndrome
5. Hemodynamics: (~CVP/ ~PCWP/~CO/↓SVR).
6. Adult Dose: 2-5 mg IV; Peds Dose: 0.1 –.02 mg/kg
7. Can precipitously drop blood pressure.

## Sodium Bicarbonate
1. Class: Electrolyte replacement
2. Mechanism: buffers existing acidosis
3. Indications: acidosis, drug intoxications (barbiturates, salicylates, methyl alcohol)
4. Contraindications: metabolic alkalosis
5. Hemodynamics: (~CVP/ ~PCWP/~CO/~SVR)

6. Dose: 1 mEq/kg slow IV, IO

### Solu-Medrol
1. Class: Corticosteroid
2. Mechanism: reduces the inflammatory response.
3. Indications: anaphylaxis, asthma, COPD
4. Contraindications: Cushing's syndrome, fungal infection, measles, hypersensitivity
5. Hemodynamics: (~CVP/ ~PCWP/~CO/~SVR).
6. Dose:
    a. Adults: 40-80mg IV
    b. Peds: 1 mg/kg (up to 60mg) IV, IO

# PART 6: MEDICAL MANAGEMENT QUESTIONS

1. A 54-year old male presents with altered mental status and an increased work of breathing. The pH is reduced, and the blood sugar is high. Which of the following conditions is the patient currently experiencing?
    a. (+) Graves' disease
    b. A mild form of HHNK
    c. Diabetic ketoacidosis
    d. (+) Hypothyroidism

2. Your adult patient complains of fatigue, malaise, constipation, and says she gets cold very fast. She reiterates that she cannot stand the cold. Which of the following medications would be most beneficial to the patient?
    a. Gram- antibiotics
    b. Gram+ antibiotics
    c. Dexamethasone
    d. Levothyroxine

3. An adult patient presents a to local ER where you will pick them up. The patient presents with jaundice, hypertension, and hematemesis. Which of the following conditions is responsible for the patient presenting to the ER?
    a. Esophageal varices
    b. Upper GI bleed
    c. Lower GI bleed
    d. Diverticulitis

4.  Responding to a small ER, you find a middle aged male patient presenting with altered mental status, hyperglycemia, and increased work of breathing. You note the following findings: HR 102, RR 32, SpO2 99%, BP 142/85, and EtCO2 of 65. Which of the following management options would best benefit the patient?
    a.  Reduce the PEEP and the FiO2
    b.  Fluid bolus and insulin infusion
    c.  Increased minute ventilation
    d.  Sodium bicarbonate and calcium

5.  Your adult patient is one-week status post massive multi-system trauma. Today the patient presents with petechial hemorrhages, high PTT, and a (+) D-dimer. Which of the following conditions is the patient most likely suffering from?
    a.  ARDS with severe metabolic acidosis
    b.  Disseminated intravascular coagulation
    c.  Vaso-occlusive crisis (sickle cell anemia)
    d.  Acute chest syndrome and hemophilia

6.  Your adult patient presents with altered mental status. Upon assessment, you note the following findings: HR 55, BP 92/50, RR 12, blood glucose 92 mg/dL, SpO2 of 96%, (-) Babinski, (+) Chvostek, and pH of 7.36. What other findings would you most likely observe with this patient?
    a.  Norm K and high CO2
    b.  Ca 7.1/ Na 136/ K 4.6
    c.  High phos and low K
    d.  PTT 12/ calcium 9.2

7.  The sending hospital staff reports that your patient has acute pancreatitis. As you review the patient's medical chart, which of the following would corroborate the report of acute pancreatitis?
    a.  Amylase of 300 u/L
    b.  Bilirubin 0.2 mg/dl
    c.  Lipase of 120 IU/L
    d.  Albumin of 3.8 g/dL

8.  Your transporting a patient with SIADH. The patient is being treated with water restriction and administration of IV fluids. The critical care transport professional evaluates that treatment has been effective when the patient experiences which of the following?
    a.  ↑ urine output, decreased serum sodium and increased urine specific gravity
    b.  ↓ urine output, increased serum sodium and decreased urine specific gravity
    c.  ↑ urine output, increased serum sodium and decreased urine specific gravity
    d.  ↓ urine output, decreased serum sodium and increased urine specific gravity

9.  A patient is being treated for acute adrenal insufficiency. Which of the following findings indicate the patient is responding favorably?
    a.  Decreasing serum sodium
    b.  Decreasing serum potassium
    c.  Decreasing blood glucose
    d.  Increasing urinary output

10. The patient you'll be transporting is suspected of having hepatitis. Which of the following lab diagnostics would be helpful in confirming this suspicion?
    a.  Elevated hemoglobin level
    b.  Low blood urea nitrogen level
    c.  Elevated serum bilirubin level
    d.  Decreased erythrocytes

11. The patient presents with an altered mental status, reduced respiratory effort, (+) hepatojugular reflex. Which of the following would support the diagnosis of severe hepatitis?
    a.  Elevated liver enzymes and low serum protein level
    b.  Subnormal clotting factors and platelet count
    c.  Elevated BUN and creatinine levels and hyperglycemia
    d.  Low serum glucose and elevated serum ammonia levels

12. You'll be transporting a patient with multiple metabolic conditions. This patient is suspected of having SIADH. Which of the following findings is most ominous?
    a.  The patient complains of a severe headache
    b.  The patient complains of severe thirst
    c.  The patient has a urine specific gravity of 1.025
    d.  The patient has a serum sodium level of 119 mEq/L

13. The sending facility is treating your patient for a lower GI bleed. Which of the following findings would support this diagnosis?
    a.  Green color and texture
    b.  Black and tarry appearance
    c.  Exhibits a clay-like quality
    d.  Bright red blood in stool

14. You arrive at a small ER to find your patient hypertensive, potentially septic, with hyperactive bowel sounds. Additionally, the patient has incredibly foul-smelling vomit. Which of the following conditions is the patient most likely suffering from?
    a.  Diverticular hemorrhage
    b.  Esophageal varices
    c.  Intestinal obstruction
    d.  Severe pancreatitis

15. You are picking up a metabolic acidosis patient from an intensive care unit and delivering them to a bigger hospital. All the patient's vital signs are normal except the EtCO2, which is 70 mmHg. You decide to increase the minute ventilation to target an EtCO2 of 45. Which of the following set of findings would you most likely anticipate with this treatment?
    a. K+ drops 1.2 mEq/L & pH increases
    b. Na+ drops 20 mEq/L & pH maintains
    c. Serum Ca+ increases by 2.1mEq/L
    d. pH increases & phosphate falls by 3.6

16. The patient you'll be transporting a sustained kidney injury in a motor vehicle crash. This diagnosis was confirmed with CT. Which of the following labs is most important to observe and this patient?
    a. Osmolality
    b. Creatinine
    c. BUN level
    d. Potassium

# PART 7: MEDICAL MANAGEMENT RATIONALES

1. **(C)** This presentation (acidosis, hyperglycemia, and tachypnea) all lead toward the diagnosis of diabetic ketoacidosis, or DKA. Remember, the biggest difference between DKA and HHNK is the fact that HHNK produces just enough insulin to prevent the cells from having to undergo anaerobic metabolism, and thus prevent acidosis.

2. **(D)** This patient is experiencing hypothyroidism: a condition of hyposecretion of the thyroid gland causing low thyroid levels in the blood that result in sluggishness, slow pulse, and often obesity. It is treated with Synthroid or Levothyroxine. These patients will continue to remain sluggish, slow and cold intolerant without this medication.

3. **(A)** The Jaundice gives away that the patient has a liver pathophysiology, and the throwing up blood in the face of liver pathology strongly suggests esophageal varices. The other three answer selections are forms of GI bleeds, but the jaundice is telltale sign in this case.

4. **(C)** This patient presents with diabetic ketoacidosis (hyperglycemia, fast respiratory rate, and altered mental status). It appears the patient is trying to breathe off the excess acid created by the DKA. In this case, the best solution is to increase the patient's minute ventilation during mechanical ventilation to help and assure enough acid is blown off. Reducing PEEP will only change the oxygenation effort; fluid and insulin may be warranted but are not a top priority. While sodium bicarb may be beneficial, calcium is not a warranted in this case; therefore, this answer selection is incorrect. The ultimate teaching point here is not to reduce the patient's compensatory respiratory effort unless you are targeting a higher than normal minute ventilation. If you paralyze patient and reduce their minute ventilation, the patient will get extremely acidotic. Always make sure you're watching your patient and making ventilator decisions based on end tidal CO2 and SpO2.

5. **(B)** To be able to answer this question, it is important to be able to differentiate hematological conditions. We can initially rule out the "ARDS" answer selection because it is not even in the ballpark relative to the information given. Hemophilia will present with increased PTT, but the patient will not have a D– dimer unless they are experiencing clotting. Hemophilia is the genetic condition caused by low clotting factors, so, this answer selection is ruled out. The sickle cell and acute chest answer selections are also incorrect because these rely on an odd shaped red blood cell.

These types of anemia present differently and typically will not spike a D-dimer. Therefore, the correct answer, in this case, is DIC.

6. **(B)** Chvostek's sign is found in hypocalcemia. Therefore, the correct answer is the answer selection with a lower than normal calcium. There are two answers with calcium, one is normal (9.2) and one is reduced (7.1). The 7.1 calcium is very low and could cause Chvostek's to manifest. Thus the "calcium 7.1" is the correct answer.

7. **(A)** The normal serum amylase level is 25 to 151 units/L. With chronic cases of pancreatitis, the rise in serum amylase levels usually does not exceed three times the normal value. In acute pancreatitis, the value may exceed five times the normal value. All other options are within normal limits.

8. **(C)** The patient with SIADH has water retention with hyponatremia, decreased urine output and concentrated urine with high specific gravity. Therefore, improvement in the patient's condition reflected by increased urine output, normalization of serum sodium, and more water in the urine, decreasing the specific gravity.

9. **(B)** Clinical manifestations of Addison's disease include hyperkalemia and a decrease in potassium level indicate improvement. Decreasing serum sodium and decreasing blood glucose indicate that treatment has not been effective. Changes in urinary output are not an effective way of monitoring treatment for Addison's disease.

10. **(C)** Laboratory indicators of hepatitis include elevated liver enzyme levels, elevated serum bilirubin levels, elevated erythrocyte sedimentation rates, and leukopenia. An elevated blood urea nitrogen level may indicate renal dysfunction. A hemoglobin level is unrelated to this diagnosis.

11. **(D)** Subnormal serum glucose and elevated serum ammonia levels. In acute liver failure, serum ammonia levels increase because the liver can't adequately detoxify the ammonia produced in the GI tract. In addition, serum glucose levels decline because the liver isn't capable of releasing stored glucose. Elevated serum ammonia and subnormal serum glucose levels depress the level of a client's consciousness. Elevated liver enzymes, low serum protein level, subnormal clotting factors and platelet count, elevated blood urea nitrogen and creatine levels, and hyperglycemia aren't as directly related to the client's level of consciousness.

12. **(D)** A serum sodium of less than 120 mEq/L increases the risk for complications such as seizures and needs rapid correction. The other data are not unusual for a patient with SIADH and do not indicate the need for rapid action.

13. **(B)** Black and tarry stools (melena) are a sign of bleeding in the upper gastrointestinal (GI) tract. As the blood moves through the GI system, digestive enzymes turn red blood to black. Bright red blood in the stool is a sign of lower GI bleeding. Green color and texture are a distractor for this question. Clay-like stools are a characteristic of biliary disorders

14. **(C)** The signs and symptoms of intestinal obstruction include pain/ tender abdomen; fowl smelling vomit; fever (septic); hyperactive bowel sounds (initially)--> absent sounds; cool- clammy skin; hypotension. One of the key features is the foul-smelling vomit.

15. **(A)** To answer this question, you must have a working knowledge of the winter's formula, or ultimately that changing end tidal CO2 also changes the potassium in the same direction. Every 10 mmHg of change with EtCO2, the potassium will change by a factor of 0.5 in the same direction. Therefore, if you were to change an EtCO2 by 25 mmHg, then you'd expect a change in potassium by 1.2 mEq/L, therefore the answer selection with this value is the correct answer.

16. **(D)** Remember, the kidneys that only remove water but also electrolytes, including potassium. If the kidneys fail because they are injured, or for any other reason, then they will not be able to remove potassium and thus potassium will be allowed to build up. If potassium can build up beyond 6.0, then clinical complications can occur. While these other three options should be monitored, the one that could cause cardiac arrest is potassium, therefore it should be monitored closely.

# CHAPTER 8: NEUROLOGICAL EMERGENCIES

## PART 1: THE NEURO ASSESSMENT

### INTRODUCTION

The neurologic examination is a skill which we must develop throughout our careers. The neurologic exam remains the most important diagnostic tool that we can employ to assess our neurologic patients because it provides insight as to our patients' improvement or decline. As with all focused assessments, our approach should be systematic and should be conducted in the same manner every time we assess a patient. Obtain the clinical history and allow it to guide assessment.

### THE REPONSIVE PATIENT

#### *ASSESS THE LEVEL OF CONSCIOUSNESS*

1. Obtain their current neurologic baseline
2. AVPU: Awake– eyes open spontaneously; Verbal- arouses to stimulation by voice; Painful– purposeful movements to painful stimuli; Unresponsive- no response to any stimuli
3. Awake alert and oriented (AAO): this simple and classic assessment identify if the patient is oriented to time, place, and person.
4. This simple method is useful because these elements of awareness disappear in this order: time, place, and then person.
5. Progression from Awake to Comatose
   a. Awake and alert (see above)
   b. Agitated- patients who are agitated have higher level of mental functioning when compared to someone who presents as sleepy or sleeping
   c. Lethargic– these patients present sleepy or sleeping
      i. Arousal to Voice: these patients are easily woken by talking to them
      ii. Arousal to Gentle Stimulation: these patients are woken by gentle touch
      iii. Arousal to Painful Stimulus: these patients are only awoken by a painful stimulation
   d. Comatose- these patients are not aroused by any stimulation whatsoever.

#### *ASSESS THE VISUAL FIELD*

1. Assess extra ocular movement in their visual field: dysconjugate gaze and nystagmous– indicates a neuro etiology
2. Identify if there are any visual field deficits
   a. These are very important findings
   b. Begin by and having the patient cover an eye, have your hand outside of their field of vision and move your fingers into their field of vision
   c. Note any dyssymmetry and where their field of vision begins
3. Identify whether the patient is experiencing any visual changes

      a. Blurry vision, double vision, loss of vision, or spots in their visual field all can indicate neuro pathology

      b. The presence of visual changes can either be transient or ongoing

## FACIAL ASSESSMENT

1. Ask the patient to smile and assess for facial symmetry: poor symmetry can indicate stroke
2. Ask the patient to stick out their tongue and say "ah".
    a. Tongue deviation to one side or the other as well as asymmetrical rise of the soft palate are also indicators of neuro pathology
3. Assess for Aphasia:
    a. Expressive: patient is unable to speak or formulates words clearly
    b. Receptive: patient is unable to understand spoken word
    c. Global: both expressive and receptive
    d. Conductive: speech is fluent but using inappropriate words

## ASSESS FOR MOTOR WEAKNESS

1. Have your patient hold arms out in front of them at shoulder length with palms up.
2. Unilateral weakness (arm drift) is an indicator of the stroke of etiology.
3. Grip strength: identify unilateral or bilateral weakness.
4. Leg strength: have patient lift legs off the bed to your resistance- identify unilateral or bilateral weakness.

## ASSESS FOR PARASTHESIAS

# THE POORLY RESPONSIVE PATIENT

## RULE OUT SEDATION OR PARALYTICS

Rule out if the patient is chemically paralyzed or sedated (obtain a report from medical crew or review chart for medications).

## Assess Glasgow Coma Scale (GCS)

1. Eye Opening: Spontaneous (4); to speech (3); to painful stimuli (2); no opening at all (0)
2. Verbal Effort: normal conversation (5); confused (4); inappropriate words (3); incomprehensible sounds (2); no verbal effort (1)
3. Motor Effort: follows commands (6); localizes pains (5); withdrawals from pain (4); decorticate posturing (3); decerebrate posturing (2); no motor effort (1)

## Assess Eye Movement and Position

1. Unequal pupils: brain herniation
2. Disconjugate gaze: focal brain lesion
3. Rowing: seizure activity
4. Blink to Threat: Wave hand towards the patient's face and assess for blinking— blinking indicates patient is awake.

## Assess for any seizure activity

## Assess for Babinski Reflex

1. Stroke the plantar surface of the foot from heel to toes with a rigid object
2. Toes that fan outward indicate a positive test and, therefore, is abnormal except in very young children; indicates a (+) upper motor neuron lesion.

### Assess for clonus

1. Grasp the plantar surface of the foot and quickly dorsiflex the ankle
2. Allow the foot to relax and if there is rhythmic jerking note how long the jerking occurs in seconds.
3. The presence of clonus indicates possible seizure activity or hyper spasticity.

### Assess the Brachioradialis Reflex

1. Once struck briskly, the muscle will contract & arm will flex at the elbow and supinate
2. This is a great reflex to practice and to use to assess deep tendon reflexes (DTRs) to ensure a patient isn't too heavily sedated (like with magnesium toxicity).

### Assess for spontaneous respirations:

Rule out if the patient is under sedation or paralytic

### Assess gag reflex

### Specific neurologic findings and their meanings

1. Blood coming from the ear canal: possible basilar skull fracture
2. Halo Sign: indicates basilar skull fracture
3. Raccoon Eyes: bruising around the eyes indicating orbital fracture
4. Battle's Sign: bruising behind the ears and indicates a basilar skull fracture
5. Head injury followed by an unconscious period, then a lucid period, and then another unconscious period: this indicates an epidural bleed
6. Concave bleed on head CT: indicates an epidural bleed
7. Convex bleed on head CT: indicates a subdural bleed
8. The complaint "worst headache of my life": indicates subarachnoid bleed
9. Cushing's Triad (widening pulse pressure, bradycardia, and abnormal respiratory patterns): indicates increasing intracranial pressure
10. Brown-Sequard: Affected side: (-) motor/ vibration; Unaffected side: (-) pain/temp
11. Anterior Cord Syndrome: Below site: (-) motor/temp/pain; (+) balance/touch/vibration
12. Central Cord Syndrome: (+) motor weakness in UPPER extremities; "can tap dance, but cannot play the piano".

### ASSESS FOR SPINAL VS. NEUROGENIC SHOCK

1. Both have the same patho, but SPINAL shock will resolve days later
2. The spinal shock will NOT present with radiographic evidence of injury, or SCIWORA (spinal cord injury without radiographic abnormality).

# PART 2: BASIC NEURO PATHOPHYSIOLOGY

## INTRODUCTION

Here we will discuss basic neurogenic pathophysiology so that the conditions section will make the most amount of sense.

## PATHOPHYSIOLOGIES

### MONROE-KELLY HYPOTHESIS
1. One of the most important neurologic mechanisms involving over compression within the cranium, as in a bleed or large tumor.
2. There is only so much space within the cranium, and it is composed generally of cerebral spinal fluid (CSF), blood, and the brain.
3. Any bleeding or growing masses will have to displace one of the above three components. This is known as the Monroe– Kellie Hypothesis.

### INTRACRANIAL PRESSURE (ICP)
1. ICP is a dynamic pressure, meaning that multiple factors act on it from moment to moment causing fluctuations of pressure within the cranium.
2. ICP is influenced by increases or decreases in cardiac contraction, respirations, straining or compressing neck veins, in addition to a multitude of others.
3. Normal: 0- 15 mmHg
4. Assume this value to be high (20mmHg) when estimating cerebral perfusion pressure in patients with intracranial masses or bleeds.

### CEREBRAL BLOOD FLOW
1. The brain demands 50% of cardiac output and utilizes 20% of the total oxygen used up by the body.
2. We, as clinicians, can affect the cerebral blood flow with ventilations
3. High $pCO_2$ (hypoventilation) $\rightarrow$ Vasoconstriction
4. Low $pCO_2$ (hyperventilation) $\rightarrow$ Vasodilation

### CEREBRAL PERFUSION PRESSURE (CPP)
1. This pressure is responsible for maintaining the forward motion of blood through the brain.
2. It is the difference between mean arterial pressure (MAP) and ICP and is expressed by the following equation: CPP = MAP - ICP.
3. Minimum CPP to maintain blood flow: 70- 100 mmHg
4. Recall that mean arterial pressure has the following equation: (systolic BP + diastolic BP + diastolic BP)/3 = MAP.
5. With higher ICPs, you will have a lower CPP. Once CPP drops below 60 mmHg, then forward blood flow will nearly be stopped. Therefore, to maintain blood flow, we need to elevate CPP and to do that we need to maintain an adequate MAP.
6. Normal MAP: 70 – 100 mmHg
7. In pathophysiologies that cause increase intracranial pressure (ICP), we must have higher mean arterial pressures (MAPs) to ensure blood flow to the brain itself.
8. Consider CPP = MAP - ICP. If we have a patient with a normal MAP of 90 mmHg who has 20 mmHg of ICP, then the CPP = 90 - 20 = 70. Therefore, we need to keep CPP above 70 mmHg.
9. Patients with intracranial pathophysiologies will compensate by increasing blood pressure to help maintain CPP; it is imperative that we do not reduce blood pressure in these patients **beyond 30%, and usually only if it is above 220/110**. There are other neurological conditions that allow for BP reduction when the BP is less than 220/110- we will discuss these later. The blood pressure is acting like a fluid scaffolding holding open the blood vessels in the brain. If we drop blood pressure to "normal" levels then the patient will suffer massive brain damage and potential death.
10. **Bottom line**: in the neuro patient, we should target mean arterial pressures of 85 to 90, especially in the closed head injury (CHI) and traumatic brain injury (TBI) patients.

11. **Indications of increasing ICP**: altered mental status/ ipsilateral pupils/ decorticate or decerebrate posturing.
12. Treatment of the ICP:
    a.  Keep head of the bed at 15-30°
    b.  Ensure EtCO2 is between 35 and 45 mmHg
    c.  Utilize sedation and paralysis to control patient
    d.  Ensure oxygenation (SpO2 > 95%) and perfusion (MAP > 85)

## TRAUMATIC BRAIN INJURY (TBI)

1.  Traumatic brain injury (TBI) can manifest from any direct blow to the head, as well as secondary type injuries that occur from poor perfusion after the initial injury.
2.  Common therapeutic goals in closed head injury and traumatic brain injury include prevention of hypoxia, hypotension, and uncontrolled EtCO2.
3.  Several masses can arise following a traumatic brain injury:
    a.  Ruptured vessels leading to enlarging hematomas
    b.  Ischemic brain tissue which begins to swell
    c.  Directly injured tissue swells from the inflammatory process
4.  The goal of the critical care clinician should be aimed at maintaining oxygenation, maintaining adequate blood pressure (MAP), and ensuring and EtCO2 between 30- 35 mmHg.

## NEUROMUSCULAR DISESASES AND SUCCINYLCHOLINE

1.  There is a multitude of neuromuscular diseases that you'll face as a critical care clinician.
2.  Succinylcholine is a medication you may routinely administer to facilitate endotracheal intubation.
3.  Patients that receive succinylcholine and who have a neuro-muscular disease, have a high potential of developing massive hyperkalemia which could lead to masseter muscle spasm, malignant hyperthermia, and death.
4.  Muscles contract when a nerve sends a neurotransmitter, acetylcholine, to the muscle's acetylcholine receptors thus activating the receptors.
5.  In any disease where the muscles do not receive nervous stimuli, the muscle itself will build hundreds of thousands more acetylcholine receptors. The body thinks the muscles aren't contracting because there is a lack of receptors.
6.  Each one of these receptors releases potassium once acetylcholine or succinylcholine stimulates the receptor.
7.  Therefore, in patients with neuromuscular diseases, or patients who have been bedridden, who received succinylcholine may develop massive hyperkalemia.
8.  We should be very cautious in administering succinylcholine to any patient that has not moved in a week or more– because it could cause a fatal HYPERKALEMIA.

# PART 3: NEUROLOGICAL CONDITIONS

## INTRODUCTION

There are a multitude of neurological conditions, and several have unique management for them. It is important to be able to identify the specific neurologic condition so that specific treatment can be administered.

# NEUROLOGICAL CONDITIONS

## Aneurysm

1. Pathophys: HTN/genetics--> weakening arterial wall in brain--> bulging spot--> rupture--> vomiting, headache, vision impairment--> increased ICP--> severe AMS/CVA
2. ASST: A headache, eye pain, visual changes, numbness/ weakness to face, altered LOC, increasing ICP; positive testing: CT/MRI & Cerebral arteriogram.  The onset can be rapid or slow.
3. MGT: support ABCs, do not lower BP unless it's >220/115- and then don't lower more than 30%, deliver to neurology; monitor ICP

## Traumatic Brain Injury (TBI):

1. Pathophys: primary trauma to brain--> caused by direct blow or penetration--> bleeding/swelling; Secondary trauma to brain--> caused by brain swelling--> compresses brain tissue--> function reduced from damage from swelling
2. ASST: battles sign/ raccoon eyes/ penetration; hematoma; Cushing reflex; AMS; pupil changes; GCS changes; CT (cerebral contusion, epidural hematoma, subdural hematoma, concussion)
3. MGT: prevent secondary injury (prevent hypoxia and hypotension); treat ICP (intubate, raise HOB, mannitol, ICP monitoring); prevent/ treat Sz (phenytoin/ benzos); possible surgery

## Intracerebral Hemorrhage

1. Pathophys: HTN (and other mechanisms)--> ruptured vessel--> bleeding into brain parenchyma--> swelling, increased ICP, AMS
2. ASST: acute onset HA--> stupor-->coma; HTN; bradycardia; abnormal pupils; CT revealing ICH
3. MGT: support ABCs; maintain pre-clinical BP; prevent/ treat Sz (phenytoin/ benzos); treat ICP (intubate, raise HOB, mannitol, ICP monitoring); reverse anticoagulation with fresh frozen plasma (FFP) if needed

## Subarachnoid Hemorrhage

1. Pathophys: ruptured blood vessel in brain--> rapidly fills subarachnoid space with blood--> the patient may experience an intense, sudden headache accompanied by nausea, vomiting, and neck pain--> brain swelling, increased ICP, AMS
2. ASST: 'worst headache of my life', radiates to neck; nuchal rigidity; photophobia; n/v; AMS
3. MGT: support ABCs; maintain normal BP; prevent/ treat Sz (phenytoin/ benzos); treat ICP (intubate, raise HOB, mannitol, ICP monitoring); reverse anticoagulation with FFP if needed

## Epidural Hematoma

1. Pathophys: fracture of temporal bone--> Rupture of the middle meningeal artery--> rapid accumulation of blood in epidural space
2. ASST: HA; LOC-lucid interval- LOC pattern; ipsilateral dilated pupil; confusion-coma; CT-concave hematoma
3. MGT: support ABCs; prevent/ treat Sz (phenytoin/ benzos); treat ICP (intubate, raise HOB, mannitol, ICP monitoring); surgery to evacuate blood (burr holes)

## Subdural Hematoma

1. Pathophys: head trauma--> venous rupture--> bleeding into subdural space--> brain edema, increased ICP
2. ASST: Mechanism (head injury); HA- slowly developing; gradual mental status changes; CT-crescent shaped (concave) hematoma
3. MGT: support ABCs; prevent/ treat Sz (phenytoin/ benzos); treat ICP (intubate, raise HOB, mannitol, ICP monitoring); surgery to evacuate blood (surgical drainage)

## Ischemic Stroke

1. Pathophys: blockage of cerebral artery (embolus or thrombus)--> anoxic injury to distal tissue--> brain swelling, increased ICP, reduced function
2. ASST: acute AMS; HA; facial paralysis, slurred speech, arm drift (Cincinnati stroke scale); confirm with CT or MRI
3. MGT: support ABCs; consider fibrinolytics and heparin; prevent/ treat Sz (phenytoin/ benzos); treat ICP (intubate, raise HOB, mannitol, ICP monitoring); treat hyperglycemia- insulin;

## Seizures

1. Pathophys: PRIMARY: occurs for unknown reasons; SECONDARY: caused by bleeding, trauma, electrolyte abnormalities, metabolic disturbances, meds/EtOH, etc
2. ASST: preceded by an aura; AMS; convulsions (tonic-clonic) or only tonic activity; posturing; status epilepticus- seizures without consciousness in between; EEG
3. MGT: support ABCs; treat causes (glucose for low BS, Narcan for opioid OD, thiamine to alcoholics); consider: benzos, Dilantin, phenobarbital, propofol

## Muscular Dystrophy

Pathophys: a category of genetically transmitted diseases characterized by progressive atrophy of skeletal muscles (Duchene's type is most common)

## Intracranial Pressure (ICP)

1. Pathophys: injury or mass in cranium--> swelling--> increases intracranial pressure
2. ASST: a severe headache; deteriorating level of consciousness; dilated or pinpoint pupils; alteration in breathing patterns; abnormal posturing (decerebrate, decorticate, flaccidity)
3. MGT: maintain B/P, prevent hypoxia, mannitol, sometimes emergency surgery is done to remove blood clot

## Myasthenia Gravis

1. Pathophys: auto-antibodies develop--> attacks acetylcholine receptors--> prevents inhibition of muscle depolarization--> muscle weakness and disability
2. ASST: fluctuating diplopia with ptosis (give away); weakness; exercise intolerance; tensilon test (edrophonium);
3. MGT: support ABCs; consider intubation with respiratory failure; consider acetylcholinesterase inhibitors, corticosteroids, IVIG, chemotherapy

## Guilian-Barre Syndrome

1. Pathophys: infection (viral usually)--> acute inflammation if the peripheral nerves --> myelin sheaths on the axons are destroyed--> resulting in decreased nerve impulses, loss of reflex response, and sudden muscle weakness.
2. ASST: weakness; numbness/tingling in arms & legs perceived to be painful; difficulty chewing & using muscles.
3. MGT: Intubate pts with respiratory compromise; IV immunoglobins are effective

## Multiple Sclerosis

1. Pathophys: autoimmune mechanism--> damages the myelin associated with nerve fibers--> poor nerve transmission--> diplopia, ataxia, paresthesias, monocular blindness and weakness, muscle weakness
2. ASST: Muscle weakness, muscle paralysis, visual disturbances, fatigue
3. MGT: Acute - high-dose steroids (methylprednisolone), Maintenance - methotrexate, interferon β, glatiramer acetate, fingolimod, natalizumab

## Meningitis

1. Pathophys: bacterial (typically) infection--> meninges become inflamed and pressure builds--> CNS functions are deranged
2. ASST: Triad (HA, fever, nuchal rigidity); AMS; Kernig sign, Brudzinski sign; photophobia; rash; seizures
3. MGT: penicillin, cephalosporin, vancomycin, droplet precaution

## Spinal Cord Injury (SCI)

1. Pathophys: Trauma to spinal cord--> bruising or severing of the spinal cord--> muscle paralysis and sensory impairment below the injury level--> vasodilation from loss of sympathetic tone--> BP drops
2. ASST: motor or sensory dysfunction below injury site; possible shock; (+) Babinski; confirm with CT or MRI
3. MGT: protect airway; correct any hypotension; prevent hypoxia; IV steroids (methylprednisolone)

## Transient Ischemic Attack (TIA)

1. Pathophys: Vascular injury/ dysfunction--> temporary reduction of brain perfusion--> sudden focal loss of neurological function that lasts < 24 hours
2. ASST: acute AMS; HA; facial paralysis, slurred speech, arm drift (Cincinnati stroke scale)- symptoms last less than 24 hours
3. MGT: protect airway; prevent hypoxia/ hypotension if present; drugs to prevent platelet aggregation (ASA, Plavix, Aggrenox Anticoags), Coumadin/Warfarin; lifestyle changes

## Ventricular Shunt

1. Used to treat increased ICP by draining CSF into peritoneum by gravity
2. Complications: Subdural hematoma, infection, stroke, and shunt failure (accumulation of abdominal fluid).

## Wernicke's Encephalopathy

1. Pathophys: thiamine deficiency--> glucose metabolism in brain reduced--> increased lactic acid in brain--> eye paralysis, gait instability, AMS
2. ASST: Hx EtOH abuse or poor nutrition; eye paralysis, gait instability, AMS
3. MGT: support ABCs; thiamine administration

## Brown-Sequard Syndrome

1. Pathophys: partial transection of the spinal cord from penetrating trauma--> motor lost on the same side, but below the injury as well as light touch, balance, and vibration--> on the opposite side pain and temperature is lost below the level of injury
2. ASST: History of penetrating trauma; Affected side: (-) motor/ vibration; Opposite side: (-) pain/temp
3. MGT: support ABCs; consider intubation with respiratory failure

## Anterior Cord Syndrome

1. Pathophys: spinal fracture--> shards of bone damages anterior spinal artery--> disruption of blood flow to the spinal cord itself --> paralysis and loss of pain below the level of injury occurs
2. ASST: motor paralysis and loss of pain into richer sensation below the level of injury occurs,
3. MGT: support ABCs; consider intubation with respiratory failure; balance/touch/vibration all intact

### Central Cord Syndrome

1. Pathophys: hypertension injury to the neck--> hemorrhage or swelling to central cervical segments--> loss of function in upper extremities with minimal loss to lower extremities
2. ASST: (+) motor weakness in UPPER exts.
3. MGT: MGT: support ABCs; consider intubation with respiratory failure

### Autonomic Dysreflexia

1. Pathophys: injury to T6 or higher--> widespread sympathetic response
2. ASST: HTN, HA, anxiety, nausea, flushing above SCI, piloerection above SCI
3. MGT: ABCs, monitor BP, supportive care

### Le Fort Fractures

This is a category system to grade facial fractures and mid-face stability. The yellow boxes below indicate fractured areas:

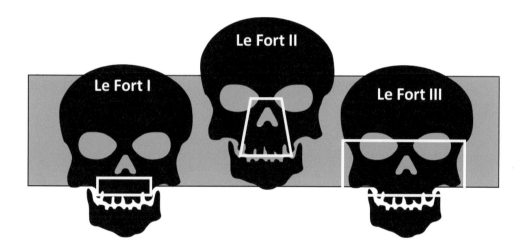

### Diffuse Axonal Injuries (DAI):

1. Pathophys: rapid acceleration- deceleration--> shearing forces damage axon--> immediate coma
2. ASST (MILD): coma 6-24 hours; begins to obey commands after 24 hours
3. ASST (Moderate): coma lasts >24hrs, no posturing; NORMAL HEAD CT with DAI
4. ASST (Severe): protracted coma and posturing; NORMAL HEAD CT
5. MGT: maximize oxygenation, Dilantin, treat ICP (HOB to at least 30, consider intubation and maintain 35mmHg EtCO2, mannitol)

## PART 4: NEUROLOGICAL PHARMACOLOGY

## INTRODUCTION

Now, let's dive into the pharmacology of neurological emergencies. There are several, and many will change hemodynamics/blood pressure. This is dangerous to most neurological patients.

## MEDICATIONS

### Phenytoin Sodium
1. Class: Antiepileptic
2. Mechanism: this is an antiepileptic that is like barbiturates. This drug reduces the chances of having a seizure (reduces seizure threshold).
3. Indications: seizures
4. Contraindications: allergy, sick sinus syndrome, seizure from hypoglycemia
5. Hemodynamics: (~CVP/ ~PCWP/ ~CO/ ~SVR)
6. Dose: 10-15 mg/kg over 30 min

### Mannitol
1. Class: Osmotic diuretic
2. Mechanism: Increases the oncotic pull of water into all vessels; therefore, more water is excreted in the form of urine
3. Indications: brain herniation; itsy lateral people change in the head injury or stroke patient
4. Contraindications: hypotension, severe dehydration, allergy
5. Hemodynamics: (~CVP/ ~PCWP/ ~CO/ ~SVR)
6. Dose: 1-2 g/ kg over 30 minutes

### Versed (midazolam)
1. Class: Benzodiazepine
2. Mechanism: Benzodiazepines are a class of agents that work on the central nervous system, acting selectively on gamma-aminobutyric acid-A (GABA-A) receptors in the brain. It enhances response to the inhibitory neurotransmitter GABA, by opening GABA-activated chloride channels and allowing chloride ions to enter the neuron, making the neuron negatively charged and resistant to excitation.
3. Indications: sedation; seizures
4. Contraindications: Allergy/ hypotension
5. Can precipitously drop blood pressure.
6. Hemodynamics: (↓CVP/ ↓PCWP/ ~CO/ ↓SVR)
7. Dose: 2-5 mg IV

### Ativan (lorazepam)
1. Class: Benzodiazepine
2. Mechanism: See above.
3. Indications: sedation; seizures
4. Contraindications: Allergy/ hypotension
5. Can precipitously drop blood pressure.
6. Hemodynamics: (~CVP/ ~PCWP/ ~CO/ ~SVR)
7. Dose: 0.05 mg/kg IV

### Ketamine
1. Class: Hypnotic
2. Mechanism: This medication provides sedation as well as hypnosis. Ketamine will help to increase BP– ideal in trauma, but not in increased ICP conditions. Ketamine also will reduce bronchospasm. Used both as an analgesia and sedation.
3. Indications: sedation; pain control, bronchodilation
4. Contraindications: Allergy/ increased ICP
5. Hemodynamics: (~CVP/ ~PCWP/ ↑CO/ ↑SVR)

6. Dose: 1-2 mg/kg IV

## Fentanyl

1. Class: Opiate
2. Indications: pain control can be used for sedative– like properties
3. Contraindications: Allergy/ History of rigid chest syndrome
4. Very safe hemodynamic profile (does not drop blood pressure much at all).
5. Can be used in the hypotensive setting when a benzodiazepine would be unsafe for perfusion.
6. Opiates drop BP because of histamine release they cause. Most opioids are administered in milligrams. Fentanyl is administered in micrograms (1000 less particles of medication), so it causes histamine release 1000 times less than that of morphine/ dilaudid, etc.
7. Hemodynamics: (~CVP/ ~PCWP/ ~CO/ ~SVR)
8. Dose: 1-3 mcg/kg IV

## Methylprednisolone (Solu-Medrol)

1. Class: Steroid
2. Indications: to decrease inflammation and swelling
3. Contraindications: known hypersensitivity, suspected fungal infections
4. This is a glucocorticoid used for its anti- inflammatory and immunosuppressive properties
5. Adult Dose: (INITIAL)- 30 mg/kg over30 minutes; (MAINTENANCE)- 5.4 mg/kg/hr for 23 hours
6. Peds Dose: 1-2 mg/kg over 2 minutes

# PART 5: BOLTS AND DRAINS

## INTRODUCTION

Any device that is placed in the patient's cranial vault for measurement of pressures and other parameters is commonly referred to as a "bolt". There are several different types ranging from incredibly invasive to not very invasive.

## DEVICES

### Ventriculostomy Drain

1. The intraventricular catheter is a soft tube placed through a burr hole into the lateral ventricle and allows for both monitoring and for therapeutic drainage of CSF to reduce the ICP.
2. This must be leveled at the Foramen of Monroe, which is found between the external opening of the auditory canal (tragus) and the corner of the eye (canthus).
3. Fluid drained must be monitored for the amount, color, and clarity at hourly intervals, and drainage can be either constant or intermittent.
4. Infection and bleeding is common complications.

### Subarachnoid Screw

1. The subarachnoid screw (or "bolt") is considered the second choice of devices placed by neurosurgeons for monitoring ICP.
2. They are relatively easy to install, but their accuracy is significantly less than the more direct ventriculostomy drain.

### Fiber Optic Monitors

1. The fiber optic device has a pressure sensor at the tip, and it can be placed into the ventricle, the subarachnoid space, etc.
2. Fiber optic monitors don't have to be leveled and recalibrated – the transducer is built into the tip of the device, and gets calibrated once just before insertion.

### Leveling and Zeroing Ventriculostomies

1. It is important that the device is leveled properly to ensure accurate readings.
2. PROCEDURE:
   a. Position your patient's HOB at 30-45 degrees for the measurement.
   b. Ensure the transducer is at the midpoint height between the tragus of the ear in the canthus of the eye; placed at the anatomical position of the Foramen of Monro.
   c. Obtain the ICP waveform on the monitor by turning the three-way stopcock nearest the patient so that the ICP waveform is visualized.
   d. Remove the transducer cap, zero the transducer, and replace the cap.
   e. In the transport environment, they should be done each time the patient is moved.

### Drainage

1. There will be times you will need to assess the drainage system associated with an ICP monitoring system.
2. Each hour, measure and record the drainage and ensure the proper waveform.
3. It is imperative that normal saline (that does not have a bacteriostatic preservative) be utilized as the fluid with the transducer.
4. The height of the drainage bag must always remain at the same level the physician prescribed. If the drainage bag is too high, then flow out of the cranium will not happen. If the drainage bag is too low, been too much flow will occur causing drastic intracranial decompression. At just the right height, flow will commence at the prescribed pressure limit.
5. Sometimes you may need to drain the system because of an increasing ICP.
6. Cerebrospinal fluid should be drained if the ICP is greater than 20 cmH2O.
7. No more than 3cc of cerebrospinal fluid should be drained at any particular time.

### Waveforms

1. The ICP tracing waveform is composed of three waves: one for the choroid plexus pulsations, one for the tidal wave as blood pushes forward through the vasculature, and one for the Dicrotic notch.

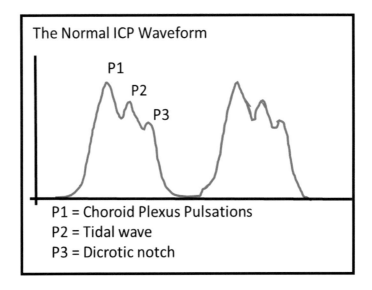

The Normal ICP Waveform

P1

P2

P3

P1 = Choroid Plexus Pulsations
P2 = Tidal wave
P3 = Dicrotic notch

2. These are labeled as P1, P2, and P3.
3. P1 should always be the tallest and P2 should be the second tallest.
4. An elevated P2 means that the intracranial compliance is probably decreasing as the ICP is rising

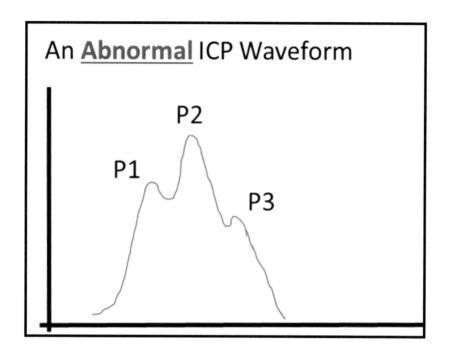

# PART 6: NEUROLOGICAL MANAGEMENT QUESTIONS

1. A 62 y/o female states she has a headache that began yesterday when she was moving furniture. Since then, she has had increasing eye pain and blurred vision. The only other symptom she has is some facial numbness. Her only history is a-fib. Vital signs are: BP 162/92, HR 52, SpO2 98%, RR 16. These symptoms are indicative of which of the following?
   a. Wernicke's encephalopathy
   b. Diffuse axonal injury
   c. Berry aneurysm
   d. Subarachnoid hemorrhage

2. A 16 y/o male was in a one car MVC where he only had a lap seat belt on and was the only back seat passenger. He complains of an inability to feel or move his lover extremities. You assess these neurological deficits to begin at the level of the umbilicus. He complains of HA, severe nausea. You notice his skin is very flushed from waist and up. V/S: BP 142/100, HR 121, RR 21, SpO2 100%. Which of these conditions does this describe?
   a. Diffuse axonal injury
   b. Traumatic brain injury
   c. Guilian-Barre syndrome
   d. Autonomic dysreflexia

3. A 19 y/o college football player was tackled and did not get up. He was taken off the field and rushed to the local hospital. He had a GCS of 6 until approximately 10 hours after his injury, where he began recovering well. Which of these conditions does this describe?
    a. Diffuse axonal injury (severe)
    b. Diffuse axonal injury (progressive)
    c. Diffuse axonal injury (moderate)
    d. Diffuse axonal injury (mild)

4. A 25 y/o was playing softball and was struck with a softball bat to the head. Upon your arrival, it is reported that he immediately went unconsciousness. Then they were just going to take him by personal car to the ER, but he became "woozy" again. Now the patient has a GCS of 6 (E1, V1, M4). He has a hematoma to the occipital region of his skull. He friends report he takes no medicines. V/S: 118/72, HR 92, RR 12, SpO2 99%. Which condition does this describe?
    a. Epidural hematoma
    b. Autonomic dysreflexia
    c. Subdural hematoma
    d. Diffuse axonal injury

5. You are assessing a patient with facial trauma, and you notice that the upper teeth and gums have been fractured. You assess for crepitus and free movement of this bone. It does move along with the nose and the orbital bones. Which Le Fort fracture is present?
    a. II
    b. I
    c. III
    d. IV

6. You are assessing a patient with facial trauma, and you notice that the upper teeth, nose, and gums have been fractured. You also notice there is a globe rupture and bilateral crepitus to the medical and lateral aspects of the orbital bones. How would you classify this per Le Fort?
    a. III
    b. I
    c. II
    d. IV

7. As you are preparing to transport a patient with a cranial drain, you are calculating what your blood pressure minimum would need to be to maintain a 70 mmHg CPP. The patient's ICP monitor is showing 59 mmHg. The patient weighs 77kg. What mean arterial pressure would you need to target to achieve this CPP?
    a. 117
    b. 129
    c. 135
    d. 109

8. You are calculating MAP on your head injury patient. Assume and ICP of 15mmHg. What is patient's CPP if your patient has a blood pressure of 120/90?
    a. 100
    b. 94
    c. 106
    d. 118

9. You are calculating MAP on your head injury patient. Assume and ICP of 15mmHg. What is patient's CPP if your patient has a blood pressure of 136/88?
    a. 103
    b. 97
    c. 89
    d. 115

10. A 57 y/o male was involved in a 1- car MVC with rollover. The patient was ejected approximately 50 feet and impacted asphalt. Upon arrival, EMS reported he was awake, alert, and reporting pain to his back. They mentioned that as they were applying a long spine board, he had on open left ankle fracture, but never complained of the pain- just back pain. EMS then noticed hypotension and priapism. The patient's blood sugar is 130 mg/dL and both pupils are 4mm and briskly reactive to light. V/S: BP 62/40, HR 109, RR 26, SpO2 88%. Which condition does this best describe?
    a. Subarachnoid hemorrhage
    b. Neurologic hyporeflexia
    c. Spinal cord injury
    d. Traumatic brain injury

11. A 27 y/o male is found unresponsive. This occurred at a class at a university. The instructor reports the patient was answering a question, trailed off, began looking upward and leftward, and then slumped to the floor. Then it is reported that the patient 'tensed up' for about a minute. The EMS report confirms a blood sugar of 83 mg/dL and pupils were at 3mm bilaterally and reactive to light. The patient slowly woke up en route to the ER per EMS. V/S: BP 122/80, HR 77, RR 20, SpO2 98%. Which condition matches this description??
    a. Seizure
    b. Meningitis
    c. Hypoglycemia
    d. Dysreflexia

12. A 31 y/o female falls off a 10-foot ladder and impacts her head on the cement. She initially exhibited an intact mental status but begins to become increasingly confused until she becomes combative. She has no history and is on no medications. Her right pupil is 3 mm larger than the left. V/S: 178/102, HR 55, RR 21, SpO2 99%. Which of the following is causing this deterioration?
    a. Ischemic stroke
    b. Intracranial pressure
    c. Diffuse axonal injury
    d. Transit ischemic attack

13. You're transporting an ICU patient with the following vital signs and findings: HR 65, BP 167/87, RR 24 and irregular, ICP monitor reads 24, CVP 18, and wedge pressure 17. Which of the following is the most appropriate action?
    a. Re-shoot a wedge pressure
    b. Drain the ventriculostomy
    c. Administer metoprolol
    d. Prepare for cardiac arrest

14. You are transporting a patient to a neuro ICU from a smaller rural hospital. The patient was struck in the head by a falling tree limb. Currently, he is awake and alert. Which of the following would best indicate increasing ICP?
    a. Developed a headache upon ascent
    b. Mentioning he is getting drowsy
    c. Complaining of spots in his visual field
    d. Answering questions inappropriately

15. Earlier tonight, your patient was in a three car MVC with rollover where your patient was ejected. Which of the following vital sign values would make you confident that you were preventing secondary brain injury?
    a. BP 92/50, SpO2 92%, EtCO2 22
    b. BP 110/56, SpO2 90%, EtCO2 35
    c. BP 167/87, SpO2 95%, EtCO2 44
    d. BP 88/66, SpO2 99%, EtCO2 46

16. An adult patient has had a massive stroke. Which of the following findings would be consistent with Cushing's Reflex?
    a. HR 46, BP 197/60, CVP 7, RR 21
    b. BP 182/57, tachypnea, EtCO2 35
    c. RR 24, HR 58, hypotensive for 2 hours
    d. EtCO2 47, hypertensive, RR 18, HR 50

17. The first responder is feverishly ventilating the patient with a bag-valve mask who recently was a victim of a car vs. pedestrian accident. The patient has facial and head trauma. You estimate that the first responder is ventilating approximately 30 times a minute. Which of the following dangerous pathophysiologies would this cause?
    a. Physiologic eucapnia
    b. Pathologic hypercapnia
    c. Systemic vasodilation
    d. Cerebral vasoconstriction

18. Your patient looks at you when you speak to her. When you ask her the date, she says "blue." You note left-sided weakness when she grips your fingers. What is her Glasgow Coma Score?
    a. 11
    b. 13
    c. 12
    d. 14

19. Your adult patient can obey simple commands and opens their eyes when they hear you speak. They can talk to you in sentences but seem a little confused and unsure of where they are. What is their current Glasgow Coma Scale score?
    a. 10
    b. 11
    c. 12
    d. 13

20. A 51 y/o homeless male is found behind a convenient store unconscious. He only groans to painful stimuli and additionally localizes the painful stimuli with his upper extremities. There is not much more history on this patient, and he doesn't have any identification. At the time of assessment, his blood sugar was 101 mg/dL and his pupils are 5mm and reactive bilaterally. V/S: BP 154/92, HR 103, RR 22, SpO2 94%. Which condition does this best match?
    a. Multiple sclerosis
    b. Guilian- Barre syndrome
    c. Wernicke's encephalopathy
    d. Myasthenia gravis

21. A 30 y/o rugby player receives a critical blow to his head in the frontal section of the skull. He complains of a small headache at the time, but he's able to continue playing. Later at dinner, he mentioned that his headache was still present, but 'not too bad.' The next morning, his wife reported he was slurring words and not answering questions (~ 20 hours s/p impact). At the time of EMS transport, his blood sugar was 74 mg/dL, and his pupils were 5mm and sluggish bilaterally. V/S: BP 144/74, HR 66, RR 22, SpO2 99%.
    a. Subarachnoid injury
    b. Epidural hematoma
    c. Spinal cord injury
    d. Subdural hematoma

22. A 21 y/o mixed martial arts fighter is complaining of severe HA after a fight. His trainer reports that about 30 min after the fight, he became increasingly sleepy. After an hour of the fight, the trainer says he became unarousable. The patient's pupils are both dilated to ~ 8mm and poorly reactive to light. During the exam, the patient begins to posture. V/S: 198/ 104, HR 48, RR 28, SpO2 99%. Blood sugar is 104 mg/dL Which of the following conditions does this describe?
    a. Ischemic stroke
    b. Intracerebral hemorrhage
    c. Wernicke's encephalopathy
    d. Severe spinal cord injury

23. Your adults, the patient, has been thrown from his car following an MVC rollover. You are picking up your patient at a local regional hospital and taking them to the level one trauma hospital in the area with neuro services. The CT shows a rightward shift of 5 mm. The patient currently has a ventriculostomy placed and indicates and ICP of 38 mmHg. Which of the following would best reduce ICP and increase cerebral perfusion pressure?
    a. Elevate the HOB and then administer a fluid bolus
    b. Increase minute volume to get ICP to 25– 30 mmHg
    c. Reduce the BP with vasodilators up to 30% of MAP
    d. Hyperventilate the patient and admin nitroglycerin

# PART 7: NEUROLOGICAL MANAGEMENT RATIONALES

1. **(C)** Aneurysms occur via a weakening of the arterial wall of a vessel in the brain which eventually ruptures. This can lead to a headache, eye pain and visual changes, numbness in weakness, altered level of consciousness as well as increasing ICP. Autonomic dysreflexia and diffuse axonal injury typically require a traumatic event. Wernicke's encephalopathy is from a thiamine deficiency. The best answer, in this case, is Berry aneurysm. Even if you don't know the specific type of an aneurysm, these are the signs and symptoms of an aneurysm.

2. **(D)** This patient has had obvious damage to his spinal cord resulting in a strange reaction by the autonomic nervous system where blood pressure increases, heart rate increases, as well as nausea and vomiting. This is called autonomic dysreflexia.

3. **(D)** Diffuse axonal injuries (DAIs) have three magnitudes: mild, moderate, and severe. Mild is categorized as being comatose for 6-24 hours while moderate is characterized as being comatose for greater than 24 hours without the presence of posturing, and severe is protracted coma with posturing. It is interesting to note that in DAI, there is no change on CT or MRI, and they presented with a normal head CT or MRI. Because this can occur within 10 hours it is considered a mild DAI.

4. **(A)** This patient presents with the classic signs of an epidural bleed. When the patient loses consciousness, has a lucid period afterwards, and then goes back unconscious, you should be highly suspicious of an epidural bleed. In this particular case, the patient gets "woozy" after his lucid period. This still qualifies and is representative of an epidural bleed.

5. **(C)** In this case, we have complete craniofacial separation; therefore, this is a Le Fort III. Le Fort fractures are fractures of the midface, which collectively involve separation of all or a portion of the midface from the skull base. Le Fort type 1: [horizontal maxillary fracture, separating the teeth from the upper face, fracture line passes through the alveolar ridge, lateral nose and inferior wall of maxillary sinus]; Le Fort type 2 [pyramidal fracture, with the teeth at the pyramid base and nasofrontal suture at its apex, fracture arch passes through posterior alveolar ridge, lateral walls of maxillary sinuses, inferior orbital rim, and nasal bones]; Le Fort type 3 [craniofacial disjunction, fracture line passes through nasofrontal suture, maxillo-frontal suture, orbital wall and zygomatic arch].

6. **(A)** The orbital bones, the nasal bones and the maxilla bones have all been fractured. This is a Le Fort III injury.

7. **(B)** This is a simple skill where we need to calculate MAP and CPP. To calculate MAP, double the diastolic pressure and add it to the systolic pressure. Take this value in divided by three. You have now arrived at your mean arterial pressure (MAP). To identify cerebral perfusion pressure (CPP) take your MAP and subtract the total ICP. That value is your cerebral perfusion pressure (CPP).

8. **(A)** This is a simple skill where we need to calculate MAP and CPP. To calculate MAP, double the diastolic pressure and add it to the systolic pressure. Take this value in divided by three. You have now arrived at your mean arterial pressure (MAP). To identify cerebral perfusion pressure (CPP) take your MAP and subtract the total ICP. That value is your cerebral perfusion pressure (CPP).

9. **(C)** This is a simple skill where we need to calculate MAP and CPP. To calculate MAP, double the diastolic pressure and add it to the systolic pressure. Take this value in divided by three. You have now arrived at your mean arterial pressure (MAP). To identify cerebral perfusion pressure (CPP) take your MAP and subtract the total ICP. That value is your cerebral perfusion pressure (CPP).

10. **(C)** There are three things that indicate spinal cord injury in this case. The patient's open ankle fracture is the first because he is not complaining of pain. The second is the priapism- damage to a male's spinal cord prevents the muscle that keeps blood out of the penis from remaining constricted. Once it is relaxed from SCI, the penis can fill with blood. Thirdly, hypertension occurs because the spinal cord injury (SCI) also relaxes the smooth muscle in vessels. Once they relax, vasodilation occurs, and hypotension follows. Subarachnoid hemorrhage and traumatic brain injury both present with altered mental status typically, it doesn't fit the profile here. Neurologic hyporeflexia not a real condition. Never choose the answer that you are unfamiliar with- Ever.

11. **(A)** The tensing up represents a tonic or tonic-clonic type seizures. You can think of seizures with hypoglycemia, but since the blood sugar is normal, the hypoglycemia selection can be ruled out.

12. **(B)** This patient has a history of a direct blow to the head and a declining mental status. Additionally, one people is enlarging indicating herniation. The symptomology is most likely due to increased intracranial pressure (ICP).

13. **(B)** The patient ICP has elevated beyond 20 mmHg; therefore, it is important to drain the ventriculostomy to prevent herniation and symptomologies of increased ICP.

14. **(B)** This patient has recently received a traumatic brain injury; therefore, it is important to look for signs of decreasing level of consciousness, posturing, and pupillary changes. The only answer here that indicates the patient is losing intubation is the selection where he is in appropriately answered questions. On the GCS scale this would be a verbal score of 3.

15. **(C)** There are two answers with hypoxia: 90% and 92%, which can cause secondary brain injury. Therefore, these answer selections are incorrect. There is one true hypotensive blood pressure: 88 systolic, therefore this could cause secondary brain injury. It is also a wrong answer selection. This is only one answer: BP 167/87, SpO2 95%, EtCO2 44.

16. **(A)** There is one answer here with a high blood pressure with lighted pulse pressure and bradycardia, which demonstrates Cushing's Reflex; therefore, it is the answer. Cushing's reflex can be identified by a very high blood pressure (with widening pulse pressure) that occurs with bradycardia. This is the result of two different physiological systems working against one another. As a patient develops increasing ICP, the body will increase blood pressure to force open vessels in the brain. This increase in blood pressure acts as a fluid scaffolding to keep the vessels opened against the increasing pressure. The heart recognizes the increase in blood pressure and thinks it's a bad thing. So the heart slows down to reduce blood pressure. Therefore, we get an increasing blood pressure and a decreasing heart rate. You also can have increased respiratory rates and irregular respiratory patterns, but it is more from the increasing the ICP rather than the blood pressure/ heart rate war.

17. **(A)** This patient is currently being hyperventilated; therefore, their carbon dioxide measurements will be low. This causes a vasoconstriction within the cerebral blood flow. This is dangerous because it limits the blood flow to the delicate and sensitive brain tissue. It is important only to hyperventilate with signs of brain herniation, instill only targeting carbon dioxide levels between 30 and 35 mmHg.

18. **(B)** The patient who looks at you earns a GCS eye-opening score of 4. A patient who answers questions inappropriately earns a GCS verbal score of 3. In this case, your patient is gripping your fingers;

therefore, she is following commands. Following commands gets you a GCS motor score of 6. E4 + V3 + M6 = GCS of 13.

19. **(D)** This patient opens their eyes not spontaneously, but only when you call their name. This earns them a GCS eye-opening score of 3. If your patient is answering questions, then they are following commands and earns them a GCS motor score of 6. The fact that they are confused indicates their verbal score is 4. E3 + V4 + M6 = GCS of 13.

20. **(C)** Wernicke's encephalopathy a condition where thiamine is deficient. Thiamine is important in facilitating glucose metabolism. Thiamine deficiencies are typically seen and people who do not take in enough vitamins or are malnourished. This is a common finding an alcoholics and homeless people.

21. **(D)** This player received a traumatic blow to the frontal skull that resulted in a small headache. The next morning, he presented one stroke like symptoms. Subdural hematomas typically arise from veins, so they have a slow progression (which matches the 20 hours from impact to current symptoms) after some impact to the head. However, they also can occur spontaneously. Epidurals usually happen rapidly because they arise from arteries. Spinal cord injuries result in motor and sensory problems which are not present in this question. Therefore, the spinal cord injury option is incorrect.

22. **(B)** The patient began having a headache directly after his flight and later became incredibly sleepy and progressed towards coma. Dilated pupils indicate that there is extensive swelling of the brain and progressing toward herniation- this is indicated by both eyes being dilated from bilateral pressure to the third cranial nerves. The blood pressure indicates that there is Cushing's reflex present: high blood pressure low heart rate and elevated respiratory rate. And ischemic stroke would present with unilateral motor changes and altered level of consciousness, encephalopathy would have presented with an altered level of consciousness and without pupil changes, spinal cord injury would have most likely presented with lower blood pressure from the base of dilation. Therefore, the correct answer selection, in this case, is the intracerebral hemorrhage.

23. **(A)** This adult MVC rollover patient has suffered a traumatic brain injury. Normal ICP should be under 20 mmHg, and there should be no midline shift on CT. This indicates increasing intracranial pressure. The best treatment for this would be to increase the head of the bed to facilitate the flow of cerebral spinal fluid out of the brain, and to provide a fluid bolus to help maintain cerebral perfusion pressure

# CHAPTER 9: TOXICOLOGICAL EMERGENCIES

## PART 1: THE TOXICOLOGICAL ASSESSMENT

### INTRODUCTION

The toxicological examination is a unique one. There's usually an index of suspicion suggested by some odd findings that just do not add up or a specific location or incident (like house fire, industrial explosion, etc). Chemicals and substances that pose a toxicological risk are found throughout the industries of our society: education, agriculture, transportation, energy, environmental, and transportation. The critical care transport professional can significantly impact patient outcomes positively by quickly recognizing when a toxicological emergency is present, and by executing the correct management strategies early.

### THE TOX INITIAL ASSESSMENT

#### *GENERAL IMPRESSION*

1. As you approach the patient, look at their body position, work of breathing and skin condition and color.
2. Their body position tells you great information: tripod means they are short of breath/ hypoxic, laying on the ground with weak muscles mean they are extremely hypoxic.
3. Normal respiratory effort indicates they are receiving adequate oxygen, but labored respirations indicates they are most likely hypoxic.
4. Normal skin color indicates adequate perfusion, but pale or mottled skin can indicate poor perfusion.

#### *ASSESS MENTAL STATUS*

1. AVPU:  Awake– eyes open spontaneously; Verbal- arouses to stimulation my voice; Painful- purpose for movements to painful stimuli; Unresponsive- no response to any stimuli
2. Assess GCS
   a. Eye Opening: Spontaneous (4); to speech (3); to painful stimuli (2); no opening at all (0)
   b. Verbal Effort: normal conversation (5);  confused (4); inappropriate words (3); incomprehensible sounds (2); no verbal effort (1)
   c. Motor Effort: follows commands (6); localizes pains (5); withdrawals from pain (4); decorticate posturing (3); decerebrate posturing (2); no motor effort (1)

#### *AIRWAY*

1. Ensure a patent airway.
2. Clear, reposition, reassess as needed.

#### *BREATHING*

1. Rate
2. Quality (normal or labored)
3. Rhythm (normal or abnormal respiratory patterns).

## CIRCULATION

1. Ensure the patient has a pulse and note the rate, strength (normal, bounding, or weak), and quality (regular or irregular).
2. Obtain and assess heart rate, blood pressure, pulse oximetry, cardiac monitoring, and labs/ images if available.

## DISABILITY

1. Assess for the ability to move, lift, and hold all 4 extremities. Assess for equal grip and pedal strength. Assess for the ability to maintain a seated posture, standing and walking. Assess for cranial nerve deficits.
2. Identify deficits that existed prior to your assessment.

## EXPOSURE

1. Expose patient
2. perform a head to toe rule out life threats.

## FOCUSED ASSESSMENT

1. For every call/ flight, you should be looking for and ruling out information that would indicate that a toxicological problem exists.
2. Indications of a Toxicological Occurrence:
    a. The scene has containers that carry toxic substances
    b. Strange odors, smells, smoke, gas clouds, or vapors.
    c. These are signs that clearly indicate a toxic substance.
    d. Multiple patients that present with similar symptoms who can all be tracked to a single area, location, or activity.
    e. Bystanders who develop symptoms that are like original patients from an area, location, or activity.
3. The Toxic Patient is Prone to Violence
    a. Your toxic patient may have tried to commit suicide or otherwise may have a history of violence.
    b. Once contaminated, chemicals can alter a person's normal mentation, making them a threat to the crew.
    c. Aggressive/ combative patients may require chemical sedation/ paralysis to prevent the patient from putting the crew in danger (such as opening an aircraft door, hitting the pilot, or injuring the nurse or paramedic).
    d. You should be aggressive in performing RSI on any patient who poses a significant threat to you, your partner, and/ or pilot (if air medical transport).
4. **Identify if any toxidromes exist**. Toxidromes are specific patterns of symptomology that indicate a medication or medication class as the toxic agent.


# PART 2: TOXICOLOGICAL SYNDROMES

## INTRODUCTION

Toxicological syndromes, also known as *toxidromes*, are a constellation of commonly seen features and exam findings that are typical for certain types of poisoning or overdoses. These toxidromes group these commonly seen vital signs and findings according to which medication or drug is the culprit. The tough part is you'll have to memorize these findings, have the forethought on scene to access this information, and then treat the patient based on this the toxidrome you suspect.

## TOXIDROMES

### OPIOID TOXIDROME

1. The toxicity caused by accidental OD or illicit use of opiate derivatives
2. Toxins: Morphine, meperidine, codeine, heroin, oxycodone, hydromorphone
3. S/S: Sedation, respiratory depression, myosis (pinpoint pupils), hypotension (seen in larger overdoses)
4. MGT/ Antidote: Narcan

### SYMPATHOMIMETIC TOXIDROME

1. The toxicity mimics the endogenous catecholamines (epinephrine/ norepinephrine).
2. Toxins: cocaine, methylphenidate, epinephrine
3. S/S: tachycardia, chest pain, hypertension, agitation, seizures, hyperthermia, mydriasis (dilated pupils), diaphoresis
4. MGT/ Antidote: 12 Lead, Benzodiazepines, active cooling

### CELLULAR ASPHYXIA

1. The toxicity inhibits oxygen from either being delivered to the cells or being utilized by the cells resulting in cellular asphyxia
2. Toxins: Carbon monoxide (CO), cyanide, methemoglobin, hydrogen sulfide (swamp gas)
3. S/S: multiple victims; near burning material; CHERRY RED SKIN; tachycardia, headache, nausea, confusion, syncope
4. MGT/ Antidote: remove from exposure location, O2, methylene blue (for methemoglobinemia), hyperbaric chamber

### CHOLINERGIC TOXIDROME

1. The toxicity caused by organophosphate or carbamate insecticides or by nerve agents
2. Toxins: organophosphates, nerve agents (sarin, ricin), pilocarpine, muscarine
3. S/S: (SLUDGE): salivation, lacrimation, urinary incontinence, diaphoresis, GI (diarrhea), emesis
4. MGT/ Antidote: atropine & 2-PAM (pralidoxime); glycopyrrolate (anticholinergic)
5. Decontamination: Use waterproof PPEs to remove patient's clothing (gown and gloves for sure if not more) will limit secondary contamination to responders

### ANTICHOLINERGIC TOXIDROME

1. The toxicity caused by tricyclic antidepressants (TCAs) and other anticholinergic medications
2. Toxins: TCAs, atropine, scopolamine, diphenhydramine
3. S/S: Mad as a hatter (psychosis); red as a beet (hot, flushed skin); dry as a bone (dry mucous membranes and urinary retention); blind as a bat (pupil dilation); hot as a hare (hyperthermia)
4. MGT/ Antidote: benzodiazepines; physostigmine

## SPECIFIC MEDICATION TOXICITIES

### ACETOMINOPHEN TOXICITY

1. Critical Value: > 50 mg/L
2. S/S Phase I: 0-24 hours; n/v, no appetite, diaphoresis, dehydration, elevated liver function tests (LFTs)
3. S/S Phase II: 24-72 hours; RUQ pain, continued elevation in liver function tests (LFTs)

4. S/S Phase III: 72-96 hours; oliguria, hepatomegaly, coagulopathy, liver failure
5. S/S Phase IV: longer than 4 days; resolution of symptoms OR multiple organ failures
6. MGT/ Antidote: ABCs; activated charcoal If within 1-2 hours after ingestion); admin acetylcysteine; poison control center

## HYDROFLUROIC ACID TOXICITY

1. HF is a highly corrosive substance, and its reaction depends on the route of exposure, acid concentration, and length of exposure.
2. S/S: Low concentrations (< 15% solution) can cause minimal effects. High concentrations (> 40%) can lead to deep tissue destruction, low Ca, high K+, arrhythmias, acidosis, and shock. Contact the poison control center (PCC)
3. MGT/ Antidote: ABCs, dermal burns—> Calcium containing gels; eyes—> copious amounts of water; inhalation—> remove from the area and protect airway; all patients should be on cardiac monitor—> watch for hyperkalemia.

## AMPHETIMINE TOXICITY

1. S/S: Hx of ingestion, hypertension, tachycardia, anxiety and hyperactivity, diaphoresis, Sz, rhabdomyolysis, myocardial ischemia, cerebral hemorrhage, (+) urine test
2. MGT/ Antidote: ABCs, activated charcoal, benzodiazepines (for sz or sedation), phenobarbital or haldol (for sedation if needed), aggressive cooling (if hyperthermic), IV fluids, vasodilators (for HTN), beta blocker (if tachycardia); contact PCC

## BENZODIAZEPINE TOXICITY

1. S/S: Hx of ingestion, CNS and resp depression, hypothermia, ataxia, slurred speech, (+) in urine
2. MGT/ Antidote: ABCs, activated charcoal, intubate; flumazenil is the reversal agent, but its usage puts pt at HIGH risk for seizure. (rather bag a pt not breathing than be able to do nothing for a seizure patient); contact PCC

## BETA BLOCKER TOXICITY

1. S/S: Hx of ingestion, hypotension, bradycardia, hypoglycemia, bronchospasm, pulmonary edema, AMS, Sz
2. MGT/ Antidote: ABCs, activated charcoal, Antidote: GLUCAGON, IV atropine or transcutaneous pacing (for bradycardia), dopamine or epi (hypotension), high dose insulin with dextrose (to clear beta blockers), consider milrinone; contact PCC
3. ECG Changes: 1st-degree heart block (long PR interval); bradycardia

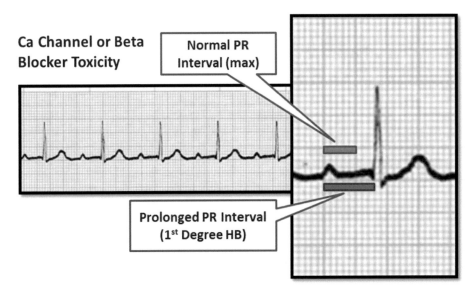

## CALCIUM CHANNEL BLOCKER TOXICITY

1. S/S: Hx of ingestion, hypotension, bradycardia, n/v, AMS, hyperglycemia, metabolic acidosis
2. MGT/ Antidote: ABCs, activated charcoal, Antidote: IV CALCIUM, glucagon/ high dose insulin/ epi (for hypotension and bradycardia), cardiac pacing (if needed), consider milrinone; contact PCC
3. ECG Changes: 1st degree heart block (long PR interval); bradycardia, high degree blocks

## CARDIAC GLYCOSIDE (DIGITALIS) TOXICITY

1. S/S: Hx of ingestion, n/v, abd pain, lethargy/ AMS/ weakness, hyperkalemia, bradycardia, conduction disturbances
2. MGT/ Antidote: ABCs, activated charcoal, glucagon, IV atropine or transcutaneous pacing (for bradycardia), lidocaine and phenytoin (for conduction disturbances), digoxin- specific antibodies (digibind) for any life-threatening arrhythmias that do not respond to normal therapy.
3. ECG Changes: Digitalis tox: Ladle sign, aka 'Dig scoping' (scooping to the right side of the QRS complex; Reverse Checkmark sign (T– wave inversion that resembles a backward checkmark).

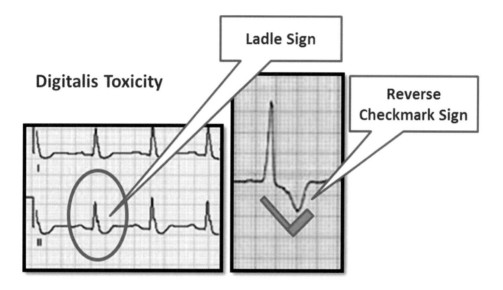

## COCAINE TOXICITY

1. S/S: Hx of ingestion, sympathetic toxidrome, chest pain, pulmonary edema, exacerbation of asthma, (+) in urine
2. MGT/ Antidote: ABCs, activated charcoal, benzodiazepines or calcium channel blockers (to relax muscle tone), IV fluids, external cooling (if hyperthermic), bicarb (if rhabdomyolysis present), vasodilators (for HTN), thrombolytics or transport for PCTA (for MI), MONA (for MI), AVOID beta blockers (causes un– contested alpha response); contact PCC

## METHANOL TOXICITY

1. S/S: hx of ingestion, lethargy/ slurred speech, "snowfield' vision or blindness, AMS, seizure
2. MGT/ Antidote: ABCs, ethanol (oral or IV); contact PCC

## SALICYLATE TOXICITY

1. S/S: hx of ingestion, tinnitus/ deafness, tachypnea, hyperthermia, AMS, n/v/d, GI bleeding, pulmonary edema, liver/ renal failure possible
2. MGT/ Antidote: ABCs, activated charcoal, monitor fluid volume and electrolytes, provide potassium replacement (if needed), bicarbonate; contact PCC

## SEROTONIN-SPECIFIC REUPTAKE INHIBITOR TOXICITY

1. S/S: hx of ingestion, AMS, n/v/d, HA, diaphoresis, shivering, hypotension, QRS prolongation, muscle rigidity, spasticity
2. MGT/ Antidote: ABCs, activated charcoal, fluids (for hypotension), benzos (for seizures); contact PCC

## ORGANOPHOSPHATE TOXICITY

1. S/S: hx of ingestion; organophosphate toxidrome
2. MGT/ Antidote: decontaminate the skin, ABCs, activated charcoal, atropine and 2 PAM (antidotes), in RSI use non- depolarizing NMBs, benzos (for seizures); contact PCC

## CHLORINE/AMMONIA GAS TOXICITY

1. S/S: hx of exposure, multiple patients, lacrimation, coughing, drooling, swelling airway, wheezing, pulmonary edema
2. MGT/ Antidote: ABCs, remove from environment, 100% humidified O2, bronchodilators, half strength bicarb via nebulizer (neutralization of mucous membranes), corticosteroids (for airway or pulmonary inflammation); contact PCC

## CAUSTICS TOXICITY

1. This results from the ingestions, inhalation, or dermal exposure to Drano, bleach, or lime.
2. S/S: hx of exposure, inhalation (throat discomfort, bronchospasm, stridor, local airway injury, wheezing, rales, pulmonary edema); Dermal (pain, redness); ingestion (nausea, vomiting, abdominal cramps, metabolic derangements
3. MGT/ Antidote: Focus on airway protection and monitoring; decontamination; flush eyes (if affected); oxygen and IV initiated; call PCC.

## TOXIC ALCOHOL TOXICITY: (Methanol, Ethylene Glycol, Isopropanol)

1. S/S: hx of ingestion, gastritis, AMS (intoxication), metabolic acidosis (from alcohol breakdown), coma, and death
2. MGT/ Antidote: ABCs, ethanol (oral or IV); contact PCC

## TRICYCLIC ANTIDEPRESSANTS (TCA) TOXICITY

1. S/S: hx of ingestion, anticholinergic toxidrome, hypotension, ventricular arrhythmias
2. MGT/ Antidote: ABCs, bicarb (for conduction disturbances, ventricular arrhythmia, or refractory hypotension), barbituates for Sz, chemical paralysis for intractable Sz (as last resort); contact PCC
3. ECG Changes: Bradycardia, QRS > 100ms in Lead II, right axis deviation.

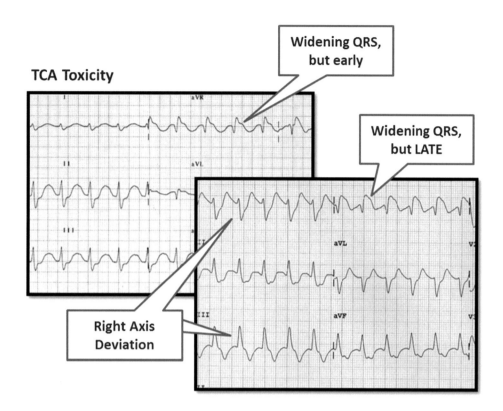

**TCA Toxicity**

Widening QRS, but early

Widening QRS, but LATE

Right Axis Deviation

# PART 3: BITES AND STINGS

## INTRODUCTION

Venomous bites and stings are responsible for significant mortality and morbidity worldwide. Interestingly, arthropods account for a higher percentage of deaths from envenomation than snakes, usually due to allergic reactions. In 2012, the American Association of Poison Control Centers (AAPCC) counted over 64,000 cases of bites and envenomation, some of which resulted in severe reactions.3 Fatalities from such exposures are typically rare, but severe systemic allergic reactions can occur. It is estimated that the incidence of anaphylaxis is approximately 50 to 2,000 episodes per 100,000 persons.

## THE CULPRITS

### SNAKES

1. There are 2 distinct types of snake which are poisonous in the United States: pit vipers (Crotalinae family which includes rattlesnakes) and coral snakes (Elapidae family).
2. Typically, pit viper bites cause tissue destruction and coagulopathy. Coral snake bites cause fasciculations and neurological deficits
3. Treatment:
    a. Monitor/ manage for airway compromise and shock
    b. IV fluids
    c. Analgesics and antiemetics
    d. Antivenin (**CroFab, ProFab**, etc.): monitor patients receiving this therapy for anaphylaxis. Antivenin is also interchangeable with *antivenom*.

## HYMENOPTERA

1. This is the portion of the animal kingdom that includes the insects **wasps, bees**, and **ants**.
2. Local reactions: edema, pain, and redness
3. Systemic reactions: airway compromise (closing throat and wheezing), anaphylaxis (throat closing, hypotension), urticaria
4. MGT:
    a. Gently remove any stinger left in the skin (to stop envenomation); use a hard, flat surface like a credit card to remove
    b. Irrigate and apply a cool pack
    c. Splint and elevate the extremity (if possible) above the level of the heart
    d. Treat for allergic reaction or anaphylactic reactions: IV, bronchodilators, antihistamines, and epinephrine

## ARTHROPODS

### Black Widow Bite
1. Presents with 2 puncture wounds, diffuse pain, muscle cramps (back and abdomen), tachycardia and high blood pressure.
2. Treatment: IV fluids, analgesics, benzodiazepines (for sedation) calcium chloride (if cardiac arrhythmias), and antivenin.

### Brown Recluse Bite
1. Presents with a bite that 1-2 days later can become necrotic leading to exudates near the site, systemic hemolysis, renal failure and death.
2. Treatment: IV fluids, analgesics, and benzodiazepines (for sedation).

### Scorpion Sting
1. These present as a neurotoxin that mimics the cholinergic toxidrome.
2. Presents with immediate pain and paresthesia, which can lead to fasciculations and paralysis. The patient may have trouble swallowing and hypersalivation.
3. Treatment: IV fluids, analgesics, and benzodiazepines (for sedation).

## POISON CONTROL

1. It should be noted that any questions about the treatment, transport, decontamination, and management of toxicological patients should be directed towards the local or national poison control center.
2. Follow your protocols or policies about toxicological patients.

# PART 4: TOXICOLOGICAL PHARMACOLOGY

## INTRODUCTION

There are a handful of pharmacological agents that should be committed to memory for the treatment of toxicological emergencies. Let's get to it.

# THE MEDICATIONS

## ACTIVATED CHARCOAL

1. Class: Absorbant
2. Mechanism: Binds, or absorbs, various chemical agents and drugs from the GI tract to restrict further absorption.
3. Indications: Poisonings following emesis or in cases where emesis is contraindicated.
4. Hemodynamics: (~CVP/ ~PCWP/~CO/~SVR).
5. Adult Dose: 50 g mixed with water
6. Peds Dose: 1 g/ kg mixed with water

## NALOXONE

1. Class: Narcotic Antagonist
2. Mechanism: Competitively binds with narcotic receptors. Basically, with a narcotic in the patient's system, this medication forces out the narcotic and temporarily removes the effects of the narcotics. Narcan has a shorter half life than its opiate counterparts, so the narcotic effect may return as the Narcan wears off.
3. Indications: Narcotics overdose, overdose unknown cause, coma or altered LOC due to unknown cause .
4. Hemodynamics: (~CVP/ ~PCWP/~CO/~SVR).
5. Adult Dose: 0.04.– 2 mg IV, may repeat q5 min. 1– 2 mg via nasal atomizer.
6. Peds Dose: 0.1 mg/kg IV, IO, or atomizer.

## ETHANOL

1. Class: Alcohol Antagonist
2. Mechanism: Competitively binds with other alcohols such as ethylene glycol, to prevent it from causing further physiologic damage.
3. Indications: alcohol intoxication (non- liquor)
4. Hemodynamics: (~CVP/ ~PCWP/~CO/~SVR).
5. Adult Dose: Loading: 10 mL/kg of a 10 percent ethanol solution in D5W ; Maintenance dose: 1 mL/kg of a 10% solution administered

## ATROPINE

1. Class: Anticholinergic
2. Mechanism: Blocks the parasympathetic receptors (slow system) thus speeding up the heart
3. Indications: bradycardia, organophosphate poisoning
4. Contraindications: hypersensitivity
5. Hemodynamics: (~CVP/ ~PCWP/↑CO/~SVR).
6. Dose:
   a. Adults: Cardiac- 1 mg IV q 3-5 minutes; organophosphate poisoning– 2-3mg IV bolus and repeat until the poisoned patient's secretions dry up.
   b. Peds: 0.01-0.03 mg/kg IV push.

## PRALIDOXIME (2-Pam)

1. Class: Cholinesterase reactivator
2. Mechanism: Deactivates certain organophosphate agents .
3. Indications: Severe organophosphate poisoning, nerve agents.
4. Hemodynamics: (~CVP/ ~PCWP/~CO/~SVR).
5. Dose: 600 mg IV or IM

# PART 5: TOXICOLOGICAL MANAGEMENT QUESTIONS

1. Your patient presents with coma, cardiac arrhythmias, hypotension, cardiac ischemia, cherry red skin, hyperthermia, and incontinence. These are assessment findings for which condition?
   a. Serotonin syndrome
   b. Amphetamine toxicity
   c. Methanol toxicity
   d. Carbon monoxide toxicity

2. Your patient has ingested a handful of pills. The pill bottle reads, "Meperidine". Which of the following signs and symptoms would you anticipate in this patient?
   a. Sedation, respiratory depression, myosis
   b. Tachycardia, hypertension, and agitation
   c. Salivation, lacrimation, and urinary issues
   d. Psychosis, hot/ flushed skin, pupil dilation

3. You are called to the scene of an industrial plant and your patient presents with huge pupils, extremely agitated, and with incredibly flushed skin. The patient's co-workers report that he is normally very calm and mild mannered. Which of the following substances is high on your differential diagnosis?
   a. Narcotic OD
   b. TCA overdose
   c. Cholinergics
   d. Alcohol OD

4. A victim of a poisoning presents with SLUDGE symptoms. Which of the following actions should be your FIRST priority?
   a. Atropine and oxygen
   b. 2-PAM and a benzo
   c. Activated charcoal
   d. RSI and intubation

5. While at a standby for a house fire, you get called over near the house to treat a firefighter. The patient has an altered mental status, bright red skin, and a pulse oximetry of 100%. Which of the following is the most appropriate action?
   a. Admin high flow O2 immediately
   b. RSI, intubate, and BVM the patient
   c. Get the patient away from house
   d. Deliver atropine and 2 PAM via IV

6.  You are handed a bottle of pills that your patient took. You look up the name on the bottle and discover it is a TCA. Which of the following signs and symptoms would you most likely find in this patient?
    a.  Drooling and copious diarrhea
    b.  Mydriasis and hyperthermia
    c.  Rhabdomyolysis and seizure
    d.  Severe respiratory depression

7.  Examine the ECG tracing below. This is from a patient you suspect has ingested a handful of pills to commit suicide. Which of the following is the patient most likely suffering from?
    a.  TCA overdose
    b.  Serotonin RI OD
    c.  Tylenol overdose
    d.  Beta blocker OD

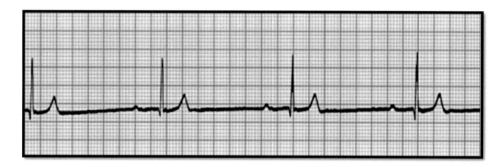

8.  Review the ECG below. This patient is an elderly woman with multiple co- morbid conditions who presented to the ER tonight with nausea and omitting and a decreasing mental status. Which of the following conditions is most likely occurring?
    a.  Acetaminophen toxicity
    b.  Cardiac glycoside toxicity
    c.  TCA/ Na blocker toxicity
    d.  Organophosphate toxicity

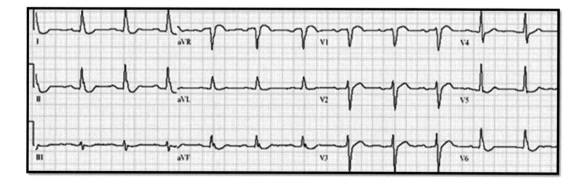

9. You are transferring a patient from a smaller hospital to a larger ICU. The patient has been there for 3 days for an acetaminophen OD. The medical staff reports (+) hepatomegaly, (+) coagulopathy, and only small, scant amounts of urine. What phase of acetaminophen toxicity is the patient experiencing?
    a. Phase I
    b. Phase II
    c. Phase III
    d. Phase IV

10. Examine the ECG tracing below. This patient has taken a handful of the drug, Elavil. Which treatment would most appropriate in this case?
    a. 1mg SQ epi
    b. 50g Glycogen
    c. Sodium bicarb
    d. Ca gluconate

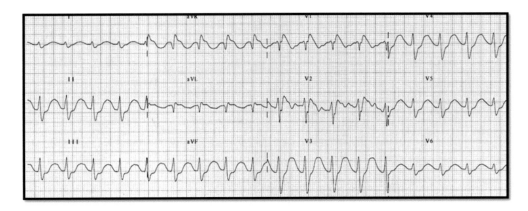

# PART 6: TOXICOLOGICAL MANAGEMENT RATIONALES

1. **(D)** The cherry red skin is a dead giveaway that these symptoms all point together to carbon monoxide poisoning.

2. **(A)** These are the signs and symptoms of opioid intoxication and meperidine is the opioid Demerol.

3. **(B)** This patient fits the profile for 2 conditions: TCA OD and CO poisoning. A big red flag is the flushed skin. Now, the question didn't read "cherry red skin" but flushed skin should still drive you to put CO poisoning high on your differential. Since, CO wasn't an answer selection. The answer here is TCA overdose/ intoxication: Mad as a hatter (agitated), Red as a beet (flushed skin), and blind as a bat (pupil dilation).

4. **(A)** This is one of those questions that make you decide on a partial treatment. Know that these are out there. To figure this question out, you'll have to identify answer selections with partially correct information. In this case, the only 2 are atropine/ oxygen and 2-PAM/ benzo. Ideally, you'd treat this patient with 2 PAM and atropine. So, look for the answer selection that has a piece of information that

isn't correct. Oxygen would be treated with all ODs, but a benzo isn't necessary here. Therefore, the answer is atropine and oxygen.

5.  **(C)** This patient is suffering from carbon monoxide poisoning. You could as the provider, suffer the same fate if you do not first get away from the house. This is a standard question set- up in toxicology because educators want you always to remember to take care of yourself first.

6.  **(B)** This patient is experiencing a TCA overdose. Blind as a bad (mydriasis- which is dilated pupils) and Hot as a hare (hyperthermia).

7.  **(D)** This patient is experiencing a beta blocker OD as evidenced by the 1st-degree heart block with sinus bradycardia. There aren't any characteristic ECG findings for serotonin or Tylenol. TCA overdoses display a widening QRS and can display right axis deviation.

8.  **(B)** This ECG is displaying the ladle sign in leads I, II, aVF, and V6, therefore, this is suggestive of a digitalis, which is a cardiac glycoside.

9.  **(A)** Remember the signs and symptoms of these phases. Phase III of acetaminophen: 72-96 hours; oliguria, hepatomegaly, coagulopathy, liver failure.

10. **(C)** This is a TCA OD ECG tracing; therefore, the most appropriate treatment would be sodium bicarbonate. Notice the wide QRS and right axis deviation.

# CHAPTER 10: OBSTETRICAL EMERGENCIES

## PART 1: THE OBSTETRICAL ASSESSMENT

### INTRODUCTION

You will be called to the obstetrical patient many times in your career. For most, these calls create a lot of anxiety. However, armed with the knowledge of the right exam questions, assessments, and management strategies, you will be able to handle these calls like a seasoned professional. It is important that you build awareness of the condition of the mother as well as the condition of the fetus. Complications can arise in one, or both. Being practiced on these assessment and management skills will best prepare you for these cases.

### INITIAL OB ASSESSMENT

#### *GENERAL IMPRESSION*

1. As you approach the patient, look at their body position, work of breathing and skin condition and color.
2. Their body position tells you great information: tripod means they are short of breath/ hypoxic, laying on the ground with weak muscles mean they are extremely hypoxic.
3. Normal respiratory effort indicates they are receiving adequate oxygen, but labored respirations indicates they are most likely hypoxic.
4. Normal skin color indicates adequate perfusion, but pale or mottled skin can indicate poor perfusion.

#### *ASSESS MENTAL STATUS*

1. AVPU:  Awake– eyes open spontaneously; Verbal- arouses to stimulation my voice; Painful- purpose for movements to painful stimuli; Unresponsive- no response to any stimuli
2. Assess GCS
   a. Eye Opening: Spontaneous (4); to speech (3); to painful stimuli (2); no opening at all (0)
   b. Verbal Effort: normal conversation (5);  confused (4); inappropriate words (3); incomprehensible sounds (2); no verbal effort (1)
   c. Motor Effort: follows commands (6); localizes pains (5); withdrawals from pain (4); decorticate posturing (3); decerebrate posturing (2); no motor effort (1)

#### *AIRWAY*

1. Ensure a patent airway.
2. Clear, reposition, reassess as needed.

#### *BREATHING*

1. Rate
2. Quality (normal or labored)
3. Rhythm (normal or abnormal respiratory patterns).
4. **Note**: mothers can have increased SOB from a compressing fetus on her diaphragm.

## CIRCULATION

1. Ensure the patient has a pulse and note the rate, strength (normal, bounding, or weak), and quality (regular or irregular).
2. Obtain and assess heart rate, blood pressure, pulse oximetry, cardiac monitoring, and labs/images if available.
3. Remember, the fetus RELIES on the pregnant patient's perfusion status. Any hypotension or poor oxygenation at all can lead to a horrible fetal outcome.

## DISABILITY

1. Assess for the ability to move, lift, and hold all 4 extremities. Assess for equal grip and pedal strength. Assess for the ability to maintain a seated posture, standing and walking. Assess for cranial nerve deficits.
2. Identify deficits that existed prior to your assessment.

## EXPOSURE

1. Expose patient
2. Perform a head to toe rule out life threats.

# FOCUSED OB ASSESSMENT

## ASSESS FOR Rh BLOOD INCOMPATIBILITY

1. Rh Incompatibility– Mom's blood can attack the baby's blood in certain circumstances, causing anemia in the newborn from RBC destruction
2. The positive (+) or negative (-) after an ABO blood type indicates the presence (positive) or absence (negative) of Rh factor.
3. If mom is Rh negative and the dad is Rh positive, then they can produce a Rh-positive baby.
4. During a Rh-negative mom's first pregnancy with a Rh-positive fetus, blood mixing during delivery sensitizes mom to the Rh-positive protein of the baby's RBCs.
5. The first pregnancy is usually free of Rh complications.
6. Subsequent pregnancies with a Rh-positive baby (and Rh-negative mom) can lead to mom's blood attacking the Rh-positive baby's blood.
7. To prevent this, a medication called Rhogam is administered to prevent mom's blood from producing antibodies for Rh positive RBCs, to prevent mom's immune system doesn't attack the baby's RBCs.
8. Therefore, each patient should be questioned on previous pregnancies and Rh status.

## ASSESS CERVIX (most likely will need MD/DO to complete this)

1. When was it last completed? It is important to know
2. because the cervix will be progressing on a moment-to-moment basis, and even if it has been 20-30 minutes since the last exam, drastic changes could have occurred.

### Effacement

1. Shortening and thinning of the cervix
2. Expressed as a percent (%)

### Dilation

1. Enlargement of the cervical opening
2. Measured 0 cm (not dilated) to 10 cm (fully dilated)

**Station**

1. Position of the presenting part of the fetus within the birth canal
2. Zero (0) is an imaginary line drawn between the Ischial spines; negative numbers (-) refer to being higher in the birth canal; positive number (+) indicates the baby is lower (almost completely delivered)
3. Measured between -5 to +5 (birth is usually +4/ +5

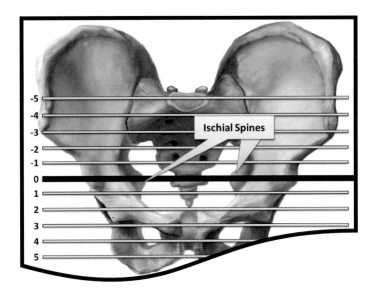

## ASSESS CONTRACTIONS AND CONTRACTION HISTORY

1. It is important to get a baseline of the contractions so you can assess if delivery is progressing slowly or quickly.
2. Onset: How long ago did the contractions start?
3. Frequency: How often do they occur?
4. Intensity: What is the magnitude of the contraction?
5. Duration: How long do the contractions last?
6. Signs of Imminent Labor:
    a. Contractions are 3-5 minutes apart over the period of an hour with each lasting approximately 30 seconds
    b. All contractions have the same, or very similar, intensity

## ASSESS EXPECTED DATE OF CONFINEMENT (EDC)

1. This is the date the fetus was conceived.
2. Calculated my multiple methods and apps (phone apps).
    a. There are other methods, but the following are 2 common ones:
    b. Naegele's Rule: add 280 days to the first day of a patient's last menstrual cycle
    c. Ultrasound: used to obtain the circumference of a fetus's head– this can be used to identify when the fetus was conceived

## ASSESS ESTIMATED GESTATIONAL AGE (EGA)

1. This is a measure of the age of a pregnancy/ fetus.
2. McDonald's Rule
    a. The fundal height in centimeters is roughly equal to the weeks gestation (most accurate between weeks 16-36)

b. Measure from the symphysis pubis (pubic bone) to the top of the fundus. cm = weeks gestation.
3. Ultrasound: used to obtain the circumference of a fetus's head– this can be used to identify when the fetus was conceived

## Assessing Fundal Height

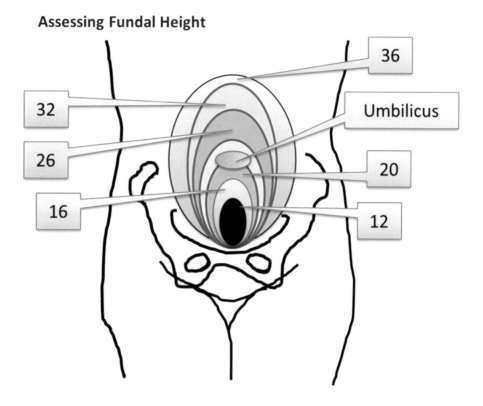

## ASSESSING DELIVERY HISTORY (GPA-TPL)
1. Gravida: Total number of all pregnancies (including the current pregnancy)
2. Para: Total number of deliveries after 20 weeks gestation
3. Abortions/ miscarriages: The number of aborted fetuses
4. Term, Full: The number of full-term infants delivered
5. Preterm: The # of preterm infants delivered
6. Living: The number of currently living children

## ASSESSING FOR HIGH RISKS AND PRIOR COMPLICATIONS
1. Experiencing problems in a prior pregnancy and in who have current high-risk conditions are reliable in predicting how the maternal patient will handle the current pregnancy.
2. High Risk OB conditions include: Preeclampsia/ HELLP/ Gestational Diabetes Mellitus/ Emboli
3. Other Conditions/ Complications: Preterm labor/ Breech presentation/ Abruption and Previa/ Shoulder dystocia/ umbilical cord prolapse/ uterine rupture/ Postpartum hemorrhage.

## ASSESS FOR RUPTURE OF MEMBRANES
1. This is the spilling of amniotic fluid from the rupture of the amniotic sac
2. This can be either normal (associated with labor) or premature (occurs before labor begins).
3. Sometimes this can cause a prolapsed cord if the fetal head isn't in the birth canal– therefore, always examine for a prolapsed cord after the patient's water breaks.

*ASSESS FOR IMINENT DELIVERY*

1. The current literature suggests NOT transporting a patient who is indicating IMMINENT DELIVERY.
2. These patients should either be taken to the OR for immediate Cesarean section or otherwise be transported by high-risk OB team or neonatal team by ground:
   a. Cervical dilation of 5 cm or more with contractions 5 minutes apart (5 at 5 rule)
   b. Less than 37 weeks gestation with ruptured membranes
   c. With ruptured membranes (any gestational age) and meconium staining

# PART 2: THE FETAL ASSESSMENT

## INTRODUCTION

Please always remember that there are two patients in every OB call. Mom must come first, but the fetus is a very close second. As with all assessments, get a baseline, so that you can be sensitive to small changes in vital signs, labs, observable signs of disease, and other diagnostic indicators.

## FETAL ASSESSMENT

### *FETAL HEART RATE MONITORING*

1. Monitoring FHR helps to identify fetal compromise.
2. NORM: 110- 160/min
3. Types:
   a. Auditory/ Doppler: "listening" to the fetal heart rate
   b. Electronic Fetal Monitoring: Usage of waveforms based on FHR trends and contraction trends
4. FHR Baseline
   a. This is the average FHR during a 10- minute period
      i. Must be a 2 minute period free of episodic changes in this 10 minutes
      ii. NORM: 110-160/ min
   b. Bradycardia
      i. FHR less than 110 for longer than 10 minutes
      ii. Caused by:
         1. Umbilical cord compression/ Maternal hypotension or hypoxia
         2. Uterine hyperstimulation
   c. Tachycardia
      i. FHR greater than 160 for more than 10 minutes
      ii. Caused by
         1. Transient fetal hypoxia/ fetal anemia/ maternal fever/
         2. Maternal or fetal fever/ sympathetic drugs (like terbutaline)

## VARIABILITY

Variability is the long and short term trending of fetal heart rate. Consider variability like Goldie Locks– too much is bad and too little is bad, but a moderate amount is just right.

## SHORT-TERM VARIABILITY

1. Fetal heart rate will fluctuate.  Suppose every 10 seconds you looked at the heart rate monitor, obtained the fetal heart rate, and wrote that number down on a piece of graph paper.  In 60 seconds, you would have six heart rates documented.  If you are to do this for several hours, you can add a long strip that looks like some form of ventricular fibrillation.  This is **short-term variability**.

2. These are beat to beat changes (over seconds) and is observed from the top graph of the toco-monitor strip. In the below picture, the 'x' mark a measured FHR at that time. Short-term variability is depicted as an up-and-down jagged line. The bottom graph represents uterine contractions.

3. Influenced by the parasympathetic NS, which is more susceptible to hypoxia than the sympathetic branch.

4. There are three types of short-term variability: normal variability, marked variability, and loss of variability.

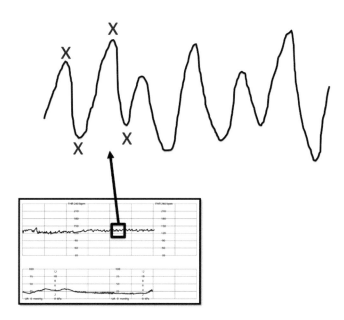

### Normal (aka Moderate) Variability

1. While I am not an expert on these by far, I have been trained by experts to recognize in the field real world problems and manage them appropriately.

2. Normal short-term variability resembles a fine-to-moderate ventricular fibrillation tracing. This is a good sign, otherwise known in the OB world as a *reassuring sign*.

273

3. Moderate (normal) variability reflects an oxygenated fetus and normally functioning fetal autonomic nervous system (it's fight or flight system). As contractions occur it stimulates the fetus which reacts with moderate variability in heart rate; this is a good sign. Moderate variability is ideal when assessing an FHR.

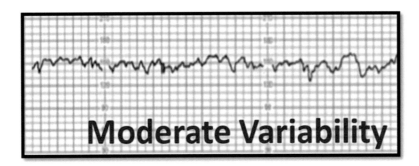

**Marked Variability**
1. Acute hypoxia or cord compression are common causes of increased variability.
2. Drastic changes in the beat to beat FHR trend is also called a saltatory pattern.
3. The presence of marked variability, when paired with decelerations, should alert the clinician to look for possible causes of acute hypoxia, as well as be alert to signs that the hypoxia is progressing to acidosis.

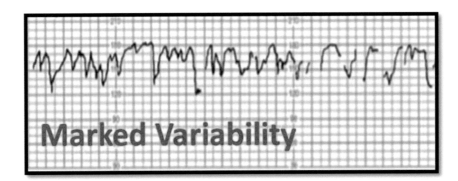

**Loss of Variability**
1. Fetal hypoxia, congenital heart abnormalities, and sustained fetal tachycardia can cause decreased variability.
2. Basically, anything that reduces fetal oxygenation for a long period will cause a loss of variability, which looks more like a "flat line".

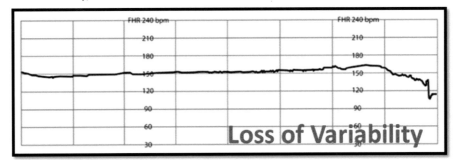

**Normal to Near-Death: A Continuum of Fetal Hypoxia**

In the below picture, we follow a normal fetus that experiences a hypoxic event, either fetal or maternal in nature. The healthy fetus will have the resources of sugar and oxygen to be able to compensate with a burst of tachycardia as evidenced by the second data set. The increased heart rate is followed by marked short-term variability, which is an indication the clinician should act by administering more oxygen, ensuring adequate blood pressure of the mother, and potentially displacing the gravid uterus in some fashion.

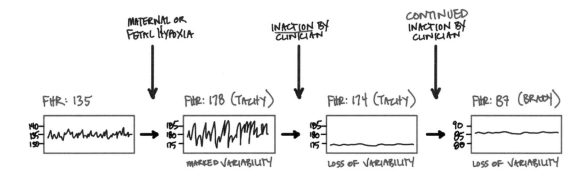

Should the clinician FAIL to act, the third data set is likely to occur. Here you see the FHR a loss of variability, an ominous sign (this means very bad in the OB world), however, the FHR is still in normal. The FHR in normal range means we still have a chance to correct the situation.

Should the clinician continue to NOT act, then the fourth data set and patient presentation may manifest. In this last data set, preceding the death of the infant essentially, the FHR is now bradycardic (89 bpm) and the loss of variability persists- both of these are signs of impending fetal death, and most OB receiving centers would rush them to surgery for emergent Cesarean section.

## *LONG-TERM VARIABILITY*
1. Long-term variability describes the increasing or decreasing trend in heart rate from baseline.
2. Fetal heart rate can elevate or dip, and then return to baseline based on physiologic or pharmacologic conditions.

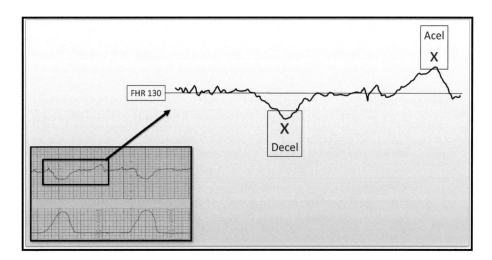

3. Long– term variability is broad swings in FHR over a minute or more and is highly Influenced by the sympathetic nervous system.
4. There are two main types of long-term variability patterns: **decelerations** (decels) and **accelerations** (acels), however, decelerations can be broken into three separate types.

## Accelerations:
1. An increase in FHR by 15 bpm above baseline lasting 15 seconds to 2 minutes.
2. With uterine contractions or fetal movement, it indicates: Intact CNS and normal fetal pH
3. Accelerations by themselves indicate fetal hypoxia.
4. Therefore, ask the mother if she felt fetal movement with all accelerations not coupled with uterine contractions. If movement was present– GOOD sign; if no movement was present with an Acel (aka A-cell which is short for acceleration and pronounced 'a-cell')- sign of fetal hypoxia.

## Decelerations:
1. A normal, gradual reduction in FHR lasting longer than 30 seconds below baseline.
2. There are three types of decelerations, or decls (aka D-cell- pronounced 'D-cells'): early, late, and variable.

### Early Decelerations:
1. This type of D-cell typically occurs as the fetus makes its way through the birth canal. The fetal head is compressed during uterine contractions resulting in vagal stimulation, and the heart rate slows. **THIS IS ALL NORMAL AND A GOOD SIGN** or known as a *reassuring sign* in the OB world.
2. This deceleration matches the contraction and is a mirror image of one another.

## Early Decelerations

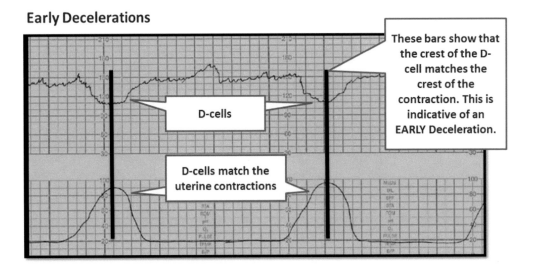

These bars show that the crest of the D-cell matches the crest of the contraction. This is indicative of an EARLY Deceleration.

D-cells

D-cells match the uterine contractions

### Late Decelerations:
1. This type of D-cell typically occurs from uteroplacental insufficiency and is worsened by contractions, which is a ***non-reassuring sign***.
2. Decreases in placental blood flow, prolonged hypoxia, or maternal hypotension will cause the fetus to react slower to the contraction. WE NEED TO FIX THIS IMMEDIATELY.
3. This is like if you were running a race and sprinting the entire time. There would be a point at which you slowed down considerably because you cannot sustain the 100% effort. This also happens to the fetus; they get fatigued (run out of oxygen and/or

sugar) and cannot keep up with the changing environment of the uterus during labor. If the hypoxia is not corrected, then the fetus will worsen and die.

4. All late decelerations are considered potentially ominous.

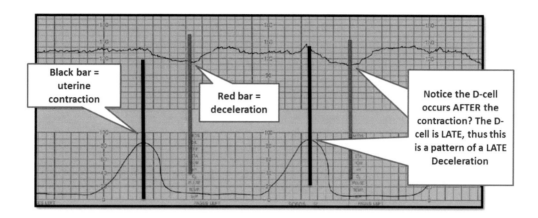

Variable Decelerations:

1. This type of deceleration is characterized by a variable duration, intensity, and timing.
2. They resemble the shapes of the letters capital U, V, or W.
3. Variable decelerations are caused by compression of the umbilical cord.
4. These decelerations can have "shoulders", which are mini- accelerations that come both before and after a deceleration.
5. As the cord is compressed, the umbilical vein is occluded, and this causes an acceleration (first shoulder). Then occlusion of the umbilical artery occurs and initiates a sharp D-cell. Finally, the recovery phase is due to relief of the compression, followed by a return to baseline. Sometimes, another mini acceleration (second shoulder)occurs after this central deceleration.

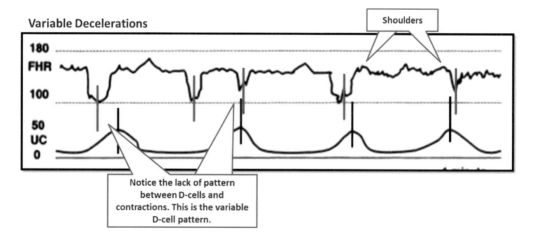

## PUTTING IT ALL TOGETHER

### Assess FHR Baseline:

1. NORM: 110– 160 beats/ minute
2. Use auscultatory, doppler, graphic or ultrasound techniques.

### Assess for ADEQUATE Variability:

1. Moderate variability- fetus is adequately oxygenated.
2. If hypervariable- could be transducer. Consider applying more conduction gel to transducer.
3. Low/poor variability- hypoxia, acidosis, mag, narcotics, or fetal sleep can all be causes.

### Assess for Accelerations:

1. These are a reassuring sign with <u>contractions</u> or <u>fetal movement</u>.
2. If they occur in the absence of fetal movement (kicking) or contractions, then look for signs of hypoxia and treat.
3. These can <u>only</u> occur in the <u>ABSENCE</u> of acidosis.

### Assess for Early Decelerations:

1. Normal with uterine contractions.
2. Continue to monitor as things can always worsen.

### Assess for Variable or Late Decelerations:

1. Cord compression is likely.
2. Perform oxygenation, perfusion, and uterine displacement procedures to improve oxygen delivery to the fetus.

### Assess for Non– Reassuring Signs:

1. Fetal tachycardia or bradycardia– without contractions or fetal movement
2. Variable D-cells w/tachycardia or bradycardia trends
3. Late D-cells w/good variability
4. Non- reassuring signs do not necessarily indicate immediate delivery but should alert you to start looking for signs of fetal hypoxia and to preventing any progress of fetal hypoxia.

### Assess for Ominous Signs:

1. Ominous signs are those that are close to warranting an emergency Caesarian section. If these are identified, medical control and directions are advised.
2. Late D-cells with loss of variability
3. Any loss of variability
4. Prolonged severe bradycardia
5. Sinusoidal pattern

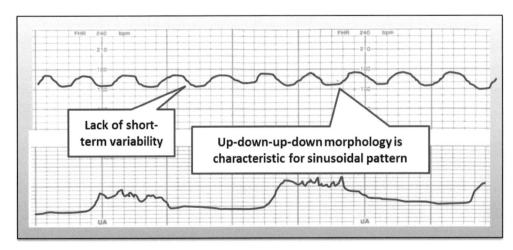

# PART 3: OBSTETRICAL CONDITIONS

## GENERAL MANAGEMENT

1. Goal: Improve uterine blood flow and fetal oxygenation.
    a. High flow O2
    b. Displace the uterus, such as using the left-lateral position. However, any position could potentially displace the uterus off the umbilical cord including on their knees and elbows, right lateral position, or even prone but with the clinician manually displacing the uterus one direction or another.
    c. Fluid boluses (20 cc/kg) until maternal hypotension is corrected
2. Perform a vaginal exam to rule out hemorrhage (as with Previa/abruption) and assess for dilation, station, and effacement; you may need a physician to conduct this for you.
3. Rule out umbilical cord prolapse or correct it (see following section )
4. Consider tocolytics.
    a. Magnesium Sulfate
    b. Terbutaline
    c. Delivery may need to be suppressed with the medications above. If the patient's water has not broken, then this is typically safe. If their water has broken, then it is recommended you ALWAYS contact med control before stopping labor. Once the water breaks, delivery shortly follows. There are times when you may need to stop delivery AFTER the rupture of membranes occur (water breaks), but again- it is highly recommended you have med control backing you up on that.
5. VEAL CHOP for FHR abnormalities:
    a. Variable d-cells = Cord compression
        i. Assess for prolapsed umbilical or nuchal cord (cord around baby's neck)
        ii. MGT: Reposition mom, support umbilical cord to ensure continued placental/ baby blood supply
    b. Early D-cells = Head compression (baby in birth canal– GOOD!)
        i. Continue routine care and monitoring– all is GOOD.
    c. Accelerations = OK if fetal movement/ contractions; hypoxia if ALONE
        i. Assess for uterine contraction
        ii. MGT: admin O2 if no contractions accompany the A-cells
    d. Late = Placental insufficiency (poor placental perfusion)
        i. Assess for maternal hypotension and oxygen saturation in addition to identifying ominous or non– reassuring signs of the fetus
        ii. MGT: reposition patient and administer oxygen; consider consult.

## OBSTETRICAL CONDITONS
### Abruptio Placenta
1. Patho: blunt/penetrating trauma Or Spontaneously--> disrupts the connections of the placenta with the uterine wall--> bleeding--> fetal demise--> mother hypotension and shock--> death
2. S/S: vaginal bleeding (only in 80% of cases), abdominal/ back pain, shock, loss of fetal heart tones or slowing fetal heart tones
3. MGT: ABCs, O2, tilt left lateral 15 degrees if > 20 weeks gestation, aggressive fluid resuscitation (target >0.5 cc/kg/hr), rapid transport

## Placenta Previa

1. Patho: Placenta positions itself in the lower third of the uterus and partially or completely blocks the cervical opening → thin placenta is ripped during uterine contractions → vaginal bleeding
2. S/S: Bright red, but painless bleeding; occurring after vaginal exam or intercourse supports the diagnosis
3. MGT: ABCs, O2, tilt left lateral 15 degrees if > 20 weeks gestation, aggressive fluid resuscitation (target >0.5 cc/kg/hr), rapid transport

## Preterm Labor

1. Patho: Uterine contractions, effacement and dilation of the cervix
2. S/S: Rhythmic uterine contractions (10 min apart or less for an hour before week 37); cervical dilation; rupture of membranes; passage of 500cc or more of blood
3. MGT: IV/O2/monitor; FHR monitor; OB assessments; pt to their left side (lowers pressure on vena cava); tocolytics (mag or terbutaline)

## Breech Delivery

1. Patho: Complete Breech- buttocks with knees bent; Frank Breech- buttocks with ankles at the face of infant; Single or Double Footling Breech- one or two feet presenting
2. S/S: Rhythmic uterine contractions (10 min apart or less for an hour before week 37); cervical dilation; rupture of membranes; passage of bloody show
3. MGT: Support maternal ABCs; Allow buttocks to deliver without added traction; Don't touch the fetus until the umbilicus delivers; Sweep legs out; Sweep arms out; Place infant in vertex position, and with an assistant, protect the infant's face and rotate the patient with the buttocks going towards the ceiling; Mauriceu Maneuver— cradle baby; insert finger into baby's mouth, bring neck to moderate flexion, pull baby body away from mom with head rotating downward.

## Shoulder Dystocia

1. Patho: Fetal shoulder stuck on pubic symphysis, and sacrum ⊠ delivery cannot continue
2. S/S: Turtle sign during vaginal delivery; failure of crowning progress
3. MGT: ABCs, O2, McRobert's Maneuver (quickly flex the legs against the abdomen); Woods corkscrew maneuver (rotate the shoulders 180*); Sweep the anterior arm (reduces shoulder width)

## Umbilical Cord Prolapse

1. Patho:
   a. Overt: Cord enters the vaginal canal (after rupture of membranes) and presents before the fetus
   b. Occult: cord slips into pelvis and is compressed by the presenting part
2. S/S: Visible cord; fetal distress: absence of short- and long-term variability, fetal bradycardia, recurrent D-cells that do not respond to positioning/ fluids/ or oxygen
3. MGT: Maternal ABCs supported; Remove pressure from the cord for the duration of transport (hand into the vagina; lift anatomy off cord; check for a pulse; wrap with warm, moist dressing; Trendelenburg or knee to chest helps; tocolytics; RAPID transport to OR for C-section.

## Uterine Rupture

1. Patho: Complete disruption of the layers of the uterine wall → Spontaneous or via trauma → bleeding into abdominal cavity → shock/ acidosis/ death
2. S/S: ACUTE onset of SEVERE abdominal pain; shock symptoms; evidence of fetal distress if uteroplacental blood flow is affected; external uterine palpation reveals a change in uterine morphology

3. MGT: Left lateral recumbent position; O2, aggressive fluid resuscitation (Target UOP of 0.5 cc/kg/hr indicates adequate intravascular volume); PRBCs; Emergent surgery required.

## Post-Partum Hemorrhage
1. Patho: 500cc blood loss with vaginal delivery; 1000cc blood loss with C- section
2. S/S: Overt blood, or no signs of bleeding with evidence of shock
3. MGT: For visible lacerations → direct pressure; IV/O2/Fluids (aggressive); Fundal massage; Oxytocin

## Pre– eclampsia
1. Patho: vasospasm (unknown cause) in renal arteries--> decreased renal blood flow--> kidneys retain sodium/ water/ proteins--> increased blood pressure
2. S/S: classic triad (hypertension, edema, proteinuria) in >20 weeks gestation; headache; visual changes; anxiety; proteinuria of > 300 mg/dL indicates PIH/ pre-eclampsia.
3. MGT: IV/O2/monitor; pt to their left side (lowers pressure on vena cava); control HTN (hydralazine, labetalol, or nitro); stop seizures- mag sulfate; (stops seizures, reduces BP, and stops contractions) OR benzos (for seizures) and terbutaline (reduces contractions) NOTE: the presence of seizure reclassifies the condition as ECLAMPSIA

## HELLP Syndrome
1. Patho: unknown cause--> clotting cascade initiated--> anemia and over-worked liver
2. S/S: triad (Hemolytic anemia, Elevated Liver enzymes, Low Platelet count); abdominal pain; vision disturbances; a headache; hyperreflexia
3. MGT: IV/O2/monitor; pt to their left side (lowers pressure on vena cava); blood transfusion (combats anemia); mag sulfate (prevents seizures)

## Thyroid Storm
1. Patho: Pregnancy/ Trauma/ Infections → Hyperthyroidism → ↑ fever/ ↑ HR/ ↑ BP/ (+) Sweating
2. S/S: ↑ fever/ ↑ HR/ ↑ BP/ (+) Sweating
3. MGT: IV/O2/monitor; Propranolol (reduces HR and decreases thyroid levels); Potassium iodine (prevents T4 and T3 from being released); Hydrocortisone (thyroid storm depletes cortisol)

## Spontaneous Abortion
1. Patho: when the fetus and placenta deliver before the 20th week of pregnancy- commonly called a miscarriage
2. S/S: uterine cramping, backache- bright red vaginal bleeding- note number of pads per hour- symptoms of shock (tachycardia, weak pulses, mottled/ pale skin, hypotension)- CBC (assess for anemia), HCG (to confirm if pregnant)
3. MGT: prevent shock (oxygen, IV, fluids, blood, pressors); IV fluids and bed rest

## Ectopic Pregnancy
1. Patho: pregnancy resulting from gestation elsewhere than in the uterus--> growing fetus disrupts structural anatomy--> bleeding
2. S/S: spotting, sudden onset of severe lower ABD pain- cramping, unilateral cramping, missed menses or (+) pregnancy test- transvaginal ultrasound- exploratory laparoscopic surgery
3. MGT: IV/O2/Monitor; Methotrexate or surgery

# PART 4: OBSTETRICAL PHARMACOLOGY

## IN GENERAL

There are a handful of useful medications to consider with your OB patients, in addition to oxygen and isotonic fluids. Unless you are with a OB/peds transport team, these medications may get forgotten unless practiced more routinely.

## THE MEDICATIONS

### Labetalol
1. Class: Beta Blocker
2. Mechanism: Causes non-selective beta blockade. Non-selective means that both beta receptors are blocked, thus, HR, AV conduction, and contractility will both be reduced, and bronchospasm is a possibility. Additionally, it partially blocks alpha 1, so vasodilation occurs. (+) slow onset and long half-life.
3. Indications: hypertensive crisis
4. Contraindications: asthma, hypotension, bradycardia, cardiac failure, high degree heart block, cocaine use (B-blocker causes uncontested alpha stimulation).
5. Hemodynamics: ($\downarrow$CVP/ $\downarrow$PCWP/$\downarrow$CO/$\downarrow$SVR).
6. Dose:
   a. 20 mg IV over 2 minutes; may repeat 40-80 mg q 10 minutes; max of 300 mg
   b. Maintenance infusion: 2 mg/min

### Hydralazine
1. Class: Vasodilator
2. Mechanism: Direct acting arterial vasodilator, but has little effect on the venous system.
3. Indications: PIH, eclampsia, CHF, pulmonary hypertension
4. Contraindications: acute coronary syndromes, valvular disease, AMI, hypersensitivity
5. Hemodynamics: ($\downarrow$CVP/ $\downarrow$PCWP/$\downarrow$CO/$\downarrow$SVR).
6. Dose: 5-40 mg over 2-3 minutes

### Propanolol
1. Class: Beta Blocker
2. Mechanism: Causes non-selective beta blockade. Non-selective means that both beta receptors are blocked, thus, HR, AV conduction, and contractility will both be reduced, and bronchospasm is a possibility. Additionally, it partially blocks alpha 1, so vasodilation occurs. (+) slow onset and long half-life. Additionally, it can REDUCE T3 and T4 levels.
3. Indications: hypertensive crisis due to THYROID STORM
4. Contraindications: asthma, hypotension, bradycardia, cardiac failure, high degree heart block, cocaine use (B-blocker causes uncontested alpha stimulation).
5. Hemodynamics: ($\downarrow$CVP/ $\downarrow$PCWP/$\downarrow$CO/$\downarrow$SVR).
6. Dose: Adult: 1-3 mg slow IV push- do not exceed push of more than 1 mg/min.

## Mag Sulfate

1. Class: Electrolyte, Muscle relaxant
2. Mechanism: decreases the excitability of muscles, therefore, relaxes skeletal and smooth muscle: reduces BP, relaxes uterine contractions, bronchodilates, slows HR.
3. Indications: ventricular tachycardia refractory to other treatments, eclampsia, tocolysis for pregnancy
4. Contraindications: Bradycardia, hypotension, heart block
5. Hemodynamics: (↓CVP/ ↓PCWP/↓CO/↓SVR).
6. Dose:
   a. Adults: 1-2 g administered IV over 10-20 minutes
   b. Peds: (peds dose located in a more relevant section)

## Calcium Chloride

1. Class: Electrolyte
2. Mechanism: Essential in neurotransmission and muscle contractions; calcium competes with magnesium, so it's given in mag overdoses.
3. Indications: Hypermagnesemia, beta blocker OD, hypocalcemia
4. Contraindications: VFib during CPR, hypercalcemia, risk for digitalis toxicity, hypophosphatemia, renal calculi; Pulseless ventricular tachycardia
5. Hemodynamics: (↑CVP/ ↑PCWP/↑CO/↑SVR)
6. Dose: 1-2 grams over 5 minutes.

## Terbutaline

1. Class: Bronchodilator, smooth muscle relaxant (uterine relaxant)
2. Mechanism: Stimulates the beta 2 receptor, which relaxes bronchiole smooth muscle which causes bronchodilation.
3. Indications: Tocolytic (stops uterine contractions); Acute bronchospasm (from COPD, asthma, allergic reaction or any other cause of bronchoconstriction)
4. Contraindications: Hypertension, tachycardia, acute coronary syndromes, hypersensitivity, concurrent digitalis therapy, congenital heart diseases
5. Hemodynamics: (↑CVP/ ↑PCWP/↑CO/↑SVR)
6. Adult dose: 0.25 mg SQ every 15 minutes to a max of 0.5 in 4 hours. Peds: (peds dose located in a more relevant section)

## Oxytocin

1. Class: Labor Inducer
2. Mechanism: Increases uterine contractions (induces labor and reduces postpartum hemorrhage after placental birth).
3. Indications: postpartum hemorrhage
4. Contraindications: Hypersensitivity; when labor is progressing normally; in cases where vaginal delivery is contraindicated
5. Hemodynamics: (~CVP/ ~PCWP/~CO/~SVR)
6. Labor Inducing Dose: 1-2 milliunits/min IV infusion; Titrate to desired level of contraction; Max: 20 milliunits/min
7. Post–partum Hemorrhage Dose: 20-40 milliunits/min IV infusion; ALTERNATIVE Dose: 10 units IM

# PART 5: OBSTETRICAL LABS

## IN GENERAL

In addition to pharmacology, there are a handful of useful OB lab values that to consider with your OB patients. This can help in both the clinical and testing realms.

## THE LABS

### Hemoglobin
1. HGB indicates oxygen carrying capacity
2. Norm: ~ 13-18 g/dL
3. Critical Value:
   a. < 8 g/dL indicates bleeding, iron deficiency, anemia
   b. > 20 g/dL indicates dehydration

### Hematocrit
1. Hematocrit, or "crit", indicates oxygen carrying capacity
2. It is the percentage of RBCs in a sample of blood.
3. Norm: 35-45% in women/ 40-50% in men
4. Critical Value:
   a. < 13% indicates bleeding, iron deficiency, anemia
   b. > 60% indicates dehydration

### Lactate
1. Produced in large amounts during anaerobic metabolism
2. Norm: 4-20 mg/dL (SI = 0.5-2 mmol/L)
3. Critical Value:
   a. > 45 mg/dL this indicates that there is ischemic disease or hypoperfusion, or both
   b. (SI >4.5 mmol/L) this indicates that there is ischemic disease or hypoperfusion, or both

### Proteinuria
1. Indicates protein is spilling into the urine from PIH, Pre– eclampsia, severe HTN
2. Norm: < 100mg/dL
3. Critical Value: > 300 mg/dL indicates PIH/ Pre-eclampsia

### Prothrombin Time (PT)
1. PT is a measure of the extrinsic pathway of coagulation, and basically tells us the clotting tendency of blood. Increased values basically tell us clotting occurs faster.
2. Normal: 11.4– 14.2 seconds
3. HIGH (longer): DIC, massive transfusion, vitamin K deficiency, warfarin therapy

### International Normalized Ratio (INR)
1. The INR is very similar to the PT value; however, it is mathematically "normalized". It is a measure of the extrinsic pathway of coagulation and tells us the clotting tendency of blood. Increased values tell us clotting occurs faster.
2. Normal:  0.9– 1.2 second(s)
3. HIGH: DIC, massive transfusion, vitamin K deficiency, warfarin

## D- dimer

1. This lab value is a degradation product of fibrin. After a clot is formed, it begins to degrade and releases D-dimer into the bloodstream. It is used primarily to rule out DVT/ PE/ thrombosis rather than confirm it. It is more reliable with a negative result than with a positive result.
2. Normal:
   a. US: 250 [ng/L]
   b. SI: 250 [mg/L]
3. HIGH: Potential DVT/PE/thrombosis/DIC
4. LOW: VERY LITTLE CHANCE OF ANY THROMBOSIS

## Platelets (Plts)

1. Platelets are self-remnants that play a fundamental role in hemostasis. Too few platelets and excessive bleeding can occur, too many platelets can cause blood clots to form and cause stroke, myocardial infarction, and pulmonary embolism.
2. Normal: 150-400 [x 109/L]
3. HIGH: Anemia, acute blood loss, preeclampsia, infection
4. LOW: DIC, HIV, blood transfusion, chemotherapy
5. Critical Values: <50 or 1000 x 109/L

## Thyroid Stimulating Hormone (TSH)

1. TSH stimulates the thyroid gland to produce T4 and T3; both of which stimulate the metabolism of almost every tissue in the body.
2. Normal: 0.5– 5.0 [nU/mL]
3. HIGH: Hypothyroidism (because the thyroid isn't producing enough T3 and T4, so the pituitary starts cranking out lots of TSH.

## Triiodothyronine (T3)

1. T3; Increases the basal metabolic rate, and, therefore, increases the body's oxygen and energy consumption.
2. Normal: 60-181 ng/dL
3. HIGH: Hyperthyroidism/ Thyroid storm
4. Low: Hypothyroidism

## Thyroxine (T4)

1. T3; Increases the basal metabolic rate, and, therefore, increases the body's oxygen and energy consumption.
2. Normal: 0.8 – 2.7 ng/dL
3. HIGH: Hyperthyroidism/ Thyroid storm
4. Low: Hypothyroidism

# PART 5: OBSTETRICAL MANAGEMENT QUESTIONS

1. The sending nurse reports that there is a blood incompatibility between the mother and the baby. She states that the Rh came back from the lab and could harm the baby. From this, what do we know about the mother and the child?
    a. Mom (+) and fetus (-)
    b. Mom (-) and fetus (+)
    c. Mom (-) and fetus (-)
    d. Mom (+( and fetus (+)

2. Your pregnant patient is experiencing labor. The sending nurse reports that your patient is at a +5 station. Which of the following is most likely the way that she would express this information?
    a. "Oh my, you have to come right now! The patient is a +5."
    b. "Hey! How are you guys? Oh don't worry, she's only a +5."
    c. "Hello there. She is dilated at +5 and appears safe to fly."
    d. "Maybe you guys should hurry up. The slacker protein is +5."

3. You receive the following information on your patient: G1P0A0, 35 weeks gestation, contractions are 5 minutes apart, and the cervix is maximally dilated and effaced. Which of the following would be most appropriate in this case?
    a. Get the patient to the helicopter quickly
    b. Prepare equipment for immediate delivery
    c. Slowly administer magnesium sulfate
    d. Prepare for the McDonald's procedure

4. You receive a report on your female patient. The patient is G5/P3/A1. What does this tell us?
    a. The patient has had 3 abortions
    b. The patient has delivered 2 times
    c. The patient is currently pregnant
    d. The patient is at risk for severe PIH

5. Your patient is in labor, and you are transporting them to a hospital with better OB receiving capabilities. Examine the fetal monitor tracing at the top of the next page and choose the most likely pathophysiology present.
    a. Significant fetal hypoxia
    b. Severe fetal alkalosis
    c. A uterine Rupture
    d. A placental previa

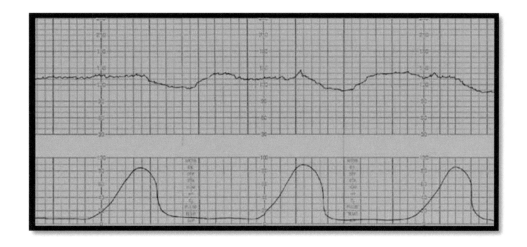

6.  In the above toco monitor tracing, how far apart are the patient's contractions?
    a.  13 minutes apart
    b.  3 minutes apart
    c.  6 minutes apart
    d.  16 minutes apart

7.  Describe the variability in the above tracing (question 5).
    a.  Marked Variability
    b.  Moderate Variability
    c.  Normal variability
    d.  Poor variability

8.  You look down at the fetal monitor strip and notice the below tracing. What is causing this particular pattern on the tracing?
    a.  Placental previa
    b.  Uterine rupture
    c.  Cord compression
    d.  Preeclampsia

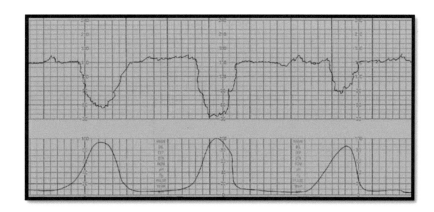

9. In the toco monitor tracing from question #8, how far apart are the patient's contractions?
   a. 13 minutes apart
   b. 3 minutes apart
   c. 6 minutes apart
   d. 16 minutes apart


10. Describe the variability in the above tracing (question 8).
    a. Marked Variability
    b. Moderate Variability
    c. Normal variability
    d. Poor variability


11. You are assessing your pregnant patient and note the following toco tracing. From this tracing, which of the following is correct regarding the condition of the fetus?
    a. The fetus is in acidosis
    b. Acute cord compression
    c. This is a healthy fetus
    d. Acute abruption placenta

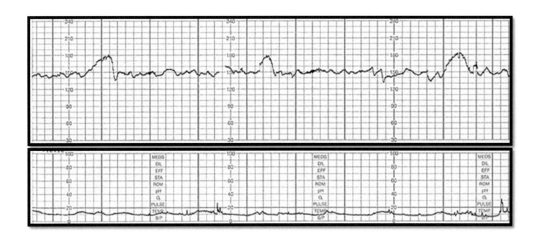

12. Describe the variability in the previous tracing (question 11).
    a. Marked Variability
    b. Moderate Variability
    c. Normal variability
    d. Poor variability


13. Your 34 week gravid patient is in labor and you are assisting to deliver. You notice "turtle sign". What maneuver should you immediately perform?
    a. McRobert's maneuver
    b. Preform an episiotomy
    c. Preform Valsalva
    d. Breech birth maneuver

14. A patient presents with a history of endometriosis and vaginal bleeding. She is 26 years old. What needs to first be ruled out?
    a. An ectopic pregnancy
    b. Pelvic inflammatory disease
    c. Toxic shock syndrome
    d. Ruptured ovarian cyst


15. Your pregnant patient is complaining of fatigue and malaise. Her first pregnancy resulted in gestational diabetes. She currently is presenting with these vital signs: HR 98, RR 22, BP 162/102, and pulse oximetry of 94%. Paired with this information, which of the following findings is consistent with PIH?
    a. 125 mg/dL of protein in urine; (+) platelets < 400
    b. 455 mg/dL of protein in urine; (+) peripheral edema
    c. (+) platelets less than 400; (+) peripheral edema
    d. High liver enzymes; (+) platelets of less than 100


16. You notice on your fetal monitoring equipment that your patient is experiencing late decelerations as well as poor variability. You recognize these two findings as being suggestive of which of the following?
    a. Nearing fetal death
    b. Strong fetal stability
    c. Acute fetal distress
    d. Fetal movement


# PART 5: OBSTETRICAL MANAGEMENT RATIONALES

1. **(B)** During a Rh-negative mom's first pregnancy with a Rh-positive fetus, blood mixing during delivery sensitizes mom to the Rh-positive protein on the baby's RBCs. Subsequent pregnancies with a Rh-positive baby (and Rh-negative mom) can lead to mom's blood attacking the Rh-positive baby's blood.

2. **(A)** Remember that station is a way to describe where the child is in the birth canal. A positive number means the child is coming closer to the vaginal opening while a negative number means they have not traveled very far from the uterus. Therefore, a positive number means that labor has begun, and that fetus is moving towards delivery. A station of +5 means that crowning probably is occurring, so they would be anxious to get help into the room.

3. **(B)** Remember that signs of imminent labor include contractions are 5-7 minutes apart over the period of an hour; all contractions have the same, or very similar, intensity; 100% effaced and fully dilated- there are all signs of imminent delivery, so you should prepare your equipment for delivery. It isn't the best idea to put this patient in your aircraft. Deliver, then arrange/ discuss transport with medical direction.

4. **(C)** Gravida: the total number of all pregnancies (including the current pregnancy); Para: the total number of deliveries after 20 weeks gestation; Abortions– the number of abortions. Therefore, this patient is currently pregnant.

5.  **(A)** A late deceleration is an indication of prolonged fetal hypoxia and possible acidosis. You are behind the oxygen 8- ball in these cases and need to act quickly to correct the fetal hypoxia. While these other conditions can cause fetal hypoxia, a late deceleration is SPECIFIC to fetal hypoxia of any etiology, therefore, "significant fetal hypoxia" is the correct answer.

6.  **(B)** Each small box represents 10 seconds, and there are six small boxes before a bold line occurs. Therefore, each bold line represents a minute. The contractions here are 3 minutes apart. .

7.  **(D)** The variability reflects the baby's fight or flight response (sympathetic response). A healthy and oxygenated fetus will have MODERATE variability and accelerations. A fetus who is being starved of oxygen for any reason will present with low (aka poor) variability and later decelerations. Moderate variability looks like course ventricular fibrillation while poor variability looks like asystole. In this case, the correct answer is poor variability.

8.  **(C)** This Tracing exhibits three decelerations that are VARIABLE because they differ in magnitude (they are all different depths and widths). This indicates the umbilical cord is being compressed.

9.  **(B)** Each small box represents 10 seconds, and there is 6 small boxes before a bold line occurs. Therefore, each bold line represents a minute. The contractions here are 3.5 minutes apart.

10. **(A)** The variability reflects the baby's fight or flight response (sympathetic response). A healthy and oxygenated fetus will have MODERATE variability and accelerations. A fetus who is being starved of oxygen for any reason will present with low (aka poor) variability and later decelerations. Moderate variability looks like course ventricular fibrillation while poor variability looks like asystole. In this case, the correct answer is poor variability.

11. **(C)** The tracing exhibits accelerations, which are ONLY possible in a well oxygenated, and non-acidotic, fetus. Therefore, the answer here is a "healthy fetus".

12. **(B)** This looks like course ventricular fibrillation; therefore, it is MODERATE variability.

13. **(A)** Turtle sign indicates shoulder dystocia. At this point, the McRoberts maneuver should be performed which involves quickly flexing the legs against the patient's abdomen- this causes the birth canal to widen slightly . The Woods' corkscrew maneuver should be performed next which involves turning the fetus by inserting your hands into the vagina, grasping its shoulders and spinning the baby 180 degrees. The fetus naturally corkscrews as it travels through the birth canal and sometimes gets a shoulder caught on the pubic bone (shoulder dystocia). By turning the baby, you mimic this corkscrew action which can free up the baby's shoulder. Another option is to pull out the baby's arm which reduces the baby's width and thus allowing delivery.

14. **(A)** The ectopic pregnancy should be ruled out first because it can cause significant bleeding and death.

15. **(B)** The classic triad of high blood pressure, proteinuria, and edema strongly indicates PIH thus, is the correct answer to this question.

16. **(A)** One of the worst tracings possible for a fetus is a persistent deceleration with poor variability. This means the baby is extremely tired and will not be able to continue fighting acidosis. Act quickly to correct or have the MD perform a C-section.

# CHAPTER 11: NEONATAL EMERGENCIES

## PART 1: THE NEONATAL ASSESSMENT

### INTRODUCTION

Once you have delivered a newborn, you must turn focus to treating both the mother and child. This can be a difficult task, but with practice and study, you can effectively assess and manage both mom and the neonate. This chapter will primarily focus on the newborn assessment and management, in addition to the devices and technology required to maintain a stable patient. A conceptual, stepwise process that is systematic, meaning you do it the same way every single time you practice, is required to be efficient at the neonatal assessment. The neonatal resuscitation program (NRP) is the gold standard with respect to assessment and management of neonatal patients and will be the backbone of this chapter.

### THE INITIAL NEONATAL ASSESSMENT

#### Step 1: Assess for Stability
1. There are essentially three questions that if answered "yes" to, then the baby can be considered stable and can remain with the mother.
   a. Term?
   b. Breathing?
   c. Good tone?
2. If all are 'YES', then provide warmth by placing the infant on the mom in skin on skin fashion, or in the isolette for routine care, APGARs, and management.
3. If there is even a single 'NO' to these three questions, then proceed with the neonatal assessment.

#### Step 2: Assess the ABCs
1. Position the head (opens airway)– suction if meconium stained
2. Dry the skin– helps prevent hypothermia
3. Stimulate the baby– triggers the baby to breathe
4. Reposition the head– maintains an open airway
5. Obtain Respiratory Rate and manage as needed
   a. Apneic→ begin positive pressure ventilations (PPVs) for 30 seconds
   b. Breathing with difficulty→ PPV or CPAP
   c. Breathing without difficulty→ Term newborns admin 21% O2; Pre-term use judicial O2 PRN
6. Obtain Heart Rate and manage as needed
   a. Less than 100 bpm →
      i. Begin positive pressure ventilations (PPVs) for 30 seconds
      ii. Reassess HR every 30– 60 seconds
      iii. Once HR rises above 100 bpm, then PPVs are stopped, unless needed for persistent cyanosis

b. Less than 60 bpm→
    i. Start chest compressions and consider intubation
    ii. Reassess HR every 30– 60 seconds
    iii. If HR remains below 60 bpm, proceed to the epinephrine step.
    iv. Once HR rises above 60 bpm, then compressions are stopped
7. Overview:
    a. Dry/ Stimulate/ Position the baby (30 seconds)
    b. Apply PPV with HR < 100 bpm (30 seconds)
    c. Apply chest compressions with HR < 60 (30 seconds)

## Step 3: Assess the need for Epinephrine

1. Continued HR greater than 60 bpm → Continue Care
    a. Maintain PPV with supplemental oxygen
    b. Maintain chest compressions
    c. Strongly consider intubation to perform best compressions and ventilations together
2. Continued HR less than 60 bpm→ Epinephrine Administration
    a. Administer 0.01-0.03 mg/kg of epinephrine
        i. Note: NRP doses in 1:10,000 epi in mL. This can be confusing. Remember, when dosing 1mg is either in a 1mL vial (1:1000), so 0.1 mg per 0.1 of epi. Or, 1mg is in 10 cc (1:10,000), so that 0.1 mg is in 1cc.
    b. Via IV, IO, umbilical vein, or endotracheal tube

## Step 4: Obtain blood sugar.

## Step 5: Assess the APGAR

1. The APGAR score is one of the first assessments of the infant's health. The baby is checked at 1 minute and 5 minutes after birth for heart and respiratory rates, muscle tone, reflexes, and color. Each area (letter of APGAR) can have a score of 0, 1, or 2, with 10 points as the maximum for the total APGAR.
2. If a baby has a difficult time during delivery, this can lower the oxygen levels in the blood, which can lower the APGAR score. APGAR scores of 3 or less often mean a baby needs immediate attention and care.
3. (A)ppearance [color]
    a. 2– Pink all over
    b. 1– Pink body, blue hands and feet
    c. 0– completely cyanotic
4. (P)ulse
    a. 2– Above 100 bpm
    b. 1– Below 100 bpm
    c. 0– Absent
5. (G)rimace [cry]
    a. 2– Crying constantly and loud
    b. 1– Weak cry that is irregular or gasping
    c. 0– Absent
6. (A)ctivity [muscle tone]
    a. 2– Moves extremities well
    b. 1– Weak extremity movement
    c. 0– Flaccid
7. (R)espiratory effort
    a. 2– Crying
    b. 1– Irregular or gasping effort
    c. 0– Absent

# THE CONTINUED NEONATAL ASSESSMENT

## Assess for Respiratory Effort

1. Work of breathing– increased WOB indicates hypoxia or cardio-pulmonary pathophysiology
2. Retractions– indicates hypoxia

## Assess for Perfusion

1. Color– cyanosis indicates hypoxia
2. NO distal pulses- indicates hypovolemia or poor cardiac output
3. Slow capillary refill (> 2 seconds)- indicates hypovolemia or other cause of hypotension

## Assess for Temperature

1. Ensure to maintain the infant's temperature, THEY WILL GET COLD, and it happens even with outstanding clinicians.
2. Use an isolette warmer, a chemical warmer, and blankets to maintain normothermia.
3. REMEMBER: hypothermia worsens any acidosis.

# PART 2: THE ISOLETTE IN TRANSPORT

## INTRODUCTION

If you transport neonates often, then you will most likely be carrying them in an isolette. The isolette is a box that isolates the infant from noise and light, also, to help maintain their temperature.

## THE ISOLETTE

### FEATURES

1. The isolette is for any infant weighing 5 kg or less.
2. Each isolette will vary from model to model. However, there are several standard features:
   a. Mounts for oxygen, medical air, or nitrous oxide tanks.
   b. ECG/ defibrillator and a transport ventilator.
   c. Patient compartment with double paned plexiglass to reduce noise and heat loss.
3. You will need to familiarize yourself with the isolette you will be using.

### APPLYING THE ISOLETTE VENTILATOR

#### A/C or SIMV

1. A/C: Each time the patient takes a breath, the ventilator will deliver a full set tidal volume. Problem– this could lead to a high minute ventilation in a poorly sedated patient.
2. SIMV: This allows the patient to take an occasional breath on their own (with or without pressure support on those breaths that you determine). Problem- this also could lead to a high minute ventilation in a poorly sedated patient.

#### Pressure or Volume

Pressure Controlled

1. Set Pressure Control between 16-20 cmH2O.
2. This is a safe mode with pediatrics because you CONTROL the highest possible pressure, thus preventing barotrauma. The drawback is that the minute ventilation will be varied so make sure you monitor the EtCO2 to ensure you are off-loading just

enough CO2 (keep EtCO2 between 35-45 mmHg)- unless metabolic acidosis is present, then provide enough minute ventilation to achieve a mid-20s EtCO2 measurement.

**Volume Controlled**

1. Set Tidal Volume between 5-7cc/kg.
3. This type of ventilation delivery guarantees a certain minute ventilation, but we can cause barotrauma. Be sure to monitor the peak inspiratory pressure values (PIP) often. Target an EtCO2 between 35-45 mmHg)- unless metabolic acidosis is present, then provide enough minute ventilation to achieve a mid-20s EtCO2 measurement.

**Set Rate: 25-35/ min**

**Set PEEP: 3-5 cmH2O**

**Set FiO2: 0.21– 1.0**

## MANAGING THE VENTILATOR NEONATE ON THE VENTILATOR

1. Maintain EtCO2 between 35-45mmHg; unless metabolic acidosis is present, then provide enough minute ventilation to achieve a mid-20s EtCO2 measurement.
2. Use rate and tidal volume (or pressure control if using pressure ventilation) to directly increase or decrease the serum CO2.
3. Target peak pressures below 35 cmH2O. Pressure control guarantees this.
4. Target plateau pressures below 30 cmH2O.

# PART 3: NEONATAL CONDITIONS

## INTRODUCTION

You should always be able to figure out the patient's condition by being provided information from any of these categories.

## GENERAL MANAGEMENT

### Maintain Airway:

1. Positioning
2. Suction
3. Endotracheal intubation.

### Maintain Breathing:

1. Supporting their effort
2. Utilize supplemental oxygen
3. Control completely with the transport ventilator.

### Maintain Circulation:

1. Ensure HR > 100 bpm, brisk capillary refill, normothermia
2. IV access: Umbilical vein, IO, IV, or endotracheal
3. Target specific pre– ductal pulse oximetry within the first 10 minutes after birth and be diligent to keep in these ranges:
    a. 1 minute: 60-65%
    b. 3 minutes: 70-75%

       c.    4 minutes: 75-80%
       d.    5 minutes: 80-85%
       e.    10 minutes: 85-95%
4. Avoid pulse oximetry greater than 95% on newborns.
5. The ductus arteriosus will be discussed in the next chapter.

## *Common Calculations in Neonatal Management*

1. Endotracheal tube size = below 28 weeks (2.5mm); 28-34 weeks (3.0mm); 34-38 weeks (3.5mm); above 38 weeks (3.5-4.0mm); QUICK: divide gestational age by 10 and round
2. Endotracheal tube depth = Kg + 6
3. Cardioversion (0.5-1 J/kg) and Defibrillation (2-4 J/kg)
4. Isotonic Fluid Bolus: 10cc/kg
5. Fluid Maintenance Formula (D10 %):
    a.   2.5- 1.5 kg  —> need 60cc/kg/day, or about 6 cc/hr.
    b.   750 g —> need 140cc/kg/day, or about 4.5 cc/hr.
6. Dextrose for Hypoglycemia: 2cc/ kg of D10
7. Normal saline (isotonic) is for fluid resuscitation boluses while D10 is for hypoglycemia and fluid maintenance.

# NEONATAL CONDITIONS

## *Apnea*

1. Patho (Primary): Born not breathing and is a result of asphyxia during the birthing process--> responds well to stimulation
2. Patho (Secondary): Characterized by the pt not breathing after the first few breaths--> only responds to assisted ventilation with supplemental oxygen
3. S/S: absence of breathing for > 20 seconds; cyanosis, pallor, hypotonia, bradycardia
4. MGT: blow by O2, then assisted ventilation if needed; 2 cc/kg D10 (if glucose is <40mg/dl); warm pt; get CBC and cultures; ampicillin and gentamycin (cultures pulled, and antibiotics started at sending facility typically)

## *Meconium aspiration syndrome*

1. Patho: fetus in distress--> expels first stool in utero--> blocks airway/ inflames lung tissue--> hypoxia/ persistent pulmonary hypertension/ delayed transition to fetal circulation/ pneumothorax
2. S/S: (+) meconium present on neonate; respiratory distress; hypoxia
3. MGT: suction trachea via endotracheal tube ONLY if meconium is seen in the airway and BEFORE stimulating the patient (prevent further meconium into the lungs); consider PPV if needed; be prepared to needle decompress a pneumothorax.

## *Pneumonia*

1. Patho: neonates have impaired immune system--> predisposes them to infections--> increased pneumonia risk
2. S/S: tachypnea, increased WOB; hypothermia; (+) chest X-ray for infiltrates; possible abnormal ABG; tough to distinguish from respiratory distress syndrome
3. MGT: NPO; ABCs; IV fluids and antibiotics (ampicillin and gentamycin); supplemental O2 and if needed, ventilatory support

## Respiratory distress syndrome

1. Patho: premature infant (<32 weeks)--> insufficient surfactant production-->poor gas exchange and increased proteins at alveolar surface--> shortness of breath
2. S/S: history of prematurity; grunting; retractions; nasal flaring; tachypnea; cyanosis; tough to distinguish from pneumonia
3. MGT: ABCs; surfactant (by qualified caregiver); monitor for improving compliance; minimize peak pressures (PIP, PEEP) as compliance improves; target SpO2 between 85-92% (prevents O2 toxicity)

## Pneumothorax

1. Patho: aggressive ventilation/ pneumonia/ meconium/ resuscitation--> simple pneumothorax--> tension pneumothorax--> respiratory/ circulatory failure
2. S/S: tachypnea; increased O2; requirements; increased WOB; tachycardia to bradycardia; cyanosis and hypotension
3. MGT: ABCs; needle decompression (22g-18g needle, 3-way stopcock, 10-20cc syringe at 2nd ICS and mid-clavicular line, 60 degrees toward apex of lung)

## Cyanosis

1. Patho: apnea/ airway obstruction/ aspiration--> poor arterial oxygenation
2. S/S: Peripheral cyanosis– only extremities are blue; Central cyanosis– extremities and the trunk are all blue.
3. MGT: ABCs; oxygen; BVM, if needed; consider transfusion if anemic

## Cyanotic congenital heart disease

1. Patho: multiple etiologies--> abnormal blood flow where deoxygenated blood is shunted from right side of heart to left side of heart--> deoxygenated blood bypasses the lungs and doesn't pick up required oxygen--> causing cyanosis
2. 5 Ts of cyanotic congenital heart disease: truncus arteriosus, transposition of the great vessels, tetralogy of Fallot, tricuspid atresia, and total anomalous pulmonary venous return
3. S/S: respiratory distress, cyanosis, pre- and post-ductal SpO2 of >10% (suspicious for PPHN); conduct 4-point BP assessment, ABGs
4. MGT: ABCs; consider prostaglandins (keeps open ductus arteriosus); manage hypotension and acidosis as needed

## Persistent pulmonary hypertension

1. Patho: elevated pressures in pulmonary vasculature ($\uparrow$ PVR) after birth--> prevents transition from fetal blood flow to normal circulation--> poor pulmonary perfusion/ hypoxemia/ R to L shunting
2. S/S: cyanosis; tachypnea; hypoxemia (but may be fluctuating)
3. MGT: ABCs; maximize oxygenation; minimize stress; maintain BP; correct any acidosis, ventilator with NITRIC OXIDE (improves oxygenation, if removed, pt can become compromised rapidly– ensure you have enough for the FULL transport).

## Metabolic Acidosis

1. Patho: Any cause (Hypoventilation/ bradycardia/ poor perfusion/ congenital heart disease/ sepsis)--> poor tissue perfusion--> lactic acid builds up--> acidosis--> prevents cells from functioning normally--> severe cell dysfunction and death
2. S/S: signs of poor perfusion (mottled- grey skin/ altered mental status/ hypotension/ slow capillary refill/ loss of peripheral pluses); ABG– profound acidosis is congenital heart issue until completely ruled out.
3. MGT: ABCs; fluids; ID and treat underlying cause; 4% bicarb if refractory to other treatments

## Shock

1. Patho: Hypovolemia (diarrhea or low fluid intake--> hypovolemia--> shock cascade); Cardiogenic (congenital heart disease/ myocardial ischemia/ tamponade--> reduced cardiac output--> shock cascade); Distributive (sepsis--> massive vasodilation--> shock cascade)
2. Shock Cascade: poor tissue perfusion--> lactic acid builds up--> acidosis--> prevents cells from functioning normally--> severe cell dysfunction and death
3. S/S: Hypotension; signs of poor perfusion; oliguria or anuria; weak pulses; cardiomegaly or hepatomegaly (end organ damage); DIC
4. MGT: ABCs; monitor blood sugar; ID and treat underlying cause; 10 cc/kg NS or blood– GIVE SLOWLY! Over 5-10 min. Fragile vessels.

## Proximal intestinal obstruction

1. Patho: an obstruction of the intestine at or above the level of the jejunum
2. S/S: bilious vomiting; minimal dilation of the abdomen; evidence of intestinal ischemia (blood mucoid stools)
3. MGT: ABCs; IV; maintain thermoregulation; ensure strict input/output

## Distal intestinal obstruction

1. Patho: a partial or complete obstruction of the distal small bowel (ileum)
2. S/S: distended abdomen; failure to pass meconium on the first 24-48 hours; bilious or non-bilious vomiting
3. MGT: ABCs; IV; maintain thermoregulation; ensure strict input/output

## Anemia

1. Patho: a reduction of the hematocrit below 38% in preterm neonates and 42% in term neonates from increased destruction, decreased production, or loss of RBCs
2. S/S: tachycardia; pallor; petechial hemorrhages; respiratory distress; shock; cyanosis; low hematocrit (< 38% in preterm/ < 42% in term neonates); positive Coombs test (shows autoimmune destruction of RBCs)
3. MGT: ABCs; IV access; fluid bolus (20cc/mL); type/ cross match and consider blood transfusion

## Choanal Atresia

1. Patho: a congenital disorder where the back of the nasal passage (choana) is blocked, usually by abnormal bony or soft tissue (membranous) due to failed recanalization of the nasal fossae during fetal development
2. S/S: CT to confirm; Retractions when attempting to breathe via nose– retractions cease when the newborn breathes through the mouth; CANNOT cry and breathe at the same time; breathing difficulty; cyanosis.
3. MGT: Aggressive ABCs including considering intubation; surgery to repair

## Diaphragmatic Hernia

1. Patho: a condition where the abdominal organs enter the chest cavity through a rupture in the diaphragm which prevents the one from growing normally
2. S/S: shortness of breath at birth; scaphoid abdomen; cyanosis; tachypnea; tachycardia; diminished breath sounds; bowel sounds in chest; positive x-ray with bowel contents seen in the chest
3. MGT: Quickly consider RSI and intubate WITH MINIMAL PPV before intubation (PPV & NIPPV will collect in stomach which is now in the thorax thus complicating intrathoracic pressures); large bore nasogastric tube; minimize PEEP to achieve O2 sat 85%; Vent: high rate/ low pressure; tolerate pH 7.25 in these pts; surgery/ ECMO center.

### Hirschsprung's disease

1. Patho: congenital abnormality--> lack of ganglion nerve cells--> normal peristalsis does not occur--> stools back up--> septic megacolon
2. S/S: decreased stooling; abdominal distention; shock (sepsis)
3. MGT: ABCs; fluid resuscitation; transport to a peds surgeon

### Acute intestinal perforation

1. Patho: the intestine becomes perforated; this can occur from necrotizing enterocolitis or spontaneously
2. S/S: progressive abdominal distention; respiratory distress; hypotension; acidosis; feeding intolerance; grossly bloody stools
3. MGT: ABCs; IV; maintain NPO; monitor for apnea; intubate if apneic; antibiotics (ampicillin, gentamycin, clindamycin); treat pH below 7.25 with 4% bicarb if acidosis is refractory to fluid boluses

### Volvulus

1. Patho: twisting of the stomach or intestine, which often has the effect of cutting off its blood supply
2. S/S: abdominal pain (fussy infant); n/v; blood in the stool
3. MGT: ABCs; NPO status; maintenance fluids; decompress the intestine with NGT; provide ↓intermittent suction; peds surg. center.

### Infectious diseases

1. Patho: bacteria/ fungus/ virus invading the tissue of the neonate
2. S/S: decreased activity of the neonate; hypo or hyperthermic; signs of poor perfusion; low BP; apnea
3. MGT: ABCs; monitor vitals; maintain normothermia; consider antibiotics; monitor glucose closely

### Hypothermia

1. Patho: temp in a neonate less than 97.5*F, which can occur in all climates
2. S/S: temp less than 97.5*F; cool skin; apnea and bradycardia; irritability; weak cry; lethargy
3. MGT: improve temp to lower limit of normal (higher than 97.5*F)

### Seizures

1. Patho: electro-neurologic derangement resulting in alteration of neurologic function
2. S/S: eye deviation; blinking; pedaling movements of the legs; tonic extension of the extremities; flexion of extremities; convulsions
3. MGT: ABCs; monitor vitals; intubate PRN; antiepileptics; sedatives

### Hypoglycemia

1. Patho: low blood sugar resulting in decreased activity and lethargy
2. S/S: decreased activity; seizures; blood glucose less than 40 mg/ dL
3. MGT: ABCs; 2 mL/kg of D10

### Esophageal atresia

1. Patho: a congenital abnormality where the esophagus is abnormally closed, thus preventing the patient from receiving nutrients
2. S/S: increased salivation; choking on feeding; non- bilious vomit; respiratory distress; inability to pass an NGT or OGT
3. MGT: ABCs; position the infant with HOB of 30*; provide intermittent suction; keep airway clear of secretions

# PART 4: CONGENITAL HEART DEFECTS

## INTRODUCTION

Approximately 1 in 100 infants will have some cardiac anomaly that prevents normal stabilization of the newborn. It is important to be proactive in the minutes after birth to ensure the newborns perfusion status is maintained.

Even though this topic is being discussed in this section, you may be sent on a pediatric call or flight involving an older infant with the same conditions. These patients can often present like the adults CHF patient: JVD, pulmonary edema, hepatojugular reflex. This is due to a poorly formed cardiac pump. Therefore, therapy is targeted to maximize an oxygenation, perfusion, and blood flow through the vasculature (improve the pump).

## MAIN TYPES

As mentioned in the hemodynamic section, the heart is a pump that facilitates the forward flow of blood through the vasculature. If there are structural lesions that allow alternate paths of blood flow, then there can exist conditions that affect blood pressure and oxygenation. We can classify these congenital heart defects as either causing cyanosis or without cyanosis (acyanosis).

### *Acyanosic Lesions*

1. These lesions cause a LEFT TO RIGHT shunt of blood resulting in oxygenated blood mixing with non-oxygenated blood typically through a whole or structural defect in the heart itself.
2. Because the left side of the heart is much stronger than the right, any hole between the atria or the ventricles will allow blood to move from the higher pressure left side into the right side of the heart; hence, a left to right shift.
3. There are three main defects that cause a left to right shunt of blood, also classified as ACYANOTIC: a patent ductus arteriosus (PDA), and atrial septal defect (ASD), and a ventricular septal defect (VSD).

#### Patent Ductus Arteriosus (PDA)

Upon the baby's first breath, oxygen triggers a halt to prostaglandin synthesis, resulting in a closure of the ductus arteriosus. Occasionally the ductus arteriosus remains patent. In

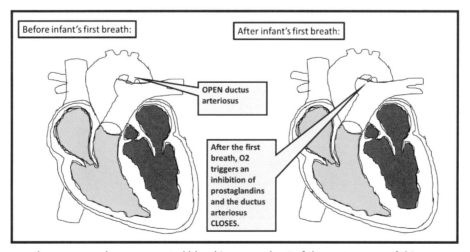

these cases, when oxygenated blood is pumped out of the aorta, some of this oxygenated blood is allowed to reenter the pulmonary artery, travel through the pulmonary vasculature, and return to the left atrium.

**Atrial Septal Defect (ASD)**

This condition is simply characterized as a hole in the septum between the left and right atria. This allows oxygenated blood from the higher pressure left atria to move into the lower pressure right atria.

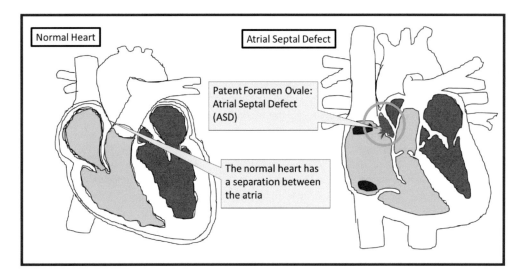

**Ventricular Septal Defect (VSD)**

This condition is simply characterized as a hole in the septum between the left and right ventricles. Just as with the ASD, oxygenated blood from the higher pressure left ventricle flows into the lower pressure right ventricle.

**Coarctation of the Aorta**

The condition is characterized by the aorta becoming abnormally narrowed. This condition makes it harder for the heart to pump blood to the body. Over time, this can lead to high blood pressure, heart failure, or other complications (see next page).

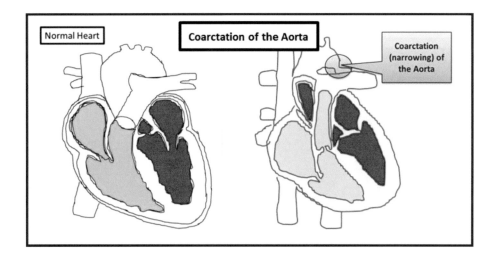

## *Cyanotic Lesions*

1. These lesions cause a RIGHT TO LEFT shunt of blood resulting in deoxygenated blood being allowed to enter the aorta and into systemic circulation, thus causing cyanosis of varying degrees.
2. There are essentially four defects that cause a right to left shunt, also classified as CYANOTIC: Tetralogy of Fallot, transposition of the great vessels, truncus arteriosus, and hypoplastic left heart syndrome.

### Tetralogy of Fallot (TOF)

1. This condition is a series of four different conditions.  When all four are present, it is the classic presentation of this condition. However, multiple variations can occur by mixing and matching any combination of these four conditions: VSD, pulmonary stenosis, a truncated (high riding) aorta, and right ventricular hypertrophy. KEEP THE PDA OPEN.
   a. VSD- as mentioned previously, this is a hole between the right and left ventricles.
   b. Pulmonary Stenosis- this is a narrowing or closing of the pulmonary artery.
   c. Truncated Aorta- the aorta normally begins in the left ventricle, and only communicates with this ventricle.  A high, or truncated, aorta is connected to both the left ventricle and the right ventricle with a very short septum that does not separate the left and right ventricles (see the figure on Truncus Arteriosus).
   d. Right Ventricular Hypertrophy- the three preceding conditions can increase the pulmonary vascular resistance (pulmonary pressure), this makes the right ventricle work harder and it increases in size.
2. The VSD and truncated aorta allow unoxygenated blood to enter the aorta and into systemic circulation, thus leading to cyanosis.  Right ventricular hypertrophy occurs because of the pulmonary stenosis and the right ventricular hypertrophy adds to the force pushing Unoxygenated blood into the aorta.  These conditions together make up the perfect storm to force unoxygenated blood into circulation.

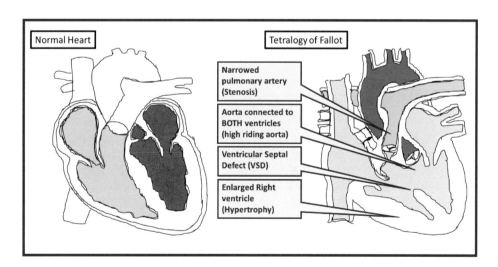

### Transposition of the Great Vessels

It is characterized by the aorta beginning in the right ventricle and the pulmonary artery beginning in the left ventricle.  This means that blood is returned to the right atrium, enters the right ventricle, enters the aorta; it enters systemic circulation, and then it is again returned to the right atria.  It essentially closes off the pulmonary circulation and left ventricle from the rest of the vasculature and heart.  This is fatal very quickly unless there is a large PDA allowing blood flow to deter pulmonary circulation for oxygenation.

Because little blood is oxygenated, cyanosis occurs. KEEP THE PDA OPEN. This the only time where pre-ductal saturation is LOWER than the post-ductal. #DEADGIVEAWAY.

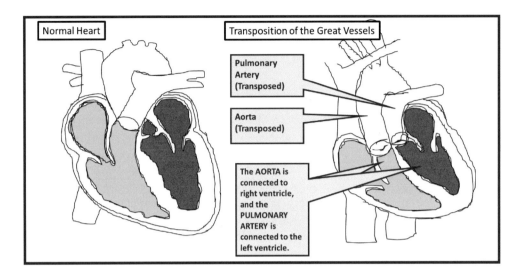

## Truncus Arteriosus

In this condition, the aorta and pulmonary artery are never formed, and instead a singular artery forms in its place. With this condition a VSD typically forms as well allowing complete communication between the left and right ventricles, the pulmonary artery, and the aorta. Because the deoxygenated blood is allowed to enter into the systemic circulation, cyanosis occurs.

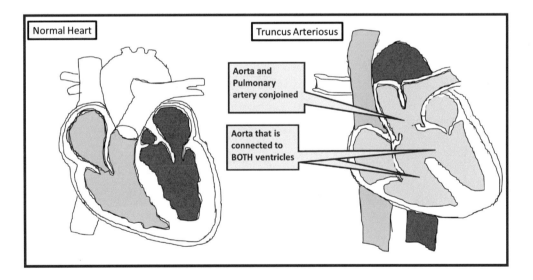

## Hypoplastic Left Heart Syndrome

In this condition, the left ventricle fails to form, as well as the failure of the mitral valve and the aortic valves to form. These patients rely on an open PDA and VSDs to deliver some oxygenated blood to the systemic circulation. KEEP THE PDA OPEN.

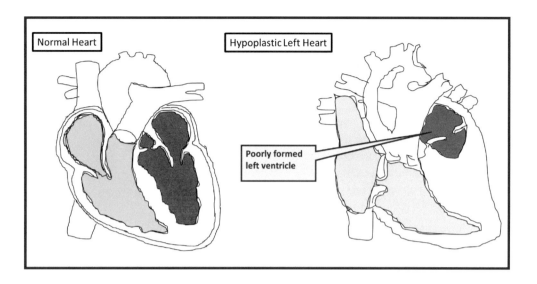

# PART 5: NEONATAL PHARMACOLOGY

## IN GENERAL

There are a handful of useful medications to consider with your neonatal patients, in addition to oxygen and isotonic fluids. Unless you are with a neonatal transport team, these medications may get forgotten unless practiced more routinely.

## THE MEDICATIONS

### Epinephrine
1. Class: Vasopressor, Sympathomimetic, bronchodilator
2. Mechanism: Markedly stimulates both the alpha and beta receptors therefore significant increases in heart rate, blood pressure, and cardiac output occur.
3. Indications: Neonates: HR < 60 after 60 seconds of positive pressure ventilation with 100% supplemental O2; ventricular fibrillation; hypotension
4. Contraindications: Hypertension, tachycardia, acute coronary syndromes, hypersensitivity
5. Hemodynamics: (↑CVP/ ↑PCWP/↑CO/↑SVR).
6. Dose: HR < 60/ Arrest: 0.01 mg/kg (0.1 mL/kg of 1:10,000) IV/IO; Hypotension: 0.1- 1.0 mg/min infusion ; Anaphylaxis:  < 6 yrs- 0.15 mg IM (0.15 mL of 1:1000); 6-12 yrs- 0.3 mg IM (0.3 mL of 1:1000); > 12 yrs- 0.5 mg IM (0.5 mL of 1:1000).
7. Hemodynamics: (↑CVP/ ↑PCWP/↑CO/↑SVR).

### Indomethacin
1. Class: NSAID
2. Mechanism: Inhibits prostaglandin synthesis.
3. Indications: Neonates: Closes a patent ductus arteriosus.
4. Contraindications: Asthma, congenital heart defects relying on the PDA to remain open to ensure adequate blood flow

5. Hemodynamics: (↑CVP/ ↑PCWP/~CO/~SVR).
6. Dose: Initial: 0.1 to 0.2 mg/kg/dose followed by 0.1 mg/kg/dose every 12 to 24 hours for 2 additional doses

## Prostaglandin E1 (PGE1)
1. Class: Prostaglandin
2. Mechanism: Keeps the ductus arteriosus open and patent.
3. Indications: Neonates: Used to keep OPEN a patent ductus arteriosus.
4. Contraindications: hypotension, tachycardia
5. Hemodynamics: (↓CVP/ ↓PCWP/~CO/~SVR).
6. Dose: Initial: 0.01 mcg/kg/minute
7. Causes APNEA– intubate if you plan on using this drug!

## Dextrose 10% (D10)
1. Class: Sugar
2. Mechanism: Supplies the cells with energy.
3. Indications: Low blood sugar; < 40 mg/dL.
4. Contraindications: Hyperglycemia
5. Hemodynamics: (~CVP/ ~PCWP/~CO/~SVR).
6. Dose: Initial: D10 2cc/kg

## Survanta
1. Class: Surfactant
2. Mechanism: Increases the surface tension in the lungs.
3. Indications:
4. Treatment of intubated infants on 30% or more oxygen whose clinical presentation and chest x-ray are consistent with RDS.
5. Prophylactic administration may be considered in infants < 26 weeks EGA
6. Premature infants
7. Contraindications: hypotension, tachycardia
8. Hemodynamics: (~CVP/ ~PCWP/~CO/~SVR).
9. Dose: 4 ml/kg in 2-4 aliquots, repeat dose as needed if responsive. Minimum: left lateral position and then in right lateral position

## Atropine
1. Class: Anticholinergic
2. Mechanism: Blocks the parasympathetic receptors (slow system) thus speeding up the heart
3. Indications: pediatric intubation, bradycardia, organophosphate poisoning
4. Contraindications: hypersensitivity
5. Hemodynamics: (~CVP/ ~PCWP/↑CO/~SVR).
6. Dose: PEDS: 0.02 mg/kg IV push, Minimum of 0.1 mg.

# PART 6: NEONATAL MANAGEMENT QUESTIONS

1. Your newborn patient currently presents with pulmonary stenosis, a high-riding aorta, and a hypertrophic right ventricle. Which of the following treatments should be avoided?
   a. Tracheal suctioning
   b. Prostaglandins
   c. Surfactant dosing
   d. High flow oxygen

2. You have medical control orders to administer prostaglandins to keep open your patient's PDA. The patient weighs 9 pounds. Which of the following the correct starting dosage for PGE1 for this patient?
   a. 0.04 mcg/min
   b. 0.2 mcg/min
   c. mcg/kg/min
   d. mcg/kg/min

3. Your neonatal patient has pale extremities and is without brachial pulses. The patient weighs 5.3 pounds. Following your initial fluid bolus, which of the following is an appropriate maintenance rate for this patient?
   a. 10 cc/hr LR
   b. 6 cc/hr D10
   c. 20 cc/hr D5NS
   d. 31 cc/hr NS

4. During the 5th minute of your newborn patient's life, you know that the pulse oximetry is 90%. The patient is intubated and being ventilated currently on pressure control of 20, PEEP of 5, rate of 29, and the FiO two of 0.75. Which of the following actions is most appropriate in this case?
   a. Reduce the FiO2 to 0.65
   b. Increase the FiO2 to 0.9
   c. Administer surfactant
   d. Administer prostaglandin

5. During transport, you notice your neonatal patient is pedaling his legs in the isolette. Which of the following treatment is most appropriate and this patient?
   a. Administer versed
   b. Administer surfactant
   c. Administer indomethacin
   d. Administer prostaglandin

6. A patient is a preemie infant delivered tonight who is approximately 7 weeks premature with persistent breathing difficulty and signs of acute acidosis. . Which of the following medications are indicated in this case?

   a. Administer versed

   b. Administer surfactant

   c. Administer indomethacin

   d. Administer prostaglandin


7. Which of the following pathophysiologies is considered a cyanotic condition?

   a. TOF

   b. VSD

   c. ASD

   d. PDA


8. You're treating your neonatal patient for hypertension that you suspect is from sepsis. Your patient weighs 8 pounds. Which of the following dosage, that method of delivery is appropriate for this patient?

   a. 26 cc over 1 minute

   b. 22 cc over 9 minutes

   c. 31 cc over 2 minutes

   d. 36 cc over 7 minutes


9. Your 33 week gestation, 3kg neonatal patient is failing to respond to additional stimulation and positive pressure ventilation. You decide to intubate the patient. Which of the following treatment regimens is most appropriate for this patient?

   a. 3.5mm tube at 8cm at the lip

   b. 2.5mm tube at 7cm at the lip

   c. 3.0mm tube at 9cm at the lip

   d. 4.0mm tube at 10cm at the lip


10. You patient was born meconium stained. Which of the following treatment regimens is most appropriate for this patient?

   a. Tracheal suctioning prior to stimulation

   b. Admin surfactant after PPV therapy

   c. Dry and warm patient, then suction

   d. Provide PPV then admin prostaglandin

# PART 7: NEONATAL MANAGEMENT RATIONALES

1. **(D)** With the provided pathophysiology, your patient presents with Tetralogy of Fallot. In this case, you should avoid high flow oxygen which could cause the ductus arteriosus to close. In these patients, the patent ductus arteriosus is the one thing keeping oxygenated blood being introduced into the systemic circulation. High oxygen or the drug indomethacin will close the PDA, which can result in the death of your patient.

2. **(A)** Prostaglandin is administered 0.01 mcg/kg/min. The patient weighs 9 pounds, which is the equivalent of 4.09 kg. Therefore, 0.01 mcg/kg/min multiplied by the patient's weight in kilograms yields 0.04 mg/min. Note, here we are just looking for the dose for this specific patient (multiplying the dose by the patient weight). If you're trying to calculate the rate of infusion, then you're premature. You obviously cannot do that here because you do not have a concentration of the medication.

3. **(B)** The patient's initial maintenance rate in this case should be 6 cc/hour of D10. The patient weighs 5.3pounds, which is the equivalent of 2.4 kg. Therefore, this patient requires about 60 cc/kg/day of D10 (by recalling that 2.5 kg patients need 60 cc/kg/day, 1.5 kg and over patients need 100 cc/kg/day. This patient is close to 2.5 kg, and thus needs about 60cc/kg/day. Therefore, 60 x 2.4 = 144, and then divide this by 24 hours in the day = 6cc/hr.

4. **(A)** During the fifth minute of life, pre-ductal pulse oximetry should be between 80 to 85%. In this case, the patient is at 90%. It is prudent to reduce the FiO2 to target 80 to 85% pulse oximetry.

5. **(A)** This patient is having a seizure. Signs and symptoms of a seizure in a neonate are as follows: eye deviation; blinking; pedaling movements of the legs; tonic extension of the extremities; flexion of extremities; convulsions. Therefore, the benzodiazepine would be appropriate in this case to stop the seizure.

6. **(B)** Premature infants may need surfactant, especially with prolonged respiratory difficulty. You can be proactive by simply identifying the gestational age of the patient and then anticipating some of the problems that can be encountered with premature infants- one of which is respiratory distress syndrome from inadequate surfactant. It should be noted that prophylaxis with surfactant is going out of vogue– there needs to be a clinical indication as well as gestational age.

7. **(A)** TOF is Tetralogy of Fallot and is characterized by several conditions which lead to a right to left shunting of blood. VSD, ASD, and PDA are all acyanotic lesions.

8. **(D)** The dosage for volume expansion is10 cc/kg. This patient weighs 8 pounds, which is equivalent to 3.63 kilograms. Therefore, the dosage should be approximately 36 cc of normal saline or blood. This should be given over 5 or 10 minutes (slowly). Remember, neonatal veins are very fragile and pushing rapidly could damage their vessels. This patient should receive 36 cc over 7 minutes.

9. **(C)** This patient is 33-week gestation, so by NRP requires a 3.0mm size endotracheal tube. The depth of the tube can be estimated by the Kg + 6, again, as per NRP. Therefore, this patient requires 2.5mm and secured at 9cm at the lip.

10. **(A)** This patient requires suctioning first BEFORE being stimulated because of the meconium.

# CHAPTER 12: PEDIATRIC EMERGENCIES

## PART 1: ANATOMICAL & PHYSIOLOGICAL DIFFERENCES

### INTRODUCTION

There are some fundamental anatomical and physiological differences in the pediatric patient when compared to the adult patient. It is important to note these differences as they often become test question topics on certification exams.

### THE DIFFERENCES

#### Cardiovascular

1. Once fetal circulation transitions into normal circulation by the oxygen triggered closure of the PDA, the circulatory system is very similar to an adult.
2. The most notable differences lie in the vital signs themselves.

| Normal Vital Signs for Pediatrics | | | |
|---|---|---|---|
| Developmental Stage | RR | HR | BP |
| Infant | 25-50 | 70-160 | >70 |
| Toddler | 20-30 | 90-150 | >80 |
| Preschool | 20-25 | 80-140 | >80 |
| School Age | 15-20 | 70-120 | >80 |
| Adolescent | 12-16 | 60-100 | >90 |

#### Respiratory System

1. Airways in children are smaller, therefore are more susceptible to collapse and obstruction.
2. Children have a larger tongue, proportionally, than do adults. This can honestly impact airway patency, therefore great care should be taken to ensure the tongue does not obstruct the airway. The tongue will equal the adult's size during adolescence.
3. The cricoid ring is the narrowest portion of the pediatric airway, unlike the adult airway where the glottic opening is the narrowest portion of the airway. This means that you might get an endotracheal past a set of pediatric vocal cords, but then hit the narrowest portion (the cricoid ring) and not be able to advance the two beyond this point.
4. Up to school age, children have a floppy and omega shaped epiglottis which can also act as an obstruction, especially when it becomes inflamed (see epiglottitis later in the section).
5. Peds also can have periodic (irregular) breathing– this is normal.

### Neurologic System

1. The anterior fontanelle closes between 16 to 18 months of age while the posterior fontanelle closes at two months of age.
2. The fontanelles should be soft and flat.
3. Crying babies and ones who only family can console are GOOD babies. Poor crying and an easily consolable child could indicate neuro compromise in infants and toddlers.

### Thermoregulation

1. The pediatric patient has increased body surface area– 4 times as exposed as an adult; however, heat production is only 1.5 times as high. Pediatrics are behind the curve when it comes to heat.
2. Additionally, pediatrics has undeveloped heat conservations systems: little adipose tissue and musculature cannot generate shivering in like older individuals. These factors also play into heat loss for an infant and pediatrics.

### Glucose

1. The pediatric patient will burn through sugar and oxygen (metabolism) rapidly since children are constantly augmenting their ow anatomy and physiology (we call this 'growing' of course).
2. There is a danger with infants and pediatrics that they may become hypoglycemic. Hypoglycemia is a real possibility in peds patients because the physiology that stores glucose, creates glucose, or signals the release of stored glucose is all immature and physiologically untrustworthy.

# PART 2: THE PEDIATRIC ASSESSMENT

## INTRODUCTION

The general goal of assessing the pediatric patient is to identify or rule out possible life threats so that emergency and routine care can be extended to the patient. You can break up the pediatric assessment into its two main themes: assessing respiratory status and perfusion status. Respiratory problems are the leading cause of death for pediatric cardiac arrest patients.

While a thorough and full assessment is important, keep in mind that pediatrics enter cardiac arrest for different reasons than do adults. Pediatrics enter cardiac arrest because of respiratory problems or shock, so great efforts should be made to prevent these states.

## THE INITIAL ASSESSMENT

### APPEARANCE

1. As you approach the patient, look at their body position, work of breathing and skin condition and color to formulate your FIRST IMPRESSION.
2. The appearance refers to the childs mental status, body position, muscle tone.
3. If the child is alert, then the patient's condition is not urgent.  However, if a child appears anything less than alert, then their condition is critical.
4. Their body position gives you great information: head bobbing means they are short of breath/ hypoxic.

## WORK OF BREATHING

1. Normal respiratory effort indicates they are receiving adequate oxygen, but labored respirations indicates they are hypoxic.
2. Watch the chest and abdomen for movement. If there's no movement of the chest or the child is visibly struggling to breathe, consider them hypoxic.
3. When retractions are noted, look at the level of the retractions in the superior– inferior plane.
4. The more anterior the site of retractions corresponds with an increasing work of breathing.
5. For example, supraclavicular retractions are worse than substernal retractions because the supraclavicular retractions are higher, thus, the patient is trying to recruit more skeletal musculature to improve ventilation.

## CIRCULATION

1. Normal skin color indicates adequate perfusion, but pale or mottled skin can indicate poor perfusion. If ever a child's skin color is pale, mottled, or blue, then begin immediate care because their situation is urgent.
2. Capillary refill should be < 2 seconds
3. Capillary refill is so important to assess for perfusion status. A good capillary refill time is a better indicator of perfusion than blood pressure in infants in my opinion.

## ASSESS MENTAL STATUS

1. AVPU: Awake– eyes open spontaneously; Verbal- arouses to stimulation by voice; Painful- purpose for movements to painful stimuli; Unresponsive- no response to any stimuli
2. Assess GCS (Adult and Child)
   a. Eye Opening: Spontaneous (4); to speech (3); to painful stimuli (2); no opening at all (1)
   b. Verbal Effort: normal conversation (5); confused (4); inappropriate words (3); incomprehensible sounds (2); no verbal effort (1)
   c. Motor Effort: follows commands (6); localizes pains (5); withdraws from pain (4); decorticate posturing (3); decerebrate posturing (2); no motor effort (1).
3. Assess GCS (Infant)
   a. Eye Opening: Spontaneous (4); to speech (3); to painful stimuli (2); no opening at all (1)
   b. Verbal Effort: coos, babbles (5); irritable cry (4); cries only to pain(3); moans to pain (2); no verbal effort (1)
   c. Motor Effort: spontaneous movement (6); localizes withdraws from TOUCH (5); withdraws from PAIN (4); decorticate posturing (3); decerebrate posturing (2); no motor effort (1).

## AIRWAY

1. Ensure a patent airway.
2. Until about four weeks old, infants are obligatory nose breathers. However, a good rule of thumb is to keep infants and toddlers noses as clear as possible to achieve optimal ventilation.
3. Gurgling- indicates fluid and airway and suction is immediately needed
4. Stridor- indicates upper airway obstruction mechanically or due to swelling
5. Snoring- indicates the tongue is on the back of the oropharynx and partially including the airway

## BREATHING & RESPIRATORY EFFORT

1. Basics
    a. Rate
    b. Quality (normal or labored)
    c. Rhythm (normal or abnormal respiratory patterns).
2. Anxious appearance/ accessory muscle use/leaning forward to inhale/ retractions/ seesaw breathing→ SIGNS OF HYPOXIA AND INCREASING WORK OF BREATHING
3. No air movement- suggests severe asthma or obstruction
4. Wheezing- suggests asthma

## CIRCULATION

1. Ensure the patient has a pulse,  and note the rate, strength (normal, bounding, or weak), and quality (regular or irregular).
2. Obtain and assess heart rate, blood pressure, pulse oximetry, cardiac monitoring, and labs/ images if available.
3. Ensure bleeding is controlled and be proactive about the potential for internal bleeding.
4. Simultaneously assess central pulse and distal pulse: a weak central pulse may indicate the compensated shock
5. Pale, mottled- suggests poor perfusion and hypoxia
6. Cyanosis– indicates hypoxemia
7. Cool skin- suggests decreased cardiac output and possibly hypoxia
8. Poor skin turgor– indicates dehydration
9. Delayed capillary refill- indicate shock
10. Fever- indicates infection

## DISABILITY (NEURO EXAM)

1. Question the parent or caregiver about the child's normal activity level, attention span, willingness to cooperate, and mood.
2. Pupils: should be equal, round, and reactive without trauma
3. Infant reflexes
    a. Palmer grasp- the infant will grab your finger when placed into their palm
    b. Rooting- the infant will turn toward the cheek that is touched with a finger
    c. Moro reflex- the infant will throw their arms and legs away from their body when startled
    d. Older children should be able to move, lift, and hold all extremities to command in with equal strength if resistance is applied.

## EXPOSURE

1. Assess the patient for evaluation but be sure to promptly cover with a blanket after assessing your patient (KEEP WARM)!
2. It is important to assess the entire body, however, be sure to protect the patient's body temperature. Even experienced clinicians will battle kids temperatures in the unpredictable and ever– changing transport environment. If you are new, please cultivate a strong will to defend your pediatric patient's temperature.
3. Remember– cold will worsen acidosis.

# PART 3: PEDIATRIC CONDITIONS

## INTRODUCTION

You should always be able to figure out the patient's condition by being provided information from any of these categories.

## PEDIATRIC CONDITIONS

### Asthma
1. Patho: a chronic inflammatory disorder of the lower airways resulting in significant inflammation, bronchospasm, and edema.
2. S/S: shortness of breath; wheezing; chest tightness
3. MGT: ABCs; admin bronchodilator (typically beta 2 agonist); admin corticosteroids; Consider CPAP/ BiPAP if they will tolerate it; With kids, keep a calm environment— help kids by conserving oxygen that is spent in increasing RR and effort in an anxious child— KEEP A CALM ENVIRONMENT!

### Croup
1. Patho: a viral infection of the upper airway that can affect the larynx, trachea, and bronchi; known for its 'barking cough'.
2. S/S: low grade fever; 'barking cough'; mild distress; stridor; STEEPLE SIGN on X-ray; Stridor at rest is more concerning than stridor with agitation
3. MGT: ABCs; cool, humidified oxygen; keep cabin cool (maybe open a window or lower cabin temperatures); administer racemic epinephrine via nebulizer (up to 3 doses); steroids (oral may not agitate them as much); intubate a compromised airway (usually done in OR); keep calm environment

### Epiglottitis
1. Patho: a bacterial infection (Hemophilus influenzae) of the upper airway most commonly affecting 3-5-year olds
2. S/S: rapid onset; drooling; tripod; stridor; obvious signs of toxicity; distress; muffled voice; high WBCs; THUMB SIGN on x-ray.
3. MGT: Ensure a calm environment; AVOID racemic epi; intubate ONLY if absolutely necessary

### Bronchiolitis
1. Patho: a viral infection most caused by the RSV, but can be caused by other agents, causing lower airway edema and bronchospasms
2. S/S: mild wheezing; tachypnea; nasal flaring; retractions
3. MGT: ABCs; supplemental oxygen and fluids; steroids; frequent suctioning; ribavirin (antivirus found to prevent kids from having to be mechanically ventilated); intubate PRN; consider CPAP/ BiPAP— but only if the patients tolerate this— avoid over agitating them keep a calm environment

### Pneumonia
1. Patho: a parenchymal lung disease caused by an infective agent or caustic substance
2. S/S: fever; grunting or cough; shortness of breath; decreased feeding or irritability; fatigue
3. MGT: ABCs; fluids; antibiotics; intubate PRN

### Acute Respiratory Distress Syndrome
1. Patho: a condition characterized by pulmonary shunting that has minimal or no response to oxygenation and can be caused by a multitude of agents
2. S/S: shortness of breath; rapid breathing; cough; fever; low BP; confusion; extreme fatigue
3. MGT: ABCs; consider albuterol; supportive care; intubation and mechanical ventilation PRN

### Seizures
1. Patho: a transient, involuntary alteration of consciousness due to excessive neuronal discharge
2. S/S: subtle sz (chewing, bicycle pedaling, eye deviation, or apnea); febrile (+ fever); status epilepticus (continuous sz lasting > 30 minutes with convulsions).
3. MGT: ABCs; Glucose, benzos, phenobarbital, fosphenytoin

### Hypovolemic Shock
1. Patho: inadequate vascular volume--> poor blood return back to the heart (low preload)--> low cardiac output--> poor tissue perfusion
2. S/S: lightheadedness; tachycardia; decreased BP; AMS; pale/ clammy skin; chest pain; diarrhea; kidney failure (low urine output)
3. MGT: ABCs; stop source of volume loss; replace lost volume (enough to improve color of skin or BP) 20cc/kg NS boluses; It is common to give multiple repeat boluses if needed to achieve a good capillary refill.

### Cardiogenic Shock
1. Patho: heart muscle or tissue damaged--> heart pumping action reduced--> low cardiac output--> poor tissue perfusion
2. S/S: signs of poor perfusion; rales and JVD ; palpable liver is likely in these patients as their cardiogenic shock isn't normally acute, but manifests over time– which also will cause the liver to enlarge (backflow problem, remember?)
3. MGT: ABCs; fluids (10- 20cc/kg boluses, however it is important to mention that judicial fluid use in the patients is highly encouraged– you can over fill their tank [vasculature] if you are not careful); inotropic support; treat primary pathologies; support cardiac function pharmacologically

### Neurogenic Shock
1. Patho: damage to spinal cord--> transmission of peripheral nervous system cut at level of spinal injury--> sympathetic tone lost--> vessels cannot constrict therefore dilate--> blood pools in these dilated vessels--> poor blood return back to the heart--> low cardiac output--> poor perfusion
2. S/S: signs of poor perfusion; red, warm skin below level of injury and cool clammy skin above injury level
3. MGT: ABCs; fluids (20cc/kg boluses); BP support

### Anaphylactic Shock

1. Patho: allergen--> elicits an immune response--> histamine release--> vasodilation--> poor blood return to the heart--> low cardiac output--> poor perfusion
2. S/S: signs of poor perfusion; general body edema; urticaria; hypotension; bronchospasm; laryngeal edema
3. MGT: High flow O2; epinephrine IM; RSI/ intubate if impending airway compromise or respiratory failure detected; diphenhydramine (H2 blocker); ranitidine (H1 blocker); albuterol; methylprednisolone

### Septic Shock

1. Patho: infection--> widespread immune response--> vasodilation with bounding pulse, but poor kidney function (warm phase)--> decreasing cardiac output, worsening perfusion, and cool extremities (cool phase)
2. S/S (warm phase): vasodilation; warm skin; bounding pulse; normal cardiac output; decreased kidney function; metabolic acidosis; AMS
3. S/S (cool phase): failing cardiac output; worsening perfusion; cool extremities to touch
4. MGT: ABCs; oxygenation and vent support; fluids; inotropic or vasoactive meds (consider dopamine for 1st line vasoactive support, epi for cold shock, and norepi for warm shock); ECMO ; broad spectrum antibiotics; anti– virials for patients < 12 weeks old.

### Meningococcal Infections

1. Patho: a deadly infection of the layers covering the brain
2. S/S: fever, chills, nuchal rigidity (+ Kernig's and + Brudzinski's signs), photophobia, HA, and irritability
3. MGT: ABCs; standard precautions; continue any antibiotics and start if not started yet; initiate droplet precautions

### Hypothermia

1. Patho: temp in an infant less than 97.5*F, which can occur in all climates
2. S/S: temp less than 97.5*F; cool skin; apnea and bradycardia; irritability; weak cry; lethargy
3. MGT: improve temp to lower limit of normal (higher than 97.5*F)

### Hypoglycemia

1. S/S: Institutions and protocols may vary, but about 55-60 mg/dL is the threshold of concern.
2. MGT: D25 2cc/kg if below


## COMMON RESUSCITATION MANAGEMENT IN CHILDREN

### ETT Size

1. Endotracheal tube size = (AGE/4) + 4mm, or [(Age + 16)/4]
2. Endotracheal tube depth = 3x tube size

### Dose of Electricity

1. Cardioversion (0.5-1 J/kg)
2. Defibrillation (2-4 J/kg)

## Fluid Resuscitation and Maintenance
1. Isotonic Fluid Bolus: 20cc/kg
2. 4/2/1 Fluid Maintenance Formula:
    a. 4cc for each kg (up to first 10 kg)
    b. 2cc for each kg between 11kg and 20 kg
    c. 1cc for every kg above 20 kg

## Dextrose for Hypoglycemia:
1. 2cc/ kg of D25 for children
2. 5cc/kg D10 for infants

# PART 4: PEDIATRIC PHARMACOLOGY

## INTRODUCTION

There are a handful of useful medications to consider with your pediatric patients, in addition to oxygen and isotonic fluids. Unless you are with a pediatric transport team, these medications may get forgotten unless practiced more routinely.

## THE MEDICATIONS
### Epinephrine
1. Class: Vasopressor, Sympathomimetic, bronchodilator
2. Mechanism: Markedly stimulates both the alpha and beta receptors therefore, significant increases in heart rate, blood pressure, and cardiac output occur.
3. Indications: anaphylaxis; ventricular fibrillation; hypotension
4. Contraindications: Hypertension, tachycardia, acute coronary syndromes, hypersensitivity
5. Hemodynamics: (↑CVP/ ↑PCWP/↑CO/↑SVR).
6. Dose: PEA/Arrest: 0.01 mg/kg; Hypotension: 0.1- 1.0 mg/kg/min ; Bradycardia: 0.01mg/kg ( Anaphylaxis: 0.01 mg/kg IM in thigh (vastus lateralis).
7. Recall that epi is either in a 1 mg/ 1mL (1:1000), or 1mg/ 10mL (1:10,000).
8. Hemodynamics: (↑CVP/ ↑PCWP/↑CO/↑SVR).

### Atropine
1. Class: Anticholinergic
2. Mechanism: Blocks the parasympathetic receptors (slow system) speeding up the heart
3. Indications: pediatric intubation, bradycardia, organophosphate poisoning
4. Contraindications: hypersensitivity
5. Hemodynamics: (~CVP/ ~PCWP/↑CO/~SVR).
6. Dose: Peds: 0.02 mg/kg IV push, minimum of 0.1 mg

## Dopamine

1. Class: Vasopressor, Sympathomimetic
2. Mechanism: stimulates the beta and alpha receptors resulting in increased contractility and myocardial workload, as well as peripheral vasoconstriction.
3. Indications: hypotension, low cardiac output, poor perfusion
4. Contraindications: Uncontrolled tachycardia, ventricular irritability, hypertension
5. Hemodynamics: (~ CVP/ ~PCWP/↑CO/↑SVR); dopamine additionally will slightly increase pulmonary vascular resistance.
6. Dose:
   a. Renal Dose: 2-5 mg/kg/min
   b. Beta Dose: 5-10 mg/kg/min
   c. Alpha Dose: 10-20 mg/kg/min
7. With the renal dosing, you'll have reduced cardiac output, but as you get into the beta (increase heart rate in contractility) and the alpha (vasoconstriction) doses, cardiac output increases.
8. Remember to always FILL THE TANK before adding a pressor. The pressor does no good if you have not adequately fluid resuscitated your patients.

## Dobutamine

1. Class: Positive Inotrope, Sympathomimetic
2. Mechanism: highly stimulates the beta 1 receptor, but also reduces afterload. But increasing contractility and decreasing SVR it makes for a fantastic medication for heart failure patients.
3. Indications: Congestive heart failure, poor cardiac output
4. Contraindications: acute coronary syndrome, tachycardia, hypertension, hypersensitivity
5. Hemodynamics: (~ CVP/ ~PCWP/↑CO/↓SVR); Note that Dobutamine reduces SVR and Dopamine increases SVR.
6. Dose: 2-20 mg/kg/min

## Diphenhydramine

1. Class: Histamine 2 (H2) blocker
2. Mechanism: competes for histamine 2 receptor sites, when these sites are blocked, the effect of histamine is reduced
3. Indications: allergic/ anaphylactic reactions
4. Contraindications: hypersensitivity
5. Hemodynamics: (~ CVP/ ~PCWP/~CO/~SVR).
6. Dose:1mg/kg IV/IO/IM

## Ranitidine

1. Class: Histamine 1 (H1) blocker
2. Mechanism: competes for histamine 1 receptor sites, when these sites are blocked, the effect of histamine is reduced
3. Indications: allergic/ anaphylactic reactions; gastric acid reducer
4. Contraindications: hypersensitivity
5. Hemodynamics: (~ CVP/ ~PCWP/~CO/~SVR).
6. Dose:1mg/kg IV/IO/IM up to 50 mg over 5 minutes

## Methylprednisolone

1. Class/ mechanism: steroid, anti– inflammatory
2. Indications: allergic/ anaphylactic reactions
3. Contraindications: hypersensitivity
4. Hemodynamics: (~ CVP/ ~PCWP/~CO/~SVR).
5. Dose: 2mg/kg IV/IO up to a max dose of 125 mg.

## Naloxone:

1. Class: Narcotic Antagonist
2. Mechanism: Competitively binds with narcotic receptors. Basically, with a narcotic in the patient's system, this medication forces out the narcotic and temporarily removes the effects of the narcotics. Narcan doesn't last long, so the narcotic effect may return as the Narcan wears off.
3. Indications: Narcotics overdose, overdose unknown cause, coma or altered LOC due to unknown cause .
4. Hemodynamics: (~CVP/ ~PCWP/~CO/~SVR).
5. Peds Dose: 0.1 mg/kg IV, IO, or atomizer.

## Adenosine

1. Class: Antidysrhythmic Class IV-Like
2. Mechanism: Blocks potassium channels which slows conduction (slows HR) and stops reentry pathways (resets SVT).
3. Indications: SVT
4. Contraindications: High degree AV block, sick sinus syndrome
5. Hemodynamics: (~CVP/ ~PCWP/~CO/~SVR).
6. Dose: 0.1 mg/kg rapid IV push with a flush; second and third doses– 0.2 mg/kg rapid IV push with a  flush.

## Dextrose (D10 or D25)

1. Class: Carbohydrate
2. Mechanism: Directly increases blood sugar.
3. Indications: Hypoglycemia
4. Contraindications: Do not infuse into a vein that could extravasate as extravasation causes tissue necrosis.
5. Hemodynamics: (~CVP/ ~PCWP/~CO/~SVR).
6. Adolescent Dose (older, bigger kids): 10-25 g (ie, 20-50 mL 50% solution or 40-100 mL of 25%.
7. Infants (> 6 months) and Children's Dose:  0.5-1 g/kg up to 25 g (2-4 mL/kg/dose of 25% solution) IV; not to exceed 25 g/dose
8. Infants less than 6 months: 0.25-0.5 g/kg/dose (1-2 mL/kg/dose of 25% solution) IV; not to exceed 25 g/dose

# PART 5: PEDIATRIC MANAGEMENT QUESTIONS

1. A three-month-old 7 kg infant has been vomiting and having watery diarrhea for two days. The child's lips and oral mucosa are dry, and his fontanel is sunken. His extremities are cool to the touch, and it's capillary refill is 5 seconds. Which the following the most appropriate management for this patient?
   a. 140 cc/kg NS
   b. 70 cc/kg NS
   c. 200 cc/kg LR
   d. 100 cc/kg LR

2. You are responding to a small hospital for a pediatric patient with sepsis. Which of the following signs and symptoms would indicate to you that the patient is in early septic shock?
   a. Bounding pulses, tachycardia, and a GCS 15
   b. HR 129, bound impulses, slow capillary refill
   c. Warm flushed skin, tachycardia, and irritability
   d. Slow capillary refill, cool skin, heart rate of 62

3. A 4 y/o has been involved in a rollover MVC. You have decided to intubate this patient to protect their airway. Which of the following formulas would you use to calculate the endotracheal tube size?
   a. (Age + 4)/16
   b. (Age x 2) + 8
   c. 4 + (4/Age)
   d. (Age/4) + 4

4. Your flight dispatch has sent you to a small hospital where a 24 months old child is having respiratory difficulty and is presenting with inspiratory retractions and stridor. Before going to bed last night, his mother reports that the child had a runny nose, a loud cough, and fever. Which of the following conditions is the child most likely suffering from?
   a. Bronchiolitis
   b. Epiglottitis
   c. (+) Croup
   d. (+) FBAO

5. This is a sign of meningitis and is considered positive when the leg is fully bent at the hip, and there exists an inability to straighten out the leg:
   a. SIDS sign
   b. Brudzinski sign
   c. Kernig sign
   d. Concussion sign

6. A 12-month-old child is being administered dopamine. The 15-pound child is receiving a low alpha dose from a pediatric concentration of dopamine (800mg/ 250cc). Which of the following flow rates is reflective of this dosage and concentration?
   a. cc/hr
   b. 0.26 cc/hr
   c. 12 cc/hr
   d. 21 cc/hr

7. You are explaining a condition to one of your new hires. You describe a condition that is characterized by the underdevelopment of the heart usually resulting in an absent or nonfunctional left ventricle and poorly formed ascending aorta:
   a. Pulmonary valve atresia
   b. Hypoplastic left heart
   c. Ventricular septal defect
   d. Mitral valve stenosis

8. You are transporting a four-month-old infant. This patient is experiencing a narrowing of the descending portion of the aorta resulting in a limited flow of blood to the lower part of the body. Which of the following conditions does this describe?
   a. Tetralogy of Fallot
   b. Coarctation of the aorta
   c. Severe aortic stenosis
   d. Patent ductus arteriosus

9. Your pediatric patient presents with a cough, low-grade fever, and Steeple 's sign. Which of the following conditions is your patient suffering?
   a. (+) Croup
   b. Epiglottitis
   c. (+) FBAO
   d. Pneumonia

10. Dorsiflexion of the large toe and fanning of other toes with plantar stimulation is known as what?
    a. Brudzinski sign
    b. Babinski reflex
    c. Stepping reflex
    d. Moro reflex

11. When a hole is present in the center of the heart between the lower chambers of the heart. This condition is called:
    a. Atrial septal defect
    b. Atrioventricular canal defect
    c. Acute tubular necrosis
    d. Ventricular septal defect

12. Your pediatric patient presents with hypoglycemia and is a 6 kg infant. You are currently mixing a 30 cc syringe of dextrose 10%. How would you arrive at the D10 concentration?
    a. Take 3 cc from D50 and mix with 27 cc NS
    b. Mix 6 grams of dextrose in 24 cc of 0.9 NS
    c. Take 6 cc from D50 and mix with 24 cc NS
    d. Mix 3 grams of dextrose in 27 cc of 0.9 NS

# PART 5: PEDIATRIC MANAGEMENT RATIONALES

1. **(A)** This patient should be treated with an infusion of 20 cc's per kilo of isotonic crystalloid and a blood glucose determination. The history of prolonged vomiting and diarrhea suggest hypovolemia. Therefore, this child must be treated with aggressive fluid resuscitation and reassessment.

2. **(C)** Tachycardia with bounding pulses; warm, flushed skin, delayed capillary refill, inherent ability are all likely findings in the pediatric patient with early septic shock. The cool phase of septic shock occurs when cardiac output drops (measurable by cardiac output itself, or a lowering trend in the blood pressure ) and the skin becomes cool to the touch.

3. **(D)** When determining the size of an endotracheal tube in a pediatric patient, there are a few different formulas. We offer these two formulas to calculate and a tracheal to a size: (AGE/4) + 4mm, or (Age + 16)/4. Therefore, in this case, the answer is (AGE/4) + 4mm.

4. **(C)** This child has croup. Foreign body airway obstruction is suspected of situations where a previously healthy, afebrile child rapidly develops signs and symptoms of respiratory distress. Epiglottitis is characterized by a rapid onset, high fever, and drooling. Bronchiolitis usually occurs in children under one year old that presents with wheezing. Therefore, the answer to this question is croup.

5. **(C)** Kernig's sign is observed in meningitis patients and is characterized by the inability to completely straighten out a leg when sitting or lying down. Brudzinski sign is also seen in meningitis; however, It is characterized by the flexion of the neck that usually causes flexion of the hip and knees.

6. **(A)** There is only one flow rate provided that would be dosing the patient within the alpha range. [(1.5 cc/hr)(800mg x 1000mcg/mg)]/ (250cc)/( 60cc/hr)/ (wt in Kg, or 6.8) = 12 mcg/kg/min. Be sure to practice your drug calculations for these exams.

7. **(B)** In hypoplastic left heart syndrome, as well as the failure of the mitral valve and the aortic valves to form. patients rely on an open PDA and VSDs to deliver some oxygenated blood to the systemic circulation. KEEP THE PDA OPEN.

8. **(B)** The narrowing of the aorta is a condition called coarctation of the aorta and is the correct answer. Tetralogy of Fallot is a is a series of four different conditions including VSD, pulmonary stenosis, a truncated (high riding) aorta, and right ventricular hypertrophy, however, is the wrong answer. A patent ductus arteriosus is a residual hole between the aorta and the pulmonary artery, and is also the incorrect answer. Severe aortic stenosis is a narrowing of the aortic valve and is also the incorrect answer.

9. **(A)** Croup is a viral infection of the upper airway that can affect the larynx, trachea, and bronchi; known for its 'barking cough'. It presents with low-grade fever; 'barking cough'; mild distress; stridor; and STEEPLE SIGN on X-ray.

10. **(B)** The Babinski reflex is obtained by stimulating the outside of the sole of the foot, causing extension of the big toe while fanning the other toes. The examiner begins the stimulation at the heel and goes forward to the base of the toes. Most newborn babies and young infants are not neurologically mature, and they, therefore, show a Babinski reflex. A Babinski reflex in an older child or an adult is abnormal and is a sign of a problem in the brain or spinal cord.

11. **(D)** A ventricular septal defect (VSD) is a hole or a defect in the septum that divides the 2 lower chambers of the heart, resulting in communication between the ventricular cavities. A VSD may occur as a primary anomaly, with or without additional major associated cardiac defects.

12. **(A)** Remember a "percent" solution means to mix that percentage of the drug with the reciprocal percentage of normal saline. In this case, we need 3g of dextrose in a 3cc syringe because three is 10% of 30. Dextrose 50 is mixed 25g in a 50 cc ampule (25 is half of 50 or 50%). This means that every cc of D50 contains 0.5g of dextrose to get 3g, we need to remove 6cc from the D50 ampule and mix it with 24cc of normal saline. That gives us 3g in 30cc or D10.

# CHAPTER 13: AIR MEDICAL FUNDAMENTALS

## PART 1: ACCREDITING AND REGULATNIG AGENCIES

### INTRODUCTION

The air medical transport realm is governed by federal agencies, non-profit accrediting agencies, independent certification agencies, as well as state and local governments. In this section we will discuss some of the most influential accrediting and regulating agencies.

### GOVERNANCE

#### Commission on Air Medical Transport Services (CAMTS)

1. CAMTS is a non-profit organization dedicated to improving the quality and safety of medical transport services, with 20 current member organizations- each of which sends one representative to the CAMTS Board of Directors.
2. The Commission offers a program of voluntary evaluation of compliance with accreditation standards demonstrating the ability to deliver service of a specific quality.
3. The Commission believes that "the two highest priorities of an air medical or ground inter-facility transport service are patient care and safety of the transport environment." (The preceding was transcribed directly from the CAMTS website.)
4. Ultimately, CAMTS is the accrediting body of the air and ground medical transport community. Air medical companies DO NOT have to become CAMTS accredited, but it shows a dedication to safety and patient care.
5. They produce the Accreditation Standards of the Commission on Accreditation of Medical Transport System. At the time this book was first published (January 2016), this document, a very important document that will help you understand the air medical environment, was in its 10th Edition.
6. This document is a list of standards, or rules to follow, that if followed will grant the participating air medical service the distinction of CAMTS accreditation.
7. The process involves the air medical service applying for accreditation, preparing for CAMTS to arrive and conduct their survey of the air medical service, and then CAMTS bases their decision on how well the standards (or rules) were followed. It is quite expensive for a flight program to become accredited, therefore the CAMTS visits are rarely taken lightly and services will prepare for months to get prepare for their official site survey.

#### Federal Aviation Regulations (FARs)

1. The FARs are a set of federal rules for pilots and companies/ agencies who operate aircraft within the United States.
2. The FARs are broken up into Parts, much like this text. There are 2 very important parts to differentiate: Part 91 and Part 135.
3. Part 91
   a. This portion of the FARs includes the regulations that define the operation of non-commercial aircraft within the US .

b. When you take off from your base, from a hospital, or from the scene WITHOUT a patient, then the pilot must follow the rules in Part 91.

4. Part 135
   a. This portion of the FARs includes the regulations that define the operation of commuter aircraft in the US.
   b. When you take off from your base, from a hospital, or from the scene and a PATIENT IS ON BOARD, then your aircraft is no longer "private" and is now considered commercial. Therefore, the pilot must follow the rules in Part 135 of the FARs.

5. CAMTS and the FARs (Part 91 and Part 135) provide a foundation of best practices– some by suggestion and some by law.

6. You will find their references throughout this chapter. It is important that you download a current copy of the CAMTS Accreditation Standards and add it to your study materials (www.camts.org). This text will mention more important concepts and standards from this document, but there are many more that will not be mentioned. You may need to look up the FARs (www.ecfr.gov) as well from time to time.

# PART 2: AIR MEDICAL BASICS

## INTRODUCTION

Critical care transport can occur in one of three different types of vehicles: a helicopter, an airplane, and an ambulance. Helicopters are also known as rotor-wing aircraft, airplanes are also known as fixed wing aircraft, and typically the ground versions are outfitted with critical care equipment and supplies.

## THE BASICS

### Flight Rules
1. These rules govern whether an aircraft can fly without the aid of instruments, or if they must, proceed with instrument- guided flight. Typically, these rules are dependent upon weather.
2. Visual Flight Rules: used when there is good visibility and high clouds.
3. Instrument Flight Rules: utilized when adverse and poor weather conditions exist (poor visibility and low cloud cover). Both a pilot and the aircraft have to be 'instrument rated' to be able to deliberately fly into bad weather.

### Weather Minimums
1. Flight minimums are in place to provide guidance on when flights can be accepted and when they should be declined.
2. These minimums are based on 4 major categories: terrain (mountainous vs. non–mountainous), light conditions (day vs. night), safety equipment (night vision goggles or without night vision goggles) and flight distance (local area vs. cross country).
3. The above values in the graphic are representative of ceiling altitude and visibility. For example, 800' and 2 mi represents 800-foot cloud cover and 2 miles of visibility.
4. While this can be confusing, I have color coded some common ceiling and visibility combinations. I wish there was a really easy way to study this, but it just takes lots of memorization.

| Condition | Non-mountainous | | Mountainous | |
|---|---|---|---|---|
| | Local | Cross-country | Local | Cross-country |
| **Day** | 800' and 2 mi | 800' and 3 mi | 800' and 3 mi | 1000' and 3 mi |
| **Night (NVG)** | 800' and 3 mi | 1000' and 3 mi | 1000' and 3 mi | 1000' and 5 mi |
| **Night (w/o NVG)** | 1000' and 3 mi | 1000' and 5 mi | 1500' and 3 mi | 1500' and 5 mi |

## *Conduct Preflight Check: Aircraft (The walk-around)*

1. When: Beginning of shift and prior to each flight
2. How:
   a. Look at ground and search for debris around aircraft. It is important to remove this debris from where you will be taking off. Failure to execute this can result in a piece of debris being pulled into the engines or rotors. This can result in fire or mechanical damage to the aircraft, in addition to potentially injuring the crew.
   b. Cords, covers, and cowlings: before taking off, also remember to remove the plugged-in cords from the aircraft, remove any covers, and ensure all cowlings are secured.
   c. Cowlings are the exterior paneling of the aircraft and mechanics remove them to get to all the various internal components of the aircraft. Sometimes, they will loosen. It is important to always ensure they are completely attached so they do not come undone in–flight.
   d. Eye contact with the pilot: When the rotors are turning, it is near impossible to verbally communicate. Communication can be accomplished by maintaining eye contact with the pilot and follow any hand motions or directions they provide.

## *Conduct Preflight Check: Equipment*

1. When: Beginning of shift and prior to each flight
2. How:
   a. Ensure that equipment is secured tightly.
   b. In the event of a crash, unsecured equipment will become missiles and injure you.
   c. It is obvious that we should prepare our equipment before flight so that it is "mission ready".

## *Main Types of Air Medical Transport*

1. Rotor-wing (helicopter)
   a. This is the most common air medical transport vehicle.
   b. Depending on the aircraft, it can cover ground up to about 60 miles and back without refueling; however, this is specific to the particular aircraft.
   c. **Advantages**: increased ability to maneuver and vertical takeoff and landing capabilities.
   d. **Disadvantages**:

      i.   most rotor-wing are not modified for instrument flight rules (IFR) (although some are) therefore most must fly under visual flight rules (VFR).

      ii.   Additionally, they are expensive to maintain and operate, have limited space in the interior patient and crew cabin, and sometimes are not able to complete a patient flight based on the weight of the patient.

2. Fixed wing (airplane)
   a. The aircraft are used typically for flights greater than 300 miles.
   b. **Advantages**: generally, it is safer than rotor-wing, can travel farther distances and is faster, can carry multiple patients, little to no weight limitations, and most have the capability of IFR flight.
   c. **Disadvantages**: just like rotor-wing aircraft there is a high operational cost, a hangar is typically required to maintain the aircraft, and a runway is required.

## *Flight Following*

1. Generally speaking, this is the tracking of the aircraft from liftoff to destination by either the EMS or aircraft communication center, or with an FAA air traffic control center.
2. In times where VFR conditions are present, a pilot must utilize the help of the ATC to maintain flight following, or the pilot can flight follow with their dispatch or communication center.
   a. Helicopter (rotor-wing): a VFR helicopter not flight following with ATC, must contact their communications center every 15 minutes.
   b. Airplane (fixed wing): a VFR airplane not flight following with ATC, must contact their communications center every 30 minutes.
   c. When transporting a patient by ground, communication lapse should not exceed 45 minutes.

## *Chain of Errors*

1. This is one of the most dangerous forms of aviation with a higher accident rate compared to other divisions of aviation.
2. Rarely do crashes occur because of a single error. Typically crashes occur from a series of mistakes that result in an event that causes a crash.
3. Crashes can be prevented by being proactive in identifying and preventing a link in the chain of error.

# PART 3: AIR MEDICAL SAFETY

## INTRODUCTION

Please understand this can be a very dangerous profession. As you are either continuing your career or embarking on a new one, this field not only offers the satisfaction of saving lives, but also dangers that must be recognized and anticipated. By being proactive in anticipating these dangers, they can safely be mitigated. This should be the daily goal as a medical flight crew member.

This is truly one of the coolest jobs in the world. It is like being Batman. Someone needs (medical) help, so they send out a distress call. You grab your helmet and gear and fly to go rescue that person. The internal satisfaction alone is immeasurable. This intense and rewarding job doesn't come without cost, however. Make no mistake, this job can kill you.

By the becoming intimately aware of your surroundings while in the air medical environment, identifying major and minor hazards, paying attention during the critical phases of flight, and by practicing good solid communication between the pilot in your partner, you will be able to overcome the perils of the air medical environment. Now let's talk some specifics.

## ELEMENTS OF SAFETY

### Assess for Safety of the Scene
1. Safety depends on not just noticing risk factors but looking for them.
2. Approaching the scene
   a. Hazards: Tall objects/loose objects/people/wires/barriers. Tall hazards (even shorter ones like fences) pose a threat to an aircraft that is on final approach for landing. Unleveled ground puts rescuers on the uphill side very close to the rotors.
   b. Landing zone
      i. (OLD WAY) Helicopter: day (minimum 60 ft x 60 ft) vs. night (minimum 100ft x 100ft).
      ii. **(NEW WAY- ~ 2015 and beyond) MOST programs now require 100ft x 100ft no matter what time of the day.**
      iii. Also, have the ground crew avoid shining lights in the pilot's eyes.
      iv. Constant direct communication between the pilot and ground crew is an optimal practice. This provides a direct communication in case the ground crew sees a hazard that the pilot fails to see.
3. Safe access to your patient- once you arrive safely on the ground, you need to achieve safe passage to your patient.
   a. Terrain— the path to and from your patient's location may occasionally take you over non— paved terrain. Snow, mud, rocky terrain, etc. can pose a fall threat. Listening to the EMS and fire crews is a smart idea as they are trained at how to keep you safe.
   b. Physical obstacles— if it is not the terrain then physical obstacles can either prevent you from reaching your patient or can prevent you from getting the patient back to the aircraft. Again, listen to rescue EMS and FD crews on scene as they can assist you access your patient.
   c. Animals-this may not come into play often, but you may be exposed to angry dogs, or wild animals such as snakes. Always keep yourself and your partner safe. Safely leave the aircraft. Be sure to keep "eyes out" of the aircraft as you are taking off to help the pilot look for hazards.
   d. Adequately instruct assistants (protect them from hazards). It is important to communicate short and simple directions to on scene rescue EMS and FD crews.
   e. Ensure no: loose clothing/hats/loose sheets/holding IV poles high (on crews or patients). Just like when you are leaving the aircraft, when you are approaching a running aircraft, avoid loose items and high objects.

### In-flight Hazards
1. The aviation environment, especially during flight, it is important we keep our eyes outside the aircraft periodically
2. We are looking for:
   a. Other aircraft

b. Tall antennae

c. Hazards (other aircraft, tall objects)

3. When alerting the pilot of a hazard, use this procedure:

   a. Location (clock method)

   b. Hazard

   c. Heading (tell pilot where to turn)

## Sterile Cockpit

1. This is the concept that everyone is quiet and looking outside the aircraft during critical phases of flight (Part 135.100).

2. This is to ensure:

   a. The pilot is free of distraction

   b. The radio channels are kept open the case ground crew needs to notify pilot of a hazard

   c. So, the pilot can hear the engines

3. **Critical phases of flight**: 1) taxi  2) take-off and 3) landing

4. The sterile cockpit rule doesn't indicate complete silence during takeoff, taxi and landing, but rather it stands as a cultural concept that once in those phases your eyes should be looking for hazards, obstacles, or anything else that could kill you.

5. The most dangerous intervals of flight are during taxi, takeoff and landing. Therefore, be diligent and cultivate a strong mental fortitude during these phases to ensure your safety.

## Safety Around the Aircraft

1. Approach the aircraft from the 12 o'clock position primarily, with alternatives of the 3 and 9 o'clock positions.

2. **NEVER** approach the aircraft from the rear (the 6 o'clock position) because of the tail rotor. People see and hear the main rotor and can forget about the tail rotor and walk right into it (especially during night operations).

3. When approaching or departing the aircraft, every few moments, look at the pilot's eyes.

4. You cannot hear any voice communication when outside the aircraft and rotors turning, therefore we need to look at the pilots frequently for nonverbal communication.

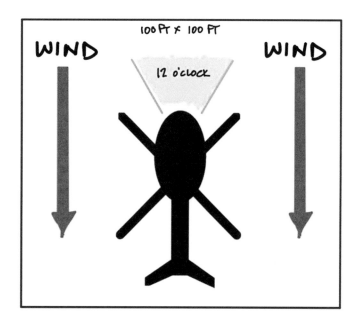

327

5. In addition to routinely looking at the pilot, it is our job to ensure that no people, debris, or objects get near the aircraft

6. Perimeter captains are individuals previously trained in establishing a landing zone who help the flight crew to keep people, debris, and objects from nearing the aircraft

### Safety Equipment In-flight

1. Seat belts: If a need arises to unbuckle, alert pilot, finish action, and re-buckle.
2. Internal helicopter communications: Always remain "plugged in" to mic
3. Make sure equipment is secured during flight
4. Scan airspace:
    a. Communicate using clock technique
    b. Communicate using high or low relative to the horizon

### Secure the Patient for Flight

1. The patient should always be strapped into the seat belt system.
2. The litter system should always be locked into place.
3. Anytime the seat belts are loosened or adjusted temporarily for patient comfort, re-secure them right away.

### Secure All Personnel and Equipment

1. Specialty teams: These may require special sleds and isolettes.
2. Families: Provide safety briefing, seat belts, communications, and hearing protection.
3. Law enforcement: Weapons may be carried by "officials or employees of a municipality or a State, or of the United States, who are authorized to carry arms" (Part 135.119).
4. VIP/ Observer: Provide safety briefing, seat belts, communications, and hearing protection

### Participating in Crew Resource Management (CRM)

1. CRM is a set of training procedures and culture used in industries where human error can have devastating effects
2. Each crewmember has a responsibility to employ and maintain the highest level of safety
3. This essentially says no matter what rank you hold in the group; you always can speak up relative to a safety concern
4. There is a specific arm of CRM that is specific to air medical transport: AMRM (air medical resource management).

### Safety Decisions for Flight

1. According to CRM, we have a responsibility to look out for the safety of ourselves and our crew
2. When it comes to us, we do not have to take any flight where we feel uncomfortable
3. Industry rule: 3 to GO, 1 to say NO.
4. Reasons to abort a flight:
    a. Bad weather– weather that puts the pilot's ability to control the aircraft in jeopardy warrants turning down a flight.
    b. Dangerous landing zone (LZ)- any landing zone that has high hazards (towers, flagpoles, telephone poles, etc), fences, un– flat ground (greater than a 10-degree grade) or loose debris warrants an abort from landing. Usually an alternative landing zone is usually identified and utilized.
    c. Real or perceived aircraft mechanical issues– anytime you feel scared, anxious, concerned, worried, or unsafe in any other vernacular, concerning a perceived issue with the aircraft mechanics at all, PLEASE SPEAK UP.

# PART 4: AIR MEDICAL SURVIVAL

## INTRODUCTION

Here you will find a several topics to ensure survival in the event of in-flight and/or post-accident situations. These are best practices and could save your life.

## SURVIVAL TOPICS AND SITUATIONS

### *Respond to In-Flight Emergencies*

1. Fire
   a. Notify pilot
   b. Utilize fire extinguisher
   c. Unplug electrical devices
2. Emergent landing
   a. Confirm emergency in the aircraft/ assist pilot.
   b. Relay info to dispatch (coordinates and description)
   c. International mayday (HELP) frequency is 121.5MHz on a VHF radio.
   d. Disable power
   e. Shut off oxygen
   f. Prepare patient and crew
   g. Crash Position: place your arms in an "X" over your chest and grasp your shoulder straps. Then keep your knees together and your feet slightly apart.
   h. The Emergency Locator Transmitter (ELT) is activated at an impact of 4G and sends out a signal the rescuers can use to identify your location.
3. Inadvertent Inclement Meteorological Conditions (IIMC)
   a. Recall that there are visual flight rules (VFR) and instrument flight rules (IFR). When a pilot experiences a change in metrological conditions mid-flight, they go from VFR to IFR, and must communicate with air traffic control.
   b. If the pilot is IFR rated, then they simply radio air traffic control and have them file an IFR flight plan with the FAA. Air traffic control will do that routinely.
   c. If a VFR pilot enters IIMC, then it can be deadly. The best action is to assist the pilot.
   d. Understand that the pilot will be very task saturated. Absolute sterile cockpit is needed.
   e. If you are to ask questions, make them brief and to the point.
   f. Alert him of any danger.
   g. Ask if there is anything you can do to help him or her out. Sometimes begin able to help them look up an 'approach plate' in the Airway manual can help tremendously.
   h. An **Airway manual** is not a medical airway manual, but rather a collection of pages that have airport specific information that can help the pilot plan a course of action once a VFR aircraft flies into IIMC.
   i. An APPRAOACH PLATE is a page in the Airway manual with different pieces of aviation information. Learn to use them and work with your pilot to be able to find and reference pieces of information out of it.

### Emergency Egress

1. Shutdown in this order: Throttle, fuel, batteries (T,F,B)
2. This reduces the chance of fire
3. Self-extrication
   a. Ensure all moving parts have stopped
   b. Identify a reference point within the aircraft
4. Meet at 12 o'clock (or 3 or 9 o'clock if 12 is not available)
5. Once primary threats are gone (fire/ explosion), return to assist with others.

### Immediate Post Accident Duties

1. Meet with survivors at designated location (12 o'clock)
2. Return to aircraft ONLY AFTER fires/ explosion threat are ruled out.
3. Assess crewmember condition and treat
4. Locate and activate ELT (emergency location transmitter)
5. Remain with the aircraft

### Shelter Building and Equipment

1. Where: Near wreckage
2. When: Right after treating crash victims
3. Materials:
   a. Fuselage, wings and stabilizers, cowlings, the doors
   b. All can be used to construct parts of shelters
4. Methods:
   a. Dig hole and use above materials as a roof
   b. Use branches/ foliage as materials with aircraft parts as a lean-to shelter
5. Where to sleep:
   a. Sleeping on aircraft fuselage can conduct your temperature to the outside environment
   b. Heat is lost this way
   c. Instead, sleep on upholstered material from the wreckage, or gather leaves and foliage to conserve heat
6. Signal fires: burn tires, fuel, transmission oil to create dark smoke used for signaling
7. Signal panels: stabilizers, doors, cowlings, batteries and lights can all be used to redirect light towards any aircraft for signaling
8. Collect water
   a. Use cowlings, plastic bags, medical packs, IV bags to collect water
   b. Usually not a factor unless rescue takes longer than 24 hours

### Initiating Survival Procedures

1. Rule of 3's: You could die within
   a. 3 hours w/o shelter
   b. 3 days w/o water
   c. 3 weeks without food
2. Survival priorities:
   a. Shelter/ fire (for heat/boil water)/ food
   b. Water does not become a factor unless the rescue takes longer than 24 hours
   c. Activate the ELT

d. Know the contents of your survival kit

e. Use IV hydration if needed

3. Fire

a. Establishes warmth and security

b. Light at night

c. Dries wet clothing

d. Build fire near wreckage but not too close to shelter

e. Consider wind direction

4. Water

a. Can drink IV hydration, also- electrolytes and glucose

b. Acquire any condensation in the morning on leaves or collect melted snow

# PART 5: AIR MEDICAL FUNDAMENTALS QUESTIONS

1. As you prepare for your day, you approach the aircraft and notice the following items. Which of these items pose a bigger danger?
   a. Rotor tie downs securely fastened to the aircraft
   b. Electrical wires rolled up neatly near socket
   c. An empty cardboard box 50 feet from aircraft
   d. Cowlings with all fasteners in locked position

2. Upon approaching the aircraft on a scene to load the patient into the aircraft with the help of assistants, which of the following should cause you to stop and correct the error?
   a. The assistant with his hat tucked inside his shirt
   b. The sheriff's deputy in his squad car and door closed
   c. The EMT with the IV bag in hand way over his shoulder
   d. Your partner who has his helmet on their head

3. Upon exiting the aircraft following a crash, which of the following would be the appropriate procedure to reduce to the chance of fire?
   a. 100 ft from the nose of the aircraft
   b. 75 ft from the right-side aircraft door
   c. 125 ft from the aircraft tail rotor
   d. 150 ft from the left side aircraft door

4. You are on a scene flight and are returning to the aircraft with fire department assistants. The aircraft is running. Which of the following actions should you take as you approach a running helicopter?
    a. Maintain the IV drips on the stretcher's IV pole
    b. Keep eye contact with the pilot as you approach
    c. Proceed to the helicopter ahead of the assistants
    d. Maintain sterile cockpit standards as you approach

5. Which of the following situations would it be reasonable to abort a flight?
    a. Crew member needing to get off on time to meet family
    b. Pilot who has 5 hours of duty time and a 1-hour flight
    c. Nighttime NVG flight with 2000ft/ 5 miles over mountains
    d. Your partner who just doesn't feel good about the flight

6. Which of the following meets minimum weather standards as per CAMTS?
    a. 800ft and 2 miles, daytime, cross country, over mountains
    b. 1000ft and 3 miles cross country over mountains at night without NVGs
    c. 1500ft and 2 miles, night, locally, over mountains, without NVGs
    d. 800ft and 3 miles locally non-mountainous at night with NVGs

7. Upon exiting the aircraft following a crash, what is the correct shutdown procedure just prior egress?
    a. Throttle, Survival Kit, Batteries
    b. Survival Kit, Throttle, Fuel
    c. Throttle, Fuel, Batteries
    d. Batteries, Throttle, Fuel

8. What are the survival priorities in order of importance?
    a. Fire, Food, Shelter
    b. Shelter, Fire, Signaling
    c. Shelter, Fire, Food
    d. Signaling, Fire, Food

# PART 6: AIR MEDICAL FUNDAMENTALS RATIONALES

1. **(C)** Prior to your shift and prior to each flight, you should do a walk around to include looking for loose debris (like this empty cardboard box near the aircraft) as well as cords, cowlings, covers to all be in their appropriate positions and locations. Cowlings should be in there locked down position. It is OK to roll up wires near a socket placed there based on FAA regulations. Rotor ties securely fastened to the aircraft is appropriate from time to time, but obviously you would need to remove these before flight.

2.  **(C)** To keep the scene safe , you will have to keep others safe who do not have the training you have.  That includes keeping the untrained from making mistakes including loose clothing, hats, lose sheets, and holding IV poles high around the aircraft while it is running.  Here the biggest concern is the EMT with the IV bag over his shoulder.

3.  **(A)** The first location to meet up after a crash is at the 12 o'clock position. As an alternative, you could meet up at the 3 and 9 o'clock positions. The 6 o'clock position is relatively unsafe as the tail rotor could still be rotating and causing a danger.

4.  **(B)** You always need to keep eye contact with the pilot while walking to the aircraft with others. Keep eye contact with the assistants as well to prevent them from doing something that could cause harm to the crew or assistants.

5.  **(D)** For any reason, real or perceived, a crew member can turn down a flight. A crew member needing to get off on time has nothing to do with safety. A 1-hour flight and 5 hours of duty time (or the remaining time the FAA says they can fly) also doesn't have anything to do with safety. The CAMTS weather minimums are safe and acceptable for a flight. The only one that is safety related is the "perceived" danger the crewmember feels. It is legitimate to decline a flight based on actual or perceived mechanical issues.

6.  **(D)** The only one that is under weather minimums is 800 ft and 3 miles locally non-mountainous at night with NVGs. It is important to know these weather minimums- you will get 1-2 questions on your exam concerning these minimums.

7.  **(C)** The correct procedure is throttle, fuel, and batteries to best reduce the chance of fire.

8.  **(C)** The correct order of post-crash priorities is shelter, fire, and then food. Water becomes an issue if the rescue takes longer than 24 hours.

# CHAPTER 14: FLIGHT PHYSIOLOGY

## PART 1: HYPOXIA

### INTRODUCTION

Hypoxia is just one of the physiological problems that can impair flight crewmembers and pilots if they are not aware of the effects of decreased oxygen pressure at altitude. Hypoxia, by definition, is the lack of enough oxygen in the blood, tissues, and/or cells to maintain normal physiological function. Breathing air at reduced barometric pressure, malfunctioning oxygen equipment at altitude, drowning, pneumonia, extremes of environmental temperatures, and carbon monoxide are just a few of the causes of oxygen deficiency in the body that results in hypoxia. The most common causes of hypoxia in aviation are flying, non-pressurized aircraft above 10,000 ft without supplemental oxygen, rapid decompression during flight, pressurization system malfunction, or oxygen system malfunction. In this chapter we will discuss 1) how our patients experience hypoxia and 2) how we experience hypoxia.

### DEFINITIONS AND BACKGROUND
1.  HYPOXIA: Lack of oxygen at the TISSUES.
2.  HYPOXEMIA: Lack of oxygen bound to hemoglobin in the BLOOD.
3.  There are 4 major locations where oxygen delivery can be derailed:
    a.  Anywhere between the ambient environment to the alveolar capillary membrane
    b.  Onto the RBC
    c.  Around the circulatory system
    d.  Across the capillary into a cell

### CAUSES OF HYPOXIA

#### Hypoxic Hypoxia
1.  Caused by higher altitudes
2.  Insufficient ventilation

#### Hypemic Hypoxia
1.  Caused by oxygen not attaching to a red blood cell
2.  Low RBCs (anemia)
3.  Low Hemoglobin (anemia)
4.  Poisoned RBCs (CO Poisoning)

#### Stagnant Hypoxia
1.  Caused by poor blood flow
2.  Heart failure
3.  Pooling of blood from sitting for a long time
4.  Pooling of blood from accelerated maneuvers

#### Histotoxic Hypoxia
1.  Caused by an inability of the cell to take in or use the delivered oxygen
2.  CO poisoning (yes it affects RBCs and tissues)
3.  Arsenic
4.  Cyanide

## THE 4 STAGES OF HYPOXIA

The stages represent the progression of the hypoxic signs and symptoms as they affect us.

### Indifferent Stage
1. 0-10K feet
2. Night vision reduced by 28%
3. HR and RR increase just a small, undetectable amount

### Compensatory Stage
1. 10-15K feet
2. Night vision reduced by 50%
3. Significant increases in HR and RR

### Disturbance Stage
1. 15-20K feet
2. Frank hypoxia is present
3. Air hunger/ HA/ nausea/ euphoria/ belligerence
4. Long list of sensory, personality, psychomotor, and mentation issues

### Critical stage
1. > 20K feet
2. Incapacitation from acute hypoxia
3. Loss of respiration and death

## EPT VS. TUC

There has been much debate and misrepresentations over these 2 terms in the last decade and a half, leading some clinicians into confusion. Ultimately, these 2 terms are synonymous and describe a period of time from exposure to low oxygen to the loss of deliberate function that could correct the situation. Ultimately, you only have a certain time of wakefulness at certain altitudes. What makes these 2 terms different is how the information was obtained.

### EFFICTIVE PERFORMANCE TIME (EPT)
1. The military first developed the timetable and concept of EPT.
2. It is based on a slow and steady ascent, or slow decompression.

### TIME OF USEFUL CONSCIOUSNESS (TUC)
1. Later, as pressurized cabin technology was developed, the military again studied the effects of hypoxia on pilots, but this time on a rapid decompression.
2. This is based on a rapid decompression event.
3. This value is roughly HALF the value of slow and steady event.

In the last 5 years, authors have begun to accept these definitions as the same and interchangeable. It is important you memorize a handful of the times in the following table below. You will have questions on upcoming exams that will ask for time you have to deliberately make a corrective action based on your altitude. These questions must state if there is an immediate depressurization (rapid decompression) or if the decompression is slow, so you can use this to your advantage. Memorize the "SLOW" column times for the given altitudes. If the question mentions a rapid decompression, then take half of the slow time. This correlates with the time in the "RAPID" column for the corresponding altitudes.

| Altitude | SLOW | RAPID |
|---|---|---|
| 18,000 ft | 20-30 min | 10-15 min |
| 20,000 ft | 10-20 min | 5-10 min |
| 25,000 ft | 3-5 min | 1-2 min |
| 30,000 ft | 1-2 min | 30-60 sec |
| 35,000 ft | 30-60 sec | 15-30 sec |
| 40,000 ft | 15-20 sec | 9-12 sec |

# PART 2: GAS LAWS

## INTRODUCTION

A working knowledge of gas laws and their relationship to physiology is vital to understanding the effects on air medical crewmembers, pilots, and patients. In this section, we will explore the various gas laws, and highlight a debate that has been going on for far too long.

## THE GAS LAWS

### Boyles's Law
1. Inverse relationship between Volume and Pressure.
2. V1P1 = V2P2
3. Higher altitudes = lower atmospheric pressure = gas expands.
4. B = Boyles = Bigger Balloon

### Henry's Law
1. Direct relationship between pressure of a gas over a liquid and the amount of gas dissolved in the liquid
2. Lower atmospheric pressure = gas wanting to come out of a solution
3. Nitrogen bubbles (with decompression illness)
4. H = Henry = Heineken

### Graham's Law
1. Premise: Lighter molecules diffuse faster than heavier molecules.
2. This is based on molecular weight and rarely plays a role in clinical practice nor in the critical care testing environment.

## Dalton's Law

1. Total pressure of a gas is equal to the sum of its individual pressures
2. If nitrogen makes up 78% of our atmosphere, then at sea level (or 760 torr) nitrogen is responsible for 78% of these 760 torr, or 592.8 torr.
3. If oxygen makes up 21% of our atmosphere, then at sea level (or 760 torr) nitrogen is responsible for 21% of this 760 torr, or 159.6 torr.
4. Remember, as you go up in altitude, the pressure gets lower, but the percentages stay the same.
5. Adjusted FiO2 Problems Seen on Exams:
   a. When we transport patients to higher altitudes than from where they were retrieved, you may have to increase the FiO2 to accommodate the higher pressures at altitude.
   b. To do this, take the starting barometric pressure and multiply it by the starting FiO2. Then divide it by the barometric pressure at the altitude of your destination. The result is the FiO2 needed to achieve the starting altitude's SpO2.
   c. EQUATION:
   $$[(Pressure_{STARTING})(FiO_{2\ STARTING})\ /\ (Pressure_{ALTITUDE})]\ =\ \textbf{FiO2 Needed at Destination.}$$
   d. Example:
      i. QUESTION: You lift off at sea level with a set FiO2 of 0.3 yielding a SpO2 of 95%. Your destination is Denver which currently has a barometric pressure of 615 mmHg (or torr). What FiO2 changes will need to be made to maintain this SpO2?
      ii. ANSWER: [(760)(0.3)/(615)] = 0.37. So, you'll need to titrate up your FiO2 to 0.37 to achieve the same SpO2.
   e. If your answer is ever > 1.0 FiO2, know that it is impossible to give more than 100% oxygen (or FiO2 of 1.0). If the patient will need more oxygen than 1.0 FiO2, then you'll need to **ADD PEEP**!
   f. Example:
      i. QUESTION: You lift off at sea level with a set FiO2 of 0.9 yielding a SpO2 of 94%. Your destination is Denver which currently has a barometric pressure of 610 mmHg (or torr). What ventilator changes will need to be made to maintain this SpO2?
      ii. ANSWER: [(760)(0.9)/(610)] =1.1. So, will not be able to maintain the same oxygen saturations by increasing the FiO2 to 1.0, therefore, you'll need to increase PEEP (start by increasing PEEP by 2 cmH2O).

## Charles's Law

1. Direct proportion of Volume and Temperature
2. As air heats up, it becomes less dense; as it cools, it becomes denser.
3. Cold air is better for a helicopter to fly in than warm air
4. C = Charles = Celsius

## Gay-Lussac's Law

1. Direct proportion between temperature and pressure
2. Higher altitudes = lower pressures = lower temperatures
3. It gets colder at higher altitudes, so bring a jacket.

## Fick's Law (my favorite)

1. Gas diffusion depends on three factors:
   a. Partial pressure of the gas
   b. Surface area of the membrane
   c. Thickness of the membrane

2. What does this mean to us?
    a. If we administer more O2→ higher FiO2 → more oxygen available for diffusion → we increase the partial pressure → higher SpO2
    b. Patient's with pathologies that reduce alveolar surface area (such as emphysema, heavy secretions, etc) → low oxygen diffusion
    c. Patients with pathologies that increase the membrane thickness slows oxygen diffusion, therefore, pulmonary edema → low oxygen diffusion → low SpO2

# PART 3: STRESSORS

## INTRODUCTION

The air medical environment exposes crewmembers, pilots, and patients to environmental, physical, and psychological stress during its operations.

## OVERVIEW

There are essentially 11 stressors of flight:

1. 5 related to ALTITUDE:
    a. Hypoxia
    b. Pressure
    c. Fatigue
    d. Thermal
    e. Dehydration
2. 6 are independent of ALTITUDE:
    a. Noise
    b. Vibration
    c. Gravitational Forces
    d. Third Spacing
    e. Spatial Disorientation
    f. Flicker Vertigo

## THE STRESSORS

### Hypoxia

1. Types
2. Stages
3. Symptomology

### Barometric Pressure

#### Low PO2

1. Remember, the percent of O2 remains the same, but the PO2 reduces as you go up in altitude. Less pressure means gases can get further apart from one another.
2. Supplemental O2

**Gases expand with altitude (Boyle's Law)**

1. Gas filled cavities and equipment will expand with increasing altitude
2. Ventilator
3. ET cuff
4. PASG

## Fatigue

1. More than a lack of sleep
2. Our cells can only store a finite amount of O2 and glucose
3. This lack of energy- producing chemicals essentially defines fatigue
4. Higher altitudes mean less O2 and less energy
5. Sick and injured people have an even less of these nutrients.

## Thermal

1. Higher altitudes mean a COLDER temperature (Gay- Lussiac's Law)
2. Hypothermia causes a left shift in oxyhemoglobin dissociation curve.
3. This means that oxygen VERY strongly sticks to the RBCs- so much (in hypothermia) that when the oxygenated RBC gets to the tissues, it doesn't let it go.

## Dehydration

1. Higher altitudes = lower temps (Gay- Lussac's) = air holds less and less moisture (humidity)
2. Therefore, the higher you go, the less moisture in the air
3. As we breathe at higher altitudes, we are essentially drying ourselves out.

## Noise

1. Elicits a sympathetic response
2. People ignore the obvious when around noise → and they can run into the rotors
3. Loud music at a concert 100-110 dB → continued listening at these levels cause hearing damage in 30 min
4. Aircraft engines: 130 dB → damage within minutes

## Vibration

1. Fatigue manifests from vibration
2. Engines cause vibration
3. The body will attempt to keep you in one spot and "fight" the vibration
4. Over several hours of flying, you will be very tired because your muscles have been working to keep you stationary.

## Gravitational Disturbances

1. Positive Gs
   a. Blood pooling in lower extremities
   b. Increased intravascular pressures
   c. Stagnant hypoxia
2. Negative Gs
   a. Stagnant hypoxia
   b. Blood pooling in upper body
   c. Headache

### Third Spacing
1. During rapid accelerations, rapid decelerations, and high velocity turns, plasma is pushed out of the vessels and into the extravascular space.
2. Third spacing exacerbates hypovolemia (because of the decrease in fluid in the vessels) and hypoxia (from the lower BP associated with loss of intravascular volume).
3. Military anti- shock garment (MASG) was developed to prevent third spacing from occurring.

### Spatial Disorientation
1. The inability to accurately orient yourself with respect to the earth's horizon.
2. We maintain spatial orientation by 3 systems: visual, vestibular (balance center in middle ears), and proprioceptive (balance center in brain).
3. In flight, we receive conflicting information so disorientation can occur easily.
4. 3 Types:
    a. Type I: pilot doesn't realize the disorientation is happening
    b. Type II: doesn't realize it is spatial disorientation, but senses something is wrong
    c. Type III: the pilot is under an illusion of intense movement of the aircraft and in turn makes drastic changes to correct the perceived problem

### Flicker Vertigo
1. Occurs when transport team members and patients are exposed to lights that flicker at a rate of 4 -20 cycles per second
2. Can cause nausea, vomiting and in severe case, seizures
3. Flickering of 4-20 per seconds can cause seizures.

### Dysbarism
1. Any syndrome caused by a pressure differential between the barometric pressure and spaces within the body.
2. Be sure to differentiate ascent vs. decent problem
3. Examples:
    a. Barotitis Media: DESCENT problem; Negative pressure middle ear unable to equalize → causes eardrum to pucker → causes microtrauma to ear drum which can rupture
    b. Delayed Ear Block: DESCENT problem; breathing 100% oxygen at altitude → middle ear absorbs O2 → decreasing middle ear pressure slowly → leading to barotitis media
    c. Barodentalgia: ASCENT; expanding gas in gums and dentition causes pain at altitude

### Atmospheres at Depth (Under water)
1. Under water, every 33ft is 1 atm.
2. At sea level you are at 1 atm
3. Therefore, at 66ft, you're at 3 atm- 1 at sea level plus the 2 depths of 33ft.

### Air vs. Ground Time Questions:
1. Add up time from liftoff to arrival at receiving hospital.
2. If it is less time than ground, rule of thumb is to go by air.
3. If ground transport is faster because of all stops and patient transitions (to aircraft, to ambulance, etc) then go by ground.

### Night Vision:
1. Takes 30 min to return (bright light)
2. Chemical rhodopsin (in rod cells) causes the "night blindness" when bright lights flash into eyes → rhodopsin flashes out and it doesn't return for 30 minutes.
3. Decreased night vision at 4000ft MSL
4. Compensatory stage of hypoxia: Night vision reduced by 50%

# PART 4: FLIGHT PHYSIOLOGY QUESTIONS

1. You have a patient that is experiencing an asthma attack and their pulse oximetry reads 88%. What type of hypoxia is present?
   a. Hypoxic
   b. Hypemic
   c. Stagnant
   d. Histotoxic

2. Your patient is a victim of a AMI with JVD, and is profoundly hypoxic. What type of hypoxia is present?
   a. Hypemic
   b. Histotoxic
   c. Stagnant
   d. Hypoxic

3. You depart for a rotor- wing mountain rescue at approximately 17,500 ft. Which of the following is true?
   a. You will have 10 minutes of EPT.
   b. You will have 20 minutes of EPT.
   c. You will have 40 minutes of TUC.
   d. You will have 5 minutes of TUC.

4. You are at 30,000 ft and you recall that your EPT is about 2 minutes. What would your TUC be should you experience a cabin decompression?
   a. 8 minutes
   b. 4 minutes
   c. 1 second
   d. 60 seconds

5. While on a flight to a high mountain rescue, your partner begins slurring his words and behaving as if they are inebriated. Fifteen minutes earlier, they were behaving fine. At what altitude range would you assess you currently were located, based on this information?
   a. Above 15K
   b. 10-14K
   c. 8-12K
   d. Below 5K

6. Your 10 kg pediatric patient is on your ventilator and shortly becomes short of breath and hypoxic enroute to the receiving facility. You discover that you are currently at 9200 ft MSL, the patient has one side of their chest larger than the other, brachial pulse is absent, and the SpO2 is suddenly 81%. Which gas law explains this change ?
   a. Charles's
   b. Dalton's
   c. Boyle's
   d. Gay-Lussac's

7. As you ascend from Oklahoma City to Denver, the barometric pressure reduces from 727 mmHg in OKC to 632 in Denver. You will use this information to calculate a corrected FiO2 for your intubated patient. What gas law does this pertain to?
   a. Boyle's
   b. Graham's
   c. Charles's
   d. Dalton's

8. You take off for a flight and realize that you forgot your jacket. A few minutes later, you are cold. Which gas law explains why you are cold?
   a. Gay-Lussacs's
   b. Charles's
   c. Fick's
   d. Henry's

9. You have been out on fixed wing flights for the entire shift and have been airborne for at least 8 of them. Which of the following stressors will affect you the greatest?
   a. Dehydration
   b. Flicker vertigo
   c. Third spacing
   d. Vibration

10. You awake patient has a history of seizures. Which of the following stressors of flight can exacerbate the patient's condition?
    a. Dehydration
    b. Flicker vertigo
    c. Third Spacing
    d. Vibration

11. After landing on a predesignated landing zone, you are waiting for EMS to arrive with your patient. Your pilot mentions his night vision seems to be impaired at this higher elevation. You know you must be at least _____ ft in altitude.
    a. 1000
    b. 2000
    c. 3000
    d. 4000

12. While in a critical phase of flight, your partner grabs their jaw and complains of a toothache. Which of the critical phases of flight would this occur?
    a. Taxiing
    b. Landing
    c. Take-off
    d. Sharp turn

# PART 4: FLIGHT PHYSIOLOGY RATIONALES

1. **(A)** An obstruction here is blocking a enough oxygen from gaining access to the alveolar capillary membrane. Therefore, this is a hypoxic problem.

2. **(C)** The problem here is a pump problem from the AMI. An AMI damages the heart and thus it cannot pump well, so fluid backs up into the jugular vein (JVD). No pulmonary edema is present so therefore it isn't a hypoxic hypoxia problem because oxygen has good access to the alveolar capillary membrane. The evidence of a poor pump indicates blood is not being pumped forward efficiently- therefore this is a STAGNANT hypoxia problem.

3. **(B)** At about 18,000 ft, you will have about 20-30 minutes of EPT and 10-15 of TUC. Therefore, the best answer is 20 minutes of EPT. Also, in rotor wing, we will always be dealing with EPT since we do not pressurize our cabins. There is no chance for "sudden" decompression.

4. D. Remember that EPT is double that of TUC. Said another way, TUC is half of the bigger value, EPT. If you half EPT, you'll arrive at a good estimate of the TUC. In this case, half of the EPT (2 minutes) is 1 minute, or 60 seconds.

5. **(A)** This patient situation is consistent with the disturbance stage of hypoxia. The patient is behaving as if he is drunk within a short time after entering a hypoxic environment. The disturbance stage is between 15-20K feet.

6. **(C)** As you go up in altitude, the weight of the atmosphere is decreasing and thus gasses begin to spread out. At sea level, the entire atmosphere is forcing gas molecules to stay close to one another. As you go up, gases expand due to the lower pressure and can cause pneumothorax and/or tension pneumothorax.

7. **(D)** Dalton's law is the law of the sum of partial pressures. So, we can use the barometric pressure of a city and multiply it by our administered FiO2 and figure out the partial pressure of oxygen we are delivering to the patient. Additionally, we can set up a simple equation (see page 42) to calculate how much to increase FiO2 at our destination to ensure we are delivering the correct partial pressure of oxygen to our patients.

8. **(A)** Gay-Lussac's law explains that as you go higher in altitude you will get colder because lower pressure translates into colder temperatures. This is commonly confused for Charles's Law which says that if you heat air up, it expands, like in a hot air balloon. So, needing a jacket is due to Gay-Lussac's law.

9. **(D)** After flying for 20 hours and being in the aircraft for 8 of those hours will incredibly fatigue the crew members due to sleep deprivation as well as vibration. Remember, vibration occurs in aircraft and your body will attempt to keep you stationary. This burns a lot of calories.

10. **(B)** In a rotor- wing aircraft, flicker vertigo is possible because light coming through the rotating blades is between 4-20/ sec. This has been shown to cause seizures in some individuals. It is important to pay close attention to seizure- risk patients during the day on helicopters.

11. **(D)** Night vision will decrease by 50% at approximately 4000ft in MSL.

12. **(C)** Barodentalgia occurs during ascent when Boyles' law says that gases expand as you go higher. Air thus expands in tooth cavities causing a great deal of pain- and this occurs during ASCENT.

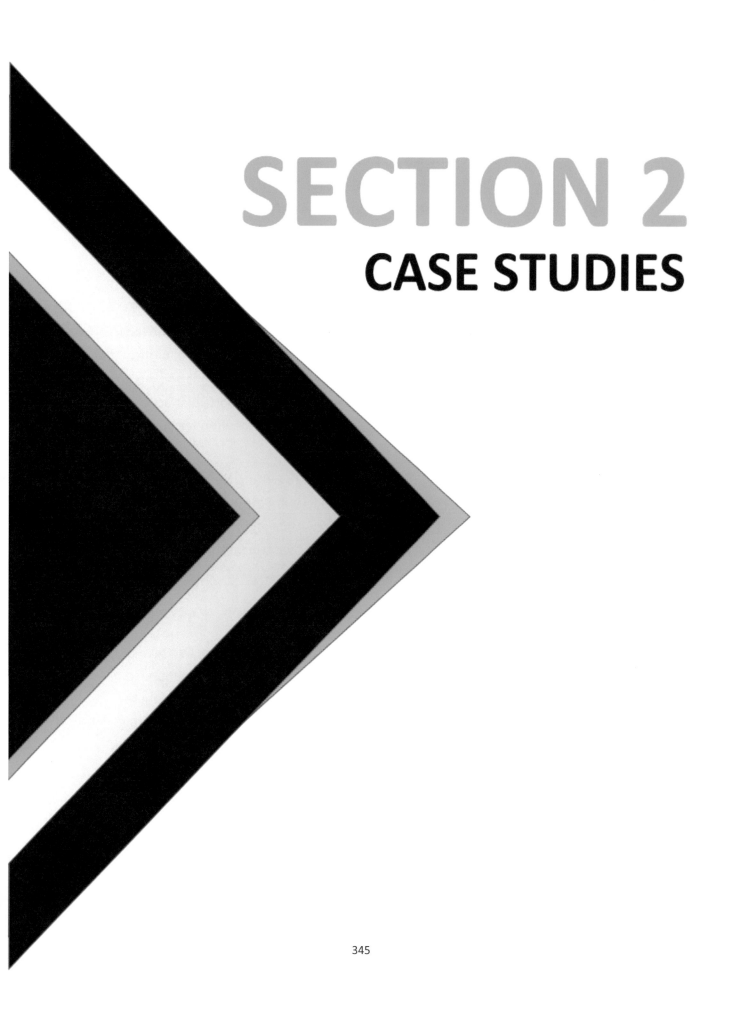

# SECTION 2
## CASE STUDIES

# Instructions for the Case Study Portion:

First off, congratulations on finishing the study portion of this text. Whether you're just starting this information for the first time, or you have done it for years and just are using it as a refresher to sharpen your knowledge and skills, it is an incredible undertaking to commit all of this material to memory. If you skip ahead without studying everything, that's OK. It might be a little more difficult and you might need to review some of the material in the earlier portions of the text.

This section is designed to test your knowledge in the form of case studies with rationales to follow each one. Your goal should be to read the scenario, and make clinical decisions based upon the information provided. There might be some information missing, but it is designed to force you to decide and to learn from that decision. Keep the answers short and almost bulleted. There is no need to write a long paragraph for each section, simply jot down the clinical action items you would perform or jot down the information you would need to execute particular actions and procedures. The rationales are on the page following the scenario for quick reference.

The scenario will be provided, and then spaces for you to write down your clinical action items. Utilize the topics below as a template to work through the scenarios. You will be provided with initial scenario information, ABCs and treatment boxes for you to jot down your management, and then updated scenario information.

## How to Use the Scenario and the Scenario Boxes

You will be given an initial set of information in the form of a narrative. Use this information to begin to filter your assessments based on the given information. Your assessments need to be all the same, and then begin to evolve to accommodate the condition the patient is experiencing. There are times you may be uncertain. During these times, figure out the top 3 most dangerous possibilities and continue assessing until you rule out as much as you can. While you are trying to make sense of the case in the initial information box, also look to the **vital signs** directly under the initial information box.

**LIFE THREATS:** Under the vital signs box there is a box labeled "Any life threats needed correcting?" In this box, you'll need to write out ANYTHING you need to fix right away that could kill the patient (like apnea, or cricothyrotomy, or needle decompression).

346

You are then given lab data, a link to an image in the appendix, or other lab information that may be needed to make a decision about management.

**MANAGEMENT PLAN**: There is a small box after the labs and imaging boxes that is for you to jot down you r management plan. This is SMALL for a reason- you should get to the point pretty quickly. Treat x with y. There is no reason to be lengthy because you won't be in the field. You need to know what to do, how to do it, and then assess for effectiveness.

**UPDATE**: After you initially manage your patient, you will be given an update in an all-black box. This will provide a page number in the book to link to for an update on the patient condition. This was designed to echo real cases that change and evolve right in front of you.

**ADDITONAL MANAGEMENT**: After the update, the 'Additional Management' page is next, and designed with brevity in mind as well. Jot down, quickly and briefly, the next few management items.

**FINAL DIAGNOSIS/PATHO:** This is the main pathophysiology in this case. Write this down so you can revisit it later. Reviewing these cases, you've gone over every so often helps to reinforce the lessons so you can stay sharp.

**[A] AIRWAY/RSI REGIMINE:** In this box, be sure to input how you would secure the airway.  Include the RSI regimen <u>every single time</u> for this type of patient, **even if this patient does not require intubation**.  The point here is to get you thinking about how to choose RSI medications and execute the intubation. **THERE WILL BE SCENARIOS THAT ACTUALLY DO NOT REQUIRE INTUBATION BUT DOESN'T MEAN YOU SHOULDN'T BE THINKING HOW YOU WOULD DO IT IF YOU HAD TO**; if you stay ready, you never have to get ready.

 **VENT SETTINGS:** In this box, briefly describe how you would manage the patient ventilation.  Include your thoughts on minute ventilation.  Additionally, identify your initial ventilator settings on this patient, **even if** they do not require ventilator management in a particular scenario. Base measurements on ideal body weight. Again, the goal is to get you to practice setting up the mechanical ventilator on every patient. Just like the RSI exercised with each patient, you should always have an idea how you would put patients on the ventilator in the case they need it. Not every scenario will require the patient to be placed on the vent but practice it anyway. **REMEMBER: If you stay ready, you never have to get ready.**

Be aware that we primarily discuss SIMV or A/C in this text to minimize confusion. Those savvy ventilation cats out there will just have to wait for my new *Ventilator Hero* text to be released. This will cover all advanced elements of ventilator

**PURFUSION STATUS:** Identify the patient's perfusion status as <u>stable</u>, <u>potentially compromised</u> or <u>compromised</u>. Also, jot down their vital signs in the left side of the box. Writing these numbers down is a kinetic learning function and ultimately makes the values more important to you, this simulated experience will be of greater value.

**HEAD-TO-TOE ASSESSMENT:** If you note anything specific about the assessment that would be valuable during your re-studying time, then jot that information down here.

**SCENARIO QUESTIONS**: You will be provided a few scenario questions at the end of the case study to consider. These are also great to return to for review of critical information.

**RATIONALES**: Once you have completed the case and are ready to have the case information revealed, turn the page and learn away. On these pages, you will be given several rationales relative to predominant pathophysiology, RSI regimen, ventilator settings, perfusion status, corrective action, labs, required management based on update, and scenario question answers. All parts of the case are explained, including the RSI and ventilator settings, which may not be needed on every patient we present. However, we try to sell you to make these assessments on every patient you ever treat and transport so that on the ones that really need it- you'll be ready.

# Case Study 1

You respond to an ER to pick up a patient who was shot while out at a bar earlier in the evening. Upon arrival, the ER staff informs you that the patient was shot at a close range with a small caliber firearm and the patient has a sealed gunshot wound to the left anterior chest. The patient is semiconscious and in obvious respiratory distress, receiving 100% oxygen via non– rebreather mask. Vitals: BP 72/48, HR 116, SpO2 88%, RR 26. (+) completely sealed occlusive dressing to the GSW. The patient is kept warm by blankets.  Pt wt: 185 lbs. Pt height: 6'1''.

## BP: 72/48 | HR: 116 | RR: 26 | SpO2: 88 | EtCO2: n/a

**ANY LIFE THREATS NEEDING ADDRESSED?**

| | | | | | |
|---|---|---|---|---|---|
| Na: | 141 | RBCs: | 3.2 | pH: | 7.36 |
| K: | 3.9 | WBCs: | 10 | pCO2: | 45 |
| Cl: | 105 | PLTs: | 132 | HCO3: | 23 |
| HCO₃: | 25 | HGB: | 9 | pO2: | 82 |
| Cr: | 8 | HCT: | 38 | BE: | XXX |
| BUN: | 0.6 | | | | |
| Glu: | 72 | | | | |

**OTHER LAB/IMAGE INFO:**

**MANAGEMENT PLAN:**

**UPDATE: Turn to page #379 for an update. Look for UPDATE #1. Use this information to continue with the case and this form.**

**ADDITIONAL MANAGEMENT:**

**FINAL DIAGNOSES/PATHO?**

**AIRWAY/RSI REGIMINE:**

**VENT SETTINGS:**

**PERFUSION STATUS:**

**HEAD 2 TOE ASSESSMENT:**

**Scenario Question 1:**
If 2 units of packed RBCs are administered, how much do you expect the HGB to increase?

**Scenario Question 2:**
What is the end sign of fluid resuscitation thus indicating that a pressor might be needed?

**Scenario Question 3:**
N/A

# CASE STUDY 1: RATIONALE

# Shot to the ~~Heart~~ Lungs

### PREDOMINANT PATHOPHYS
GSW resulting in tension pneumothorax with associated hypotension and hypoxia

### RSI REGIMEN
Consider RSI (sedative: ketamine, etomidate, or fentanyl- to prevent a further drop in BP; paralysis: Sux or Roc; continued sedation with ketamine or fentanyl). Goal with this patient is to prevent hypotension or perihypotension.

### VENTILATOR SETTINGS
Ideal body weight (IBW): 80kg; SIMV or AC on volume ventilation; Target a minute ventilation of 8 L/min (RR ~17; TV ~480cc- or any combination of RR and Vt to achieve a VE of 8 L/min)-normal VE used because the patient doesn't present acidotic...YET); I:E 1:2; PEEP 3-5 cmH2O; FiO2 1.0.

### PERFUSION STATUS: COMPROMISED

### CORRECTIVE ACTION NEEDED
This patient needs to have his airway immediately controlled: oral adjunct and BVM with supplemental oxygen at first, then consider RSI. There is no evidence for acidosis, so a normal minute ventilation is acceptable for this patient. A PEEP valve applied to the BVM would increase oxygenation as well as increased FiO2. The BP needs attention ASAP. Correcting the BP would make the EtCO2 and pulse oximetry trustworthy. Low BP can cause falsely low EtCO2 and pulse oximetry. Additionally, the wound should be sealed on three sides, not completely sealed. Then a significant fluid bolus (1-2 L of NS) should be administered right away. Consider blood products early.

### LABS
Mild anemia (low hemoglobin and hematocrit. ABG: Normal but displaying a separation of the pH and pCO2 with a low pO2– indicating poor perfusion. In healthy or compensated patients, the numbers after the decimal of a pH will usually match the numbers of the pCO2 (ex. A healthy male with pH of 7.41 would be expected to have a pCO2 of close to 41 mmHg).

### REQUIRED MANAGEMENT CHANGES BASED ON UPDATE
Anytime there is a drop in both pulse oximetry and BP, you must consider a tension pneumothorax. Consider decompression.

### QUESTION 1
One unit of PRBCs will increase the HGB by 1g/dL and HCT by 3%.

### QUESTION 2
Taping it on four sides prevents escaping air from leaving the thoracic cavity. Allowing one side to left untapped, air can rush out when pressure begins to build up and thus can prevent a tension pneumothorax. If the seal is taped on three sides, then air can build up and cause tension.

# Case Study 2

INITIAL: A mother finds her son in his bedroom asleep and she cannot awaken him. The mother calls 911 and EMS arrives, begins management, and transports the patient to the local ER. Upon your arrival, you receive the following report: 25 year old found with an empty bottle of hydromorphone which was prescribed to his mother 4 days ago, the patient is found obtunded with a GCS of 7 (E1,V2,M4), (+) miosis bilaterally, and the patient's vital signs are noted below while on 100% oxygen via BVM. The patient's intrinsic respiratory rate is 6/min. The medical staff has initiated 2 large bore IVs and administered a single NS bolus of 500cc. No other treatment has been conducted. Pt wt: 230 lbs. Pt height: 5'10''.

## BP: 82/50 | HR: 62 | RR: 6 (14 via BVM) | SpO2: 96 | EtCO2: 62

ANY LIFE THREATS
NEEDING ADDRESSED?

| | | | |
|---|---|---|---|
| Na: | 138 | RBCs: 4.8 | pH: 7.31 |
| K: | 4.1 | WBCs: 9 | pCO2: 64 |
| Cl: | 100 | PLTs: 201 | HCO3: 22 |
| $HCO_3$: | 22 | HGB: 14 | pO2: 81 |
| Cr: | 9 | HCT: 47 | BE: -1 |
| BUN: | 0.7 | | |
| Glu: | 102 | | |

OTHER LAB/IMAGE INFO:

MANAGEMENT PLAN:

UPDATE: Turn to page #380 for an update. Look for UPDATE #2. Use this information to continue with the case and this form.

ADDITIONAL MANAGEMENT:

FINAL DIAGNOSES/PATHO?

RSI REGIMINE:

VENT SETTINGS:

PERFUSION STATUS:

HEAD 2 TOE ASSESSMENT:

**Scenario Question 1:**
If Narcan is given, how long will Narcan last relative to opiates or opioids?

**Scenario Question 2:**
What is the endpoint of fluid resuscitation thus indicating that a pressor might be needed?

**Scenario Question 3:**
N/A

## CASE STUDY 2: RATIONALE

# Mama Said Knock You Out

### PREDOMINANT PATHOPHYS
Narcotic OD; Hemodynamic control

### RSI REGIMEN
Consider RSI (sedative: ketamine, etomidate, or fentanyl; paralysis: Sux or Roc; continued sedation with ketamine or fentanyl)

### VENTILATOR SETTINGS
IBW: 73 kg; ; SIMV or AC on volume ventilation; Target minute ventilation that is 8.7 L/min, alternatively, 8.5 -9.0 L/min is acceptable. To achieve this VE: RR 17-24 and TV 360-510 cc. I:E 1:2; PEEP 3-5 cmH2O; FiO2 1.0.

### PERFUSION STATUS: COMPROMISED

### CORRECTIVE ACTION NEEDED
Need to control airway (GCS 7 with BVM and oral adjunct and assisted ventilations). Consider RSI. Need to correct BP with fluids (1-2 L to begin)

### LABS
Serum: Normal. ABG: Acute respiratory acidosis with hypoxia.

### REQUIRED MANAGEMENT CHANGES BASED ON <u>UPDATE</u>
Need to correct: I:E to 1:2 (no reason to suspect air trapping/ auto PEEPing in this case); reduce the FiO2 to 0.8- 0.9 (titrate down the FiO2 to lowest possible setting to keep the SpO2 above 95%); increase minute volume (currently, your MV is 6.7 from an f 14 ad Vte 480, therefore, increase the MV somewhere between 7-9 L/min would drive DOWN the current EtCO2 of 55 mmHg. You want it much closer to 45 mmHg); Consider Narcan, but if you do, be prepared for the patient waking up if there is only a narcotic on board as the sedative. If you fix the BP and control the ventilation, then avoiding Narcan is a prudent and rational clinical decision.

### QUESTION 1
Narcan has a shorter half-life relative to opiates and opioids, so the Narcan will wear off over time, and CNS depression will recur. Be ready for a return of lower HR, BP, and RR if this is the case.

### QUESTION 2
Where there is rales or pulmonary edema, you have topped the patient out on fluids, and BP support should be switched to pressors. Choose a pressor that compliments the HR. If the patient is already tachycardic, then use something like neosynepherine that will not increase HR much. If the HR is normal or slower, then consider a pressor that causes an increase in HR.

# Case Study 3

**INITIAL:**

Your patient is a three-month-old who is being transferred to a higher level of care for respiratory distress. The patient is breathing approximately 61 times per minute, has a heart rate of 149, SpO2 87%, EtCO2 of 58, has pink skin and extremities, and appears very weak (unable to lift their own extremities). Patient has congestion in lower lobes of the lungs. Currently, there is blow by O2 via facemask and an IV in place. No other treatment completed. The vitals and ABG can be found below. Pt weight: 6 kg.

## BP: pink extremities | HR: 149 | RR: 61 | SpO2: 87 | EtCO2: 58

**ANY LIFE THREATS NEEDING ADDRESSED?**

| | | | | | |
|---|---|---|---|---|---|
| Na: | 136 | RBCs: | 6 | pH: | 7.29 |
| K: | 3.9 | WBCs: | 10 | pCO2: | 57 |
| Cl: | 104 | PLTs: | 156 | HCO3: | 23 |
| HCO₃: | 23 | HGB: | 16 | pO2: | 58 |
| Cr: | 18 | HCT: | 48 | BE: | -2 |
| BUN: | 0.6 | | | | |
| Glu: | 98 | | | | |

**OTHER LAB/IMAGE INFO:**

**MANAGEMENT PLAN:**

**UPDATE: Turn to page #381 for an update. Look for UPDATE #3. Use this information to continue with the case and this form.**

**ADDITIONAL MANAGEMENT:**

**FINAL DIAGNOSES/PATHO?**

**RSI REGIMINE:**

**VENT SETTINGS:**

**PERFUSION STATUS:**

**HEAD 2 TOE ASSESSMENT:**

**Scenario Question 1:**
Why did the patient decompensate en route?

**Scenario Question 2:**
What are the 2 most common reasons that pediatric patients develop cardiac arrest?

**Scenario Question 3:**
If your frequency is ever higher than the set RR on the vent, what must be done?

# CASE STUDY 3: RATIONALE

# Stairway to Heaven

### PREDOMINANT PATHOPHYS
Respiratory Failure/ Altitude associated tension pneumothorax

### RSI REGIMEN
Consider RSI (sedative: ketamine [bronchodilation effect with sedative properties], versed or fentanyl; paralysis: Sux [contraindicated in peds with the neuromuscular disease] or Roc; continued sedation with versed or fentanyl).

### VENTILATOR SETTINGS
IBW: 6kg (given); PRESSURE CONTROL 15 cmH2O to start. This may result in low Vte- simply increase the PC setting if low or if Vte is higher than their targeted Vt, then reduce as needed or adopt the higher Vte and recalculate the new RR by dividing the target VE by the their current Vte. SIMV or AC. Target a minute ventilation of about 2 L/min: RR 26-32; I:E 1:5– 1:7; Peep 3-5 cmH2O; FiO2 1.0.

### PERFUSION STATUS: POTENTIALLY COMPROMIZED

### CORRECTIVE ACTION NEEDED
First off, 61 breaths per minute is way too fast. The longer this can occur, the more tired the child gets. The more tired they are, the less they will be able to keep up that breathing rate and effort. It costs a lot of energy (made from sugar and OXYGEN) that depletes O2 levels and further worsens the child's condition. Securing the airway and ventilating appropriately is paramount. RSI would help the child out by forcing them to stop using extra respiratory muscles to breathe (thus reducing oxygen consumption). A PEEP valve with BVM ventilation along with 100% supplemental O2 would both increase the pulse oximetry while intubation and mechanical ventilation are being prepared.

### LABS
(+) Acute respiratory acidosis with hypoxia (acidic pH and pCO2 with a normal bicarb, and low pO2).

### REQUIRED MANAGEMENT CHANGES BASED ON UPDATE
Use DOPE acronym to rule out probable causes of the drop in BP and O2 sats. Tension pneumo is the case here. Immediate needle decompression (18g to 2nd/ 3rd intercostal space midaxillary) is required. Then have the pilot fly at the lowest and safest level. Continue en route management (recycle ABC vital signs, vent readings, and ECG monitoring).

### QUESTION 1
The patient decompensated because the pilot flew too high, gases expanded in the child's chest, and a tension pneumothorax formed causing the patient to become hemodynamically compromised.

### QUESTION 2
Respiratory insufficiency and shock. By aggressively managing these 2 conditions, you can prevent cardiac arrest in the pediatric patient.

### QUESTION 3
The patient is over breathing the ventilator and must be sedated or paralyzed so that ventilation and oxygenation can be controlled.

# Case Study 4

**INITIAL**:

You arrive to transport a 59 y/o with ST elevation in leads V1-V4. Currently, there is a systolic murmur. He has developed altered mental status, despite a pulse oximetry of 100% and a blood sugar of 102 mg/dL. The patient has received MONA, is currently on a NRB 15 L/min, and has these other findings: BP 102/75, HR 104, RR 24, and a GCS 7 (E1,V1,M5). The patient has a history of HTN (normally 150s systolic) and smoking. See Appendix A, ECG #1 and use as this patient's 12 lead ECG. Pt wt: 325 lbs. Pt height: 6'3''.

## BP: 102/75 | HR: 104 | RR: 24 | SpO2: 100 | EtCO2: 26

**ANY LIFE THREATS NEEDING ADDRESSED?**

| | | | | | |
|---|---|---|---|---|---|
| Na: | 141 | RBCs: | 5.2 | pH: | 7.42 |
| K: | 4.2 | WBCs: | 7 | pCO2: | 42 |
| Cl: | 99 | PLTs: | 174 | HCO3: | 24 |
| HCO$_3$: | 24 | HGB: | 17 | pO2: | 245 |
| Cr: | 16 | HCT: | 49 | BE: | 2 |
| BUN: | 0.5 | | | | |
| Glu: | 99 | | | | |

**OTHER LAB/IMAGE INFO:**

**MANAGEMENT PLAN:**

**UPDATE: Turn to page #379 for an update. Look for UPDATE #4. Use this information to continue with the case and this form.**

**ADDITIONAL MANAGEMENT:**

**FINAL DIAGNOSES/PATHO?**

**RSI REGIMINE:**

**VENT SETTINGS:**

**PERFUSION STATUS:**

**HEAD 2 TOE ASSESSMENT:**

**Scenario Question 1:**
Which coronary artery would you suspect is the culprit in this patient's acute myocardial infarction?

**Scenario Question 2:**
What medication would help push blood forward, increasing cardiac output (and BP) as well as reducing SVR from vasodilation?

**Scenario Question 3:**
N/A

## CASE STUDY 4: RATIONALE

# Earl Had to Die

### PREDOMINANT PATHOPHYS
Anteroseptal AMI; papillary muscle rupture

### RSI REGIMEN
Consider RSI (sedative: Etomidate, or fentanyl; paralysis: Sux [no history suggesting hyperkalemia; current K+ 3.9, which is normal] or Roc; continued sedation with versed or fentanyl). Avoid versed in this case due to relative hypotension.

### VENTILATOR SETTINGS
IBW: 84.5kg; Target a minute ventilation of about 8.5 L/min (normal because there is no evidence of acidosis); SIMV or AC; (Vt ~ 510cc) or pressure ventilation (PC 15); RR about 17- if you use different RR and Vt, just make sure they are targeting the minute ventilation of 8.5 for this patient; I:E 1:2; PEEP 3-5 cmH2O; FiO2 0.8-1.0 (you can consider reducing FiO2 because of the patient's 100% O2 sats and pO2 is 245- just ensure when you reduce FiO2, the SpO2 does not change).

### PERFUSION STATUS: COMPROMISED

### CORRECTIVE ACTION NEEDED
The patient is experiencing an anteroseptal AMI, and the murmur indicates a papillary muscle rupture (worsening the acute heart failure). The patient is hypotensive- his normal is 150s and now he is 100s. Further evidence of acute heart failure. The patient needs to be intubated due to a declining mental status and the potential for cardiac collapse. The patient should be placed on the ventilator targeting a normal minute ventilation as there isn't significant evidence of acidosis.

### LABS
Troponin and CK-MD are elevated. All other values are within normal limits. ABG: Hyperoxia, but otherwise normal.

### REQUIRED MANAGEMENT CHANGES BASED ON NEW INFORMATION
The vent needs to be adjusted: there is rate and frequency mismatch (meaning the patient is over breathing the vent), a high minute ventilation (from set rate/ frequency mismatch), and a very long E– time  (shown by an I:E ratio of 1:5).  The patient needs to be adequately sedated (the increased frequency means the patient is over breathing the vent– consider fentanyl or ketamine do avoid dropping his BP). The I:E needs to be changed to 1:2 since there is no evidence of air trapping. The low BP means the patient needs fluid and perhaps an inotrope- for better/ stronger contractions helping to shovel out blood from the heart alleviating the fluid back up (failure).  If BP continues to drop with the nitro, be sure to consider a pressor that has few beta-1 properties (which would increase HR- bad for a heart patient). Don't remove the nitro– support the BP so the patient benefits from the properties of nitro.

### QUESTION 1
Mainly, the LEFT ANTERIOR DECENDING (LAD), with a little influence from the left circumflex.

### QUESTION 2
Dobutamine. Increases squeeze, thereby ↑CO while causing a ↓ SVR from vasodilation.

# Case Study 5

**INITIAL**: You respond to a trauma scene flight where your 25 y/o female patient was entrapped for 50 minutes in 30°F weather. As you land on scene, the FD is delivering the patient to you packaged (spinal immobilization) and ready for transport. They report the patient is hypotensive and hypoxic, which developed 2 minutes before they got the patient on the stretcher. Other findings and vitals include: HR 117, RR 26, GCS 8 (E2,V2,M4), carotid pulse present but no radial pulse, and thoracic trauma noted (ecchymosis to the anterior chest wall). You're unable to hear any breath sounds or heart tones because your helicopter's engines are currently on. Patient's temp: 34.4°C, weight: 185 lbs, and height: 5'8".

## BP: unknown | HR: 124 | RR: 27 | SpO2: n/a | EtCO2: 26

**ANY LIFE THREATS NEEDING ADDRESSED?**

| | | | | | |
|---|---|---|---|---|---|
| Na: | 138 | RBCs: | 4.3 | pH: | 7.35 |
| K: | 4.1 | WBCs: | 6 | pCO2: | 37 |
| Cl: | 102 | PLTs: | 174 | HCO3: | 22 |
| CO2: | 25 | HGB: | 16 | pO2: | 99 |
| Cr: | 12 | HCT: | 43 | BE: | 0 |
| BUN: | 0.7 | | | | |
| Glu: | 102 | | | | |

**OTHER LAB/IMAGE INFO:**

**MANAGEMENT PLAN:**

**UPDATE: Turn to page #380 for an update. Look for UPDATE #5. Use this information to continue with the case and this form.**

**ADDITIONAL MANAGEMENT:**

**FINAL DIAGNOSES/PATHO?**

**RSI REGIMINE:**

**VENT SETTINGS:**

**PERFUSION STATUS:**

**HEAD 2 TOE ASSESSMENT:**

**Scenario Question 1:**
What ECG pattern would you expect to find with this patient?

**Scenario Question 2:**
If this patient were to develop cardiac arrest, when should drugs be administered?

**Scenario Question 3:**
What would you do if BP drops after increasing the PEEP to a higher than normal value on an almost hypotensive patient?

# CASE STUDY 5: RATIONALE

# Funky Cold Medina

### PREDOMINANT PATHOPHYS

Tension pneumothorax; Hypothermia; Multi-system trauma

### RSI REGIMEN

Consider RSI (sedative/ analgesia: ketamine or fentanyl (both have sedative and analgesic properties); paralysis: Sux or Roc; continued sedation/analgesia with ketamine or fentanyl).

### VENTILATOR SETTINGS

IBW: 64kg; SIMV or AC; Target a minute ventilation of about 6.5 L/min (normal because there is no evidence of acidosis); volume ventilation (TV ~ 385– 510 cc based on 64 kg IBW) or pressure ventilation (PC 15-20); RR 10– 16 but if you use different RR and Vt, just make sure they are targeting the minute ventilation of 6.5 for this patient; I:E 1:2; PEEP 3-5 cmH2O; FiO2 1.0.

### PERFUSION STATUS: COMPROMISED

### CORRECTIVE ACTION NEEDED

The sudden change in BP and pulse oximetry from what it was before to now (hypoxic and hypotensive) is a clinical indication for tension pneumothorax. You're under the rotors, so you cannot hear the lung sounds. You cannot wait for tracheal tugging or JVD because they are late indicators. If they have a tension pneumothorax, and you do not decompress, then they could die. If they do not have a tension pneumothorax, but you decompress them, know you won't hurt them if you puncture the appropriate site. The patient is not only hypotensive and hypoxic but also hypothermic. It is important to maintain BVM ventilations with 100% oxygen, remove the patient from the cold, and then begin to passively warm the patient. The patient has a decreased mental status; therefore, airway needs to be secured. Initially, BVM with an oral adjunct is acceptable. However, you should be moving towards rapid sequence intubation with this patient.

### LABS

Serum: normal. ABG: normal but displaying high normal for O2 and CO2 levels with low normal pH levels; common hypothermic findings.

### REQUIRED MANAGEMENT CHANGES BASED ON NEW INFORMATION

It appears the patient has stabilized hemodynamically, so now we need to maximize ventilation and oxygenation as well as to continue to support and maintain BP (hemodynamics). Sedation with fentanyl or ketamine would be ideal here, since the f is out of control relative to the set RR (RR = 14 vs. f = 21). By reducing the frequency, you will reinstate a normal ventilation and thus the low EtCO2 should correct- just keep an eye on it to be sure. Improve oxygenation by increasing PEEP to 5 or 6 cmH2O since we want our pulse oximetry 95% or above. Correct the I:E to 1:2 from its set 1:5 since there is no evidence of air trapping. Support BP with fluid boluses if needed.

### QUESTION1

You would expect to see an Osborne wave with hypothermia. As the patient is warmed, the Osborne wave should resolve.

### QUESTION 2

Once the patients are rewarmed to > 30°C, then medications can be administered. Defibrillation/ cardioversion should never be withheld, however.

### QUESTION 3

Once you apply PEEP to improve oxygenation and hypoxia is resolved, then maintain that PEEP. Do not let a lowering BP scare you. If BP drops, fix it with fluids or pressors to support the BP.

# Case Study 6

**INITIAL:**

You are transporting a 27-year-old female who is 39 weeks gestation. The report you receive from the sending facility is that she is currently 3 cm dilated, having contractions approximately 10 minutes apart, and her water broke. She is showing accelerations on the fetal heart rate monitor, and the tocometer readout is consistent with the contractions the patient is having. FHTs are moderately variable and about 150s. Pt weight: 155 lbs; pt height: 5'4''. Use FHT #3 in Appendix C.

## BP: 132/88 | HR: 98 | RR: 22 | SpO2: 97 | EtCO2: 40

**ANY LIFE THREATS NEEDING ADDRESSED?**

| | | | | | |
|---|---|---|---|---|---|
| Na: | 136 | RBCs: | 4 | pH: | 7.38 |
| K: | 3.9 | WBCs: | 6 | pCO2: | 41 |
| Cl: | 104 | PLTs: | 212 | HCO3: | 23 |
| HCO$_3$: | 25 | HGB: | 13 | pO2: | 92 |
| Cr: | 13 | HCT: | 41 | BE: | 1 |
| BUN: | 1.2 | | | | |
| Glu: | 122 | | | | |

**OTHER LAB/IMAGE INFO:**

**MANAGEMENT PLAN:**

**UPDATE: Turn to page #381 for an update. Look for UPDATE #6. Use this information to continue with the case and this form.**

**ADDITIONAL MANAGEMENT:**

**FINAL DIAGNOSES/PATHO?**

**RSI REGIMINE:**

**VENT SETTINGS:**

**PERFUSION STATUS:**

**HEAD 2 TOE ASSESSMENT:**

**Scenario Question 1:**
In the presence of post-partum hemorrhage, which medication would you administer, why, and in what dosage?

**Scenario Question 2:**
Briefly describe the difference between late decelerations and early decelerations.

**Scenario Question 3:**
Assume the fetus delivers with 1 minute APGAR of 5 with minimal respirations. What is your best course of action?

# CASE STUDY 6: RATIONALE

# Happy Birthday, Baby

### PREDOMINANT PATHOPHYS
Labor; imminent delivery; shoulder dystocia

### RSI REGIMEN
Consider RSI (sedative: versed, or fentanyl; paralysis: Sux or Roc; continued sedation with versed or fentanyl). Avoid ketamine because the patient is already hypertensive.

### VENTILATOR SETTINGS
IBW: 55kg; SIMV or AC; Target a minute ventilation of about 5.5 L/min (no evidence of acidosis); Volume (328– 438 TV) or pressure (18– 22 cmH2O); RR 13-20- but if you use different RR and Vt, just make sure they are targeting the minute ventilation of 5.5 for this patient; I:E 1:2; PEEP 3-5 cmH2O; FiO2 1.0.

### PERFUSION STATUS: STABLE

### CORRECTIVE ACTION NEEDED
The patient is it labor (noted by the contractions, and the dilation.). Her water breaking means the patient could have a prolapsed cord, potentially even around the fetus's neck (nuchal cord). The accelerations with contractions indicate the patient is receiving adequate oxygen. Moderate variability is desired, and the FHT is ideal for the fetus. This is a stable mother and child experiencing a healthy pregnancy so far. Administer low flow oxygen to maintain a high pulse oximetry, but always be ready to intubate via RSI should an acute condition occur and threaten the mother and child. Be ready for imminent delivery (know where equipment is, cycle in your mind the common conditions and how to identify and treat them, discuss with the pilot the plan to land temporarily while the baby is birthed should a critical condition occur while in flight).

### LABS:
Serum Slightly hyperglycemia (watch for PIH). ABG: Normal.

### REQUIRED MANAGEMENT CHANGES BASED ON NEW INFORMATION
Consider landing so you have the freedom of movement (you and the patient) allowing you access to the patient and child. Ensure high flow oxygen to the mother and monitor her vital signs as well as the FHTs. Crowning with an inability to progress forward (with or without turtle sign) indicates shoulder dystocia. Perform McRobert's maneuver, suprapubic pressure, Wood's corkscrew maneuver, and forward arm sweep to resolve the shoulder dystocia. Consider diverting to the nearest appropriate hospital if it cannot be resolved. FHTs are dropping and late decelerations are occurring due to the child trapped in the birth canal. Be prepared to measure APGARs, handle post- partum hemorrhage, and provide neonatal resuscitation.

### QUESTION 1
Oxytocin; to cause uterine contraction which will reduce bleeding; 20-40 milliunits/min IV infusion; ALTERNATIVE Dose: 10 units IM.

### QUESTION 2
Early decelerations is a good and reassuring sign. Late decelerations mean the contraction happens, and then there is a drop in the FHT- this indicates the baby is tired and not acting as quickly to the contraction as they should be. In cases of late decelerations, its most likely hypoxia or placental insufficiency. Administer high flow O2 and turn mother onto her left or right side.

### QUESTION 3
The most specific action would be to apply PPV with 21%O2 and see if that influences the infant to breathe.

# Case Study 7

**INITIAL:** You are retrieving an adult patient from an ICU and transporting them to the local level one hospital. The patient currently has the diagnosis of sepsis, and the medical staff is having difficulty keeping the blood pressure and pulse oximetry in normal ranges. One week ago, the patient had laparoscopic GI surgery. After he had sent home, he developed belly pain and nausea (two days ago). The patient presented to the ER with altered mental status and low blood pressure. Currently, the patient is receiving 300 mL NS per hour and just finished a round of antibiotics. Vent settings: A/C RR 18, TV 550, Vte 525, f 24, I:E 1:3, PEEP 3, FiO2 1.0, PIP 50 & Pplat 42. The patient received versed 15 minutes prior (5 mg). Pt weight: 88 kg. Ht: 6'2''.

## BP: 88/58 | HR: 101 | RR: 18-vent | SpO2: 89 | EtCO2: 66

**ANY LIFE THREATS NEEDING ADDRESSED?**

| | | | | | |
|---|---|---|---|---|---|
| Na: | 145 | RBCs: | 5 | pH: | 7.29 |
| K: | 4.7 | WBCs: | 18 | pCO2: | 34 |
| Cl: | 105 | PLTs: | 465 | HCO3: | 15 |
| HCO$_3$: | 14 | HGB: | 16 | pO2: | 52 |
| Cr: | 15 | HCT: | 47 | BE: | -2 |
| BUN: | 1.3 | | | | |
| Glu: | 287 | | | | |

**OTHER LAB/IMAGE INFO:**

**MANAGEMENT PLAN:**

**UPDATE: Turn to page #379 for an update. Look for UPDATE #7. Use this information to continue with the case and this form.**

**ADDITIONAL MANAGEMENT:**

**FINAL DIAGNOSES/PATHO?**

**RSI REGIMINE:**

**VENT SETTINGS:**

**PERFUSION STATUS:**

**HEAD 2 TOE ASSESSMENT:**

**Scenario Question 1:**
What condition can be present in sepsis that can prevent vasopressor medications from being effective?

**Scenario Question 2:**
How is this condition (in question 1) corrected?

**Scenario Question 3:**
When should pressors be administered from a hemodynamic standpoint?

# CASE STUDY 7: RATIONALE

# ICU Trippin'

## PREDOMINANT PATHOPHYS

Sepsis; Adrenal insufficiency

## RSI REGIMEN

(Already intubated, but if they hadn't been…) Sedation: ketamine or fentanyl Avoid etomidate due to adrenal insufficiency); Paralysis: Roc (cautious with Sux– hyperkalemia); continued sedation: ketamine/fentanyl.

## VENTILATOR SETTINGS

IBW: 82kg. Adjust vent to: PC 20-22 (dangerous PIP and Pplat), target a minute ventilation of ~ 11-12 L/min by adjusting PC to achieve a Vte of ~ 650 and a of about RR 20, I:E 1:2, PEEP 5-7 (be ready to further support slowly dropping BP from increasing PEEP), FiO2 1.0.

## PERFUSION STATUS: COMPROMISED

## CORRECTIVE ACTION NEEDED:

The diagnosis of sepsis should trigger you to recall the septic symptoms: bounding HR, high CO, and low O2sats (if warm sepsis) and weak pulse, cold extremities, with low BP, low CO, and poor sats (if cold sepsis). The patient is hypoxic and hypotensive- so we will need to take control of the airway, ensure enough PEEP and FiO2 are applied (for oxygenation), as well as adequate minute ventilation (as directed by the patient's EtCO2). Vent changes: increase PEEP to 5-7; increase MV to 11-12 L/min, because this is the patient's underlying effort (f x Vte). The frequency is high, so the patient is over breathing the vent. Ketamine or fentanyl would be prudent here. Also- the PIP is high, and so is Pplat, therefore we have a lung compliance issue (high PIP and Pplat). We need to immediately switch to pressure control ventilation because every breath at that pressure (PIP 50 and Pplat 42) is damaging the lung further and increasing mortality. Change to PC 20- then target a Vte of 650cc by adjusting PC. If we increase the BP we will be able to trust our EtCO2 values.

## LABS:

Glucose, WBC, and platelets are all high– common pattern with sepsis. ABG: partially compensated metabolic acidosis with hypoxia.

## REQUIRED MANAGEMENT CHANGES BASED ON NEW INFORMATION:

This patient will need more fluid and a pressor- look at the BP and the hemodynamics. Low SVR is suggestive of distributive shock- like sepsis- so administer more fluids (this is supported by a upper– normal CVP and PCWP– thus not yet fluid overloaded). Additionally, PEEP needs to be increased to elevate oxygenation (pulse oximetry), and MV needs to increase. Even though we have reduced our EtCO2, we are not at the finish line until we get to the range of 35-45 mmHg. Increase MV in this case by increasing the RR or PC. RR is already high, so the best choice would be to go with increasing PC (say from 20-22) and then look at the Vte to see if there was an increase after the change. Otherwise provide routine critical care en route.

## QUESTION 1

Adrenal insufficiency. If a pressor is administered and there is no significant effect, HIGHLY consider adrenal insufficiency.

## QUESTION 2

IV administration of 50-100mg of hydrocortisone.

## QUESTION 3

If your CVP is normal, but your BP is persistently low (MAP <65) then it is time for pressors.

# Case Study 8

INITIAL:

A seven-year-old 60lb boy tripped near a propane-fueled burner while a group of family members was cooking outside. The contents spilled on his legs and abdomen, and he is being transferred to the regional burn center. As you arrive at the local hospital, you find the following: HR 118, RR 22, BP 112/ 72 O2 99%. You note second-degree burns over the entire anterior surface of both legs as well as to his entire abdomen (anterior only). Silvadene has been applied to the burns as well as a damp blanket.

## BP: 112/72 | HR: 118 | RR: 22 | SpO2: 99 | EtCO2: 42

ANY LIFE THREATS
NEEDING ADDRESSED?

| | | | | | |
|---|---|---|---|---|---|
| Na: | 138 | RBCs: | 3.9 | pH: | 7.4 |
| K: | 44 | WBCs: | 5 | pCO2: | 41 |
| Cl: | 97 | PLTs: | 162 | HCO3: | 24 |
| HCO$_3$: | 25 | HGB: | 14 | pO2: | 102 |
| Cr: | 12 | HCT: | 48 | BE: | 0 |
| BUN: | 0.3 | | | | |
| Glu: | 84 | | | | |

OTHER LAB/IMAGE INFO:

MANAGEMENT PLAN:

UPDATE: Turn to page #380 for an update. Look for UPDATE #8. Use this information to continue with the case and this form.

ADDITIONAL MANAGEMENT:

FINAL DIAGNOSES/PATHO?

RSI REGIMINE:

VENT SETTINGS:

PERFUSION STATUS:

HEAD 2 TOE ASSESSMENT:

**Scenario Question 1:**
When administering fluid resuscitation, what urine output should we target?

**Scenario Question 2:**
If this patient would have had thermal burns circumferentially around his thorax, how would you know when to perform an escharotomy?

## CASE STUDY 8: RATIONALE

# Blister in the Sun

### PREDOMINANT PATHOPHYS
Thermal burn; Burn fluid resuscitation

### RSI REGIMEN
Sedation: Versed or Etomidate; Paralysis: Sux or Roc; Continued sedation: versed; Pain management: fentanyl. Remember succinylcholine is ok here because you are not 24 hours AFTER the burn.

### VENTILATOR SETTINGS:
IBW: 27kg; Pressure control (PC 18-22) or Volume control (TV 130-200 cc); Target VE: 5 L/min (no acidosis); normal minute ventilation for a 27 kg child is approximately 5 L/min (@ 200 mL/kg/min); RR 20-30 (but if you use different RR and Vt, just make sure you are targeting the minute ventilation of 5 L/min for this patient), I:E 1:2– 1:3; PEEP 3-5; FiO2 1.0.

### PERFUSION STATUS: STABLE

### CORRECTIVE ACTION NEEDED
Since this is a fluid/thermal burn that does not affect his airway, then we can assume if he's talking, his airway is patent. If his oxygenation is 95% or better, then we can assume that he's oxygenating well. His vital signs indicate he is hemodynamically stable, with a little bit of tachycardia- most likely from the pain of the burn. Therefore, our treatment will be aimed at removing the wet blanket applying dry sheets, initiating an IV, and providing fluid resuscitation and pain medication. Percent body surface area of 2nd° burns: 21.5% (both anterior surfaces of legs = one full leg = 12.5%; Front of abdomen equals 9%). Therefore, the patient needs 1170cc (21.5 x 27.2 x 2 = 1170 cc) in 24 hours (Consensus Formula). Therefore, they need half of this (584 cc) in the first 8 hours and thus need 73cc/ hr to achieve these fluid rates. Consider pain management: fentanyl or morphine or equivalent.

### LABS
Serum: Normal. ABG: normal, except for slight hyperoxia.

### REQUIRED MANAGEMENT CHANGES BASED ON NEW INFORMATION
The patient has been over fluid resuscitated- one thing that increases mortality. To correct this, we subtract the volume already administered from the volume to be infused over the first 8 hours. Then divide the result by number of hours remaining for the first 8 hours (since burn to get the NEW fluid resuscitation infusion rate). It goes like this: total in 24 hours needed: 1170 cc. Divide this by 2 (1170/2 = 584). Subtract the fluid administered since the burn by 584 cc (584-300= 284). Therefore, 284cc should be administered in the remaining 5 hours. So, 284/5 = 57 cc/hr (new maintenance infusion rate). Additionally, if the child is still in pain, then administer more pain medication. A pain that is 'not bad' is still a pain. Provide pain medication often as needed pending no hemodynamic or respiratory compromise.

### QUESTION1
1-2 cc/kg/hr; this tells us that we have adequate intravascular volume.

### QUESTION 2
This should be performed when there is little to no chest rise and fall, sudden hypoxia, increased PIP (in mechanically ventilated patients) and obviously in the presence of a circumferential thoracic thermal burn.

# Case Study 9

**INITIAL:**

An 8 y/o 52 lbs child was at a creek swimming hole with his family when he dove off of a high branch and then didn't resurface for 6-7 minutes. The child's family performed CPR until a fire EMS unit arrived and took over CPR and C-spine. Upon your arrival, your patient presents with a GCS 6 (E1,V1,T4), a fixed leftward and upward gaze, is in PEA, and has a fire-medic performing CPR and BVM ventilations. Vitals: HR 44 (PEA), BP 0, RR 20 (assisted with BVM), O2 unreadable, and EtCO2 8mm.

## BP: none | HR: 44 (PEA) | RR: 20 (BVM) | SpO2: 0 | EtCO2: 7

**ANY LIFE THREATS NEEDING ADDRESSED?**

| | | | | | |
|---|---|---|---|---|---|
| Na: | XXX | RBCs: | XXX | pH: | 7.21 |
| K: | XXX | WBCs: | XXX | pCO2: | 78 |
| Cl: | XXX | PLTs: | XXX | HCO3: | 15 |
| HCO3: | XXX | HGB: | XXX | pO2: | 39 |
| Cr: | XXX | HCT: | XXX | BE: | -6 |
| BUN: | XXX | | | | |
| Glu: | XXX | | | | |

**OTHER LAB/IMAGE INFO:**

**MANAGEMENT PLAN:**

**UPDATE: Turn to page #381 for an update. Look for UPDATE #9. Use this information to continue with the case and this form.**

**ADDITIONAL MANAGEMENT:**

**FINAL DIAGNOSES/PATHO?**

**RSI REGIMINE:**

**VENT SETTINGS:**

**PERFUSION STATUS:**

**HEAD 2 TOE ASSESSMENT:**

**Scenario Question 1:**
Per PALS, what should the EtCO2 increase to by the third minute of CPR if adequate chest compressions are administered?

**Scenario Question 2:**
What is the dose of epinephrine in pediatric PEA?

# Born on the Bayou

**PREDOMINANT PATHOPHYS**
Drowning; PALS

**RSI REGIMEN**
(Assume the patient wasn't in arrest and was hemodynamically stable, then...): sedative: versed, or fentanyl; paralysis: Sux or Roc; continued sedation with versed or fentanyl.

**VENTILATOR SETTINGS**
IBW: 24kg; SIMV or AC on volume ventilation (Vt ~ 150-200 cc) or pressure ventilation (PC 15-20 cmH2O); Target a minute ventilation of ~ 5-6 L/min is a good starting point (assume acidosis from prolonged poor perfusion from cardiac arrest); RR 25-35/min; I:E 1:2; PEEP 5-8 cmH2O (need more PEEP due to drowning); FiO2 1.0. Some clinicians have mentioned they'd like even higher PEEPs in this case (with drownings). Be aware that you may need to increase PEEP much beyond normal ranges (upwards beyond 15 cmH2O is normal in these cases)–then be sure to support BP should it drop due to PEEP.

**PERFUSION STATUS: COMPROMISED.**

**CORRECTIVE ACTION NEEDED**
Every time you are going to take over care from another team, it is important to ensure for certain whether the patient was being treated adequately. (Note- I didn't say be a jerk about it, but you need to know if the patient is heading in the right direction or if they have been heading in the wrong direction). In this case, we have two mechanisms: drowning and possible neck/ head injury. The crew has been doing CPR, but has it been effective? NO- evidenced by the low EtCO2. Direct the CPR givers to either improve the compressions or switch rescuers. After compressions have been fixed, apply your defibrillator pads and assess for a shockable rhythm (don't wait for the CPR cycle to end). You'd shock if needed and quickly resume CPR if not. The plan needs to be to start an IV or IO and to get the child intubated (they'll need lots of PEEP as a drowning patient).

**LABS**
ABG: Mixed acidosis with hypoxia.

**REQUIRED MANAGEMENT CHANGES BASED ON NEW INFORMATION**
First, the BP is low, so we will need to administer a fluid bolus. Because the patient experienced cardiac arrest resulting in lower perfusion (from poor CPR), then it is safe to assume acidosis has occurred. The heart will not want to beat because all that acid is around it (along with every other organ) and it will not want to beat as strongly, therefore we need to add an inotrope (epi, norepi, dopamine). Next, the patient's minute ventilation is too low: f x Vte = MV= 4.9 L/min. We know this is too low because the EtCO2 is 71. Next, we can see that the RR setting is too low, but luckily the patient is over breathing the vent- which is a saving grace in this case. Sedate or paralyze the patient, so you are controlling the ventilator effort- otherwise you are not controlling your patient's ventilation and FAILING to control their physiology. Additionally, the patient has a dead space problem shown by their low Vte and it not closely matching the set TV. Typically this is due to either leak or dead space. Increase the TV setting to ensure the Vte (the volume coming out of the patient's lungs) matches the set TV (the volume you want going into the lungs). In this case, increase the TV setting to 350 so that the Vte number gets higher and closer to the TV you want the patient to receive. Then, reassess to ensure the new RR and TV combination (minute ventilation) are adequate (indicated by a lowering EtCO2). Consider increasing the I:E to 1:4-5 because it is pediatric. Finally, increase PEEP to improve the pulse oximetry.

**QUESTION 1**
With adequate chest compressions, the EtCO2 should increase from ~ < 10 mmHg at the beginning of cardiac arrest to 12.5- 20 mmHg by the third minute.

**QUESTION 2**
0.01 mg/kg IV/IO every 3-5 minutes (1:10,000), or 0.1 mg/kg via ETT (1:1000).

# Case Study 10

## BP: 128/79 | HR: 108 | RR: 21 | SpO2: 98 | EtCO2: 43

**ANY LIFE THREATS NEEDING ADDRESSED?**

| | | | | | |
|---|---|---|---|---|---|
| Na: | 144 | RBCs: | 2.8 | pH: | 7.37 |
| K: | 6.6 | WBCs: | 9 | pCO2: | 44 |
| Cl: | 99 | PLTs: | 202 | HCO3: | 22 |
| HCO$_3$: | 23 | HGB: | 12 | pO2: | 92 |
| Cr: | 24 | HCT: | 42 | BE: | 0 |
| BUN: | 2.1 | | | | |
| Glu: | 152 | | | | |

**OTHER LAB/IMAGE INFO:**

**MANAGEMENT PLAN:**

**UPDATE: Turn to page #379 for an update. Look for UPDATE #10. Use this information to continue with the case and this form.**

**ADDITIONAL MANAGEMENT:**

**FINAL DIAGNOSES/PATHO?**

**RSI REGIMINE:**

**VENT SETTINGS:**

**PERFUSION STATUS:**

**HEAD 2 TOE ASSESSMENT:**

**Scenario Question 1:** What RSI medications should be avoided in this trauma patient?

**Scenario Question 2:** Is Cushing's Sign being observed in this case?

**Scenario Question 3:** When BP, pulse oximetry, and EtCO2 all drop together acutely in a trauma patient, what is high on your differential diagnosis?

# CASE STUDY 10: RATIONALE

# Hi, Por que!?

**PREDOMINANT PATHOPHYS**
AMS from closed head injury; dialysis patient (fistula present) therefore, (+) hyperkalemia.

**RSI REGIMEN**
AVOID SUX!!! Sedative: versed, or fentanyl; pain: fentanyl; Paralysis: Roc; continued sedation with versed or fentanyl). Administering succinylcholine will trigger massive hyperkalemia —> malignant hyperthermia or masseter muscle spasm.

**VENTILATOR SETTINGS**
IBW: 82kg; SIMV or AC on volume ventilation (Vt about 500 cc) or pressure ventilation (PC 15-20); Target a minute ventilation of ~ 8 L/min is a good starting point (no reason to assume acidosis); RR about 17- but if you use different RR and Vt, just make sure you are targeting the minute ventilation of 8 L/min for this patient; I:E 1:2; Peep 3-5 cmH2O; FiO2 1.0 (wean down if possible).

**PERFUSION STATUS: STABLE**

**CORRECTIVE ACTION NEEDED**
This patient has suffered a closed head injury; so, we need to be mindful of primary and secondary intracranial insult. We need to prevent even one episode of hypoxia and hypotension. Spinal precautions, high flow oxygen, preparing to intubate (to protect airway and crew), ensure patency on two large bore IVs, and prevent further hyperkalemia from avoiding SUX. This patient is a dialysis patient (exhibited by the fistula) and thus has a high chance of having hyperkalemia. Hyperkalemia is also confirmed in the labs (K+ 5.7).

**LABS**
Serum: (+) hyperkalemia with a potassium of 5.7 mmol/L. ABG: normal.

**REQUIRED MANAGEMENT CHANGES BASED ON NEW INFORMATION**
In this scenario, the clinician administered succinylcholine, which then sent the patient into further hyperkalemia, thus causing cardiac arrest. Hopefully, you wanted to avoid sux. Should you ever experience this situation (giving sux to someone hyperkalemic, here is the treatment: administer calcium to be cardio-protective, administer sodium bicarbonate to buffer the acid created and to alkalize the serum, administer glucose with insulin. The potassium sticks to the big glucose molecules, and the insulin forces the glucose–potassium mixture into the cells and out of the blood. Dantrolene is an ideal drug for malignant hyperthermia, but it is impractical because of cost and availability.

**QUESTION 1**
The only medication that should be avoided is succinylcholine. The patient is a dialysis patient and should not be administered sux.

**QUESTION 2**
No. Crushing's sign would present with high BP and low heart rate. The high BP is the body's effort to hold open cerebral blood vessels (higher pressure means vessel remains open). Our heart thinks something is wrong and slows HR down to bring down BP. The heart doesn't realize what the brain is doing. In this case we have both tachycardia and hypertension, so no, Cushing's is not occurring.

**QUESTION 3**
In trauma, it is hard not to add tension pneumothorax to a differential diagnosis. In the air, you cannot hear breath sounds, so being aware of your BP, EtCO2, and pulse oximetry is important. If they all fall together, then a tension pneumothorax is a strong frontrunner as the cause.

# Case Study 11

You are responding to a rural hospital for a 56 y/o seizure patient. Upon arrival, the RN staff informs you that wife reports going to bed and being awoken by the patient who was violently convulsing. He has no medical history. The patient has been administered 5mg of Valium (30 minutes ago), has had an IV placed as well as a Foley. Within minutes of your arrival, the patient begins seizing again (tonic- clonic) and you notice one side of the patient's body has more violent jerking motions than the other. The vitals are listed below, and a nurse hands you the lab work. Pt wt: 210 lbs; height: 6'1".

## BP: 118/70 | HR: 108 | RR: 20 | SpO2: 93 | EtCO2: 38

**ANY LIFE THREATS NEEDING ADDRESSED?**

| | | | | | |
|---|---|---|---|---|---|
| Na: | 141 | RBCs: | 4 | pH: | 7.36 |
| K: | 3.8 | WBCs: | 7 | pCO2: | 38 |
| Cl: | 99 | PLTs: | 256 | HCO3: | 23 |
| CO2: | 23 | HGB: | 14 | pO2: | 99 |
| Cr: | 8.1 | HCT: | 42 | BE: | 0 |
| BUN: | 0.8 | | | | |
| Glu: | 121 | | | | |

**OTHER LAB/IMAGE INFO:**

PTT 58s

INR: 3.1

**MANAGEMENT PLAN:**

**UPDATE: Turn to page #380 for an update. Look for UPDATE #11. Use this information to continue with the case and this form.**

**ADDITIONAL MANAGEMENT:**

**FINAL DIAGNOSES/PATHO?**

**RSI REGIMINE:**

**VENT SETTINGS:**

**PERFUSION STATUS:**

**HEAD 2 TOE ASSESSMENT:**

Scenario Question 1:
What is a common epidural bleed pattern on head CT?

Scenario Question 2:
What is a common subdural bleed pattern on head CT?

Scenario Question 3:
What is a common subarachnoid bleed pattern on head CT?

# Shake It Like a Polaroid Picture

## PREDOMINANT PATHOPHYS
Altered mental status, seizure, brain herniation

## RSI REGIMEN
Sedative: versed (for sedative and anticonvulsant properties); Pain: fentanyl; Paralysis: Succinylcholine or rocuronium; continued sedation with versed.

## VENTILATOR SETTINGS

IBW: 80kg. SIMV or AC; volume ventilation (TV ~ 480 cc) or pressure ventilation (PC 15-20); Target a minute ventilation of ~ 8 L/min is a good starting point (no reason to assume acidosis); RR 17- but if you use different RR and Vt, just make sure you are targeting the minute ventilation of 8 L/min for this patient; I:E 1:2; PEEP 3-5 cmH2O; FiO2 1.0 (wean down if possible).

## PERFUSION STATUS: STABLE

## CORRECTIVE ACTION NEEDED
Obviously, we need to protect the patient from hitting anything or falling off gurney during the seizure. Support ABCs (high flow O2, assisted ventilations with any shallow effort producing pulse oximetry < 95%). You should be preparing to intubate (altered metal status, aspiration risk) with RSI. Also, you should be preparing medications to stop seizures (luckily, benzos are also anticonvulsants). The real question is why the seizure is occurring and why there are more violent convulsions on one side of the body. This is because the patient's seizure is most likely due to a hemorrhagic stroke (perhaps a subarachnoid hemorrhage, or SAH, from a ruptured vessel). Does the patient have any labs to confirm this?- yes. His coagulation labs are abnormally high (meaning it takes a long time to coagulate). This can lead to an SAH. RSI: Sedative: versed (for sedative and anticonvulsant properties); Pain: fentanyl; Paralysis: Succinylcholine or rocuronium; continued sedation with versed.

## LABS
Serum PTT and INR are HIGH– suggest increased bleeding. ABG: normal.

## REQUIRED MANAGEMENT CHANGES BASED ON NEW INFORMATION
The CT reflects a subarachnoid hemorrhage. This expanding mass will be displacing the brain tissue causing herniation, therefore, keep an eye on pupils- when one pupil becomes fixed and dilated, that means herniation is occurring at that moment. Treat the patient with seizure prophylaxis and Mannitol (if herniation is present). The PTT and INR indicate longer clotting times, therefore, could be the cause of the hemorrhage. Consider vitamin K (clotting factor) to correct this.

## QUESTION 1
Convex in nature because the bleed is outside the dura trapped between the bone and the covering of the brain. The epidural blood cannot typically cross suture lines within the cranial anatomy.

## QUESTION 2
Concave in nature because the bleed follows the curve of the brain and looks like a flattened pancake.

## QUESTION 3
Starfish pattern and an illuminated Circle of Willis. Blood collects in the subarachnoid space and is seen in this particular pattern.

# Case Study 12

**INITIAL:**

You're responding to a local 10 bed ICU where a 60 y/o man presents with severe chest pain. He was admitted 6 days prior for pneumonia but has remained awake the entire time. The patient is being treated for on- going nonspecific chest pain. Upon arrival, you note you patient to have sweaty, pale skin; respiratory difficulty; and he is anxious. Vital signs are in the box below, and the 12-Lead can be found in Appendix A, ECG #7. The patient becomes increasingly hypoxic and then passes out. Pt wt.: 315 lbs.; Ht: 5'11''.

## BP: 132/77 | HR: 65 | RR: 18 | SpO2: 88 | EtCO2: 41

**ANY LIFE THREATS NEEDING ADDRESSED?**

| | | | | | |
|---|---|---|---|---|---|
| Na: | 145 | RBCs: | 4 | pH: | 7.39 |
| K: | 4.8 | WBCs: | 8.2 | pCO2: | 42 |
| Cl: | 97 | PLTs: | 352 | HCO3: | 34 |
| HCO$_3$: | 42 | HGB: | 13 | pO2: | 110 |
| Cr: | 9.3 | HCT: | 46 | BE: | 0 |
| BUN: | 1.1 | | | | |
| Glu: | 134 | | | | |

**OTHER LAB/IMAGE INFO:**

**MANAGEMENT PLAN:**

**UPDATE: Turn to page #381 for an update. Look for UPDATE #12. Use this information to continue with the case and this form.**

**ADDITIONAL MANAGEMENT:**

FINAL DIAGNOSES/PATHO?

**RSI REGIMINE:**

**VENT SETTINGS:**

**PERFUSION STATUS:**

**HEAD 2 TOE ASSESSMENT:**

**Scenario Question 1:**
List the 3 main criteria of Sgarbossa Criteria.

**Scenario Question 2:**
Which vasoactive medication(s) would have increased contractility and cause vasoconstriction?

**Scenario Question 3:**
After the administration of dobutamine, how would you expect your hemodynamic parameters to change?

# CASE STUDY 12: RATIONALE

# Achy Breaky Heart

## PREDOMINANT PATHOPHYS
AMI, Sgarbossa criteria

## RSI REGIMEN
sedative: versed, or fentanyl; paralysis: Sux or Roc; continued sedation with versed or fentanyl).

## VENTILATOR SETTINGS
IBW: 75 kg; SIMV or AC;  Volume ventilation (Vt ~ 450cc) or pressure ventilation (PC 15-20); Target a minute ventilation of ~ 7.5 L/min is a good starting point; RR about 17- but if you use different RR and Vt, just make sure you are targeting the minute ventilation of about 7.5 L/min for this patient; I:E 1:2; PEEP 3-5 cmH2O; FiO2 1.0.

## PERFUSION STATUS: STABLE

## CORRECTIVE ACTION NEEDED
Did you catch the Sgarbossa criteria? There is concordant (same side) QRS complex and ST-elevation > or = 1 mm in V2, and discordant (opposite side) ST segment elevation > or =  1/4 the depth of the S wave of the QRS in V1.  Every time there is left bundle branch block (LBBB) present on the 12 lead, you should look for Sgarbossa criteria. When present, Sgarbossa criteria can strongly indicate the presence of an AMI in the presence of LBBB.  Additionally, the patient passes out right in front of you. You'll need to establish an airway and maintain clinically appropriate ventilations. This patient is experiencing an AMI, and, therefore, will need to be cathed ASAP. Begin treating with MONA and highly consider a nitroglycerin drip. Also, consider heparin. Normally a beta blocker is indicated, but not in this case because the patient is hypotensive.

## LABS
Serum: (+) hyperglycemia  ABG: other than hyperoxia, it is normal.

## REQUIRED MANAGEMENT CHANGES BASED ON NEW INFORMATION
Blood pressure must be corrected because the diastolic pressure feeds the coronary arteries.  With hypoperfusion in AMI, patients die due to poor myocardial perfusion. You can bypass the fluid in this case because the CVP and wedge pressure indicate there is fluid overload. Therefore, you need some type of pressor or inotrope. In this case, your SVR is very high which would mean your heart has to work hard to pump against it, so a medication that causes a little vasodilation would help this patient. Additionally, better pumping power would help this patient. Dobutamine would perform both mechanisms: vasodilation and increase contractility. Also, the patient needs to be sedated (look at how high the frequency is- he is waking up). You can address low pulse oximetry by first fixing blood pressure (to be able to trust your pulse oximetry and end tidal CO2), then max out FiO2 followed by increasing PEEP should pulse oximetry still be low.

## QUESTION 1
List the 3 main criteria of Sgarbossa criteria.: 1) concordant ST segment elevation > or = 1 mm with the QRS complex; 2) concordant ST segment depression > = 1 mm in leads V1- V3; and 3) discordant ST segment elevation > or =1/4 the depth of the S wave.

## QUESTION 2
Dopamine, epinephrine, norepinephrine

## QUESTION 3
CVP, wedge pressure should reduce, and SVR should reduce while CO should increase.

# Case Study 13

You are transporting a 24-year-old male who was in a bar altercation earlier this evening involving a broken beer bottle. As you arrive at the patient's bedside, you find the following: 4 cm laceration of the scalp, 7-inch laceration on the left arm at the deltoid, and a small puncture wound on the right side of the abdomen at the level of the umbilicus. You find the patient on the hospital stretcher, awake alert and answering questions, with the following vital signs: BP 91/50, HR 112, RR 21, pulse oximetry 92%, and an EtCO2 32. The patient has a normal carotid pulse but has no radial pulse. Pt wt.: 185 lbs.; Ht: 6'3".

## BP: 89/50 | HR: 112 | RR: 21 | SpO2: 92 | EtCO2: 50

**ANY LIFE THREATS NEEDING ADDRESSED?**

| | | | | | |
|---|---|---|---|---|---|
| Na: | 137 | RBCs: | 2.8 | pH: | 7.34 |
| K: | 4.3 | WBCs: | 6.2 | pCO2: | 51 |
| Cl: | 100 | PLTs: | 277 | HCO3: | 22 |
| $CO_2$: | 22 | HGB: | 6.5 | pO2: | 78 |
| Cr: | 8.2 | HCT: | 28 | BE: | -1 |
| BUN: | 0.6 | | | | |
| Glu: | 99 | | | | |

**OTHER LAB/IMAGE INFO:**

**MANAGEMENT PLAN:**

**UPDATE: Turn to page #379 for an update. Look for UPDATE #13. Use this information to continue with the case and this form.**

**ADDITIONAL MANAGEMENT:**

FINAL DIAGNOSES/PATHO?

**RSI REGIMINE:**

**VENT SETTINGS:**

**PERFUSION STATUS:**

**HEAD 2 TOE ASSESSMENT:**

**Scenario Question 1:**
At what point is it prudent to administer a pressor to a trauma patient?

**Scenario Question 2:**
How much do you anticipate the hematocrit rising after 3 units of PRBCs?

**Scenario Question 3:**
At what hemoglobin level should blood products be started?

## CASE STUDY 13: RATIONALE

# Keep Bleedin' Love

### PREDOMINANT PATHOPHYS
Trauma, knife stabbing, shock

### RSI REGIMEN
Sedation (ketamine, fentanyl); pain (fentanyl); paralysis (succinylcholine or rocuronium); continued sedation (fentanyl or ketamine); roc for continued paralysis if needed.

### VENTILATOR SETTINGS
IBW: 84.5kg; SIMV or A/C; PC (15-20 cmH2O) or volume control (Vt approximately 510 cc); targeting a VE of 10 L/min; RR approximately 20- but if you use different RR and Vt, just make sure you are targeting the minute ventilation of about 10 L/min for this patient; I:E 1:2; PEEP 3-5; FiO2 1.0.

### PERFUSION STATUS: UNSTABLE

### CORRECTIVE ACTION NEEDED
This patient is experiencing class III shock, also known as decompensated shock, from one of the bleeding sources. Even though they have a 91 systolic blood pressure, they do not have a radial pulse, which means he is not perfusing all of his distal tissues. This is the definition of decompensated shock. Step one is to ensure we have adequate oxygen delivery. Therefore, we need an open airway (confirmed with speech and following commands) and a high FiO2 (O2 on non-rebreather). Second, we need to make sure that the patient is no longer bleeding. We need to look at all of the bleeding sites and ensure they have been stopped. Additionally, we can get a baseline H/H to identify of bleeding is still occurring. We also need to support the BP with fluid blouses and packed red blood cells. We should be targeting a MAP of 90 mmHg as well as a return of distal pulses.

### LABS
Serum: Anemic (low H/H) ABG: Acute respiratory acidosis with hypoxia.

### REQUIRED MANAGEMENT CHANGES BASED ON NEW INFORMATION
Anytime you have the H/H information available to you in a bleeding patent, especially one you're going to be administering blood to, it is a good idea to use it to identify if bleeding is still occurring. Remember, for each unit of PRBCs you administer, HGB should go up 1 g/dL and should increase HCT 3%. If you have the original H/H data, then you can use to compare to the blood you give in route. If the new H/H doesn't increase as expected based on the blood you gave, then bleeding is still going on, and you may need to be more aggressive with blood administration.

### QUESTION 1
When there is evidence of fluid overload (rales, high CVP) and hypotension is risking further acidosis.

### QUESTION 2
Three (3) units of PRBCs is expected to raise the hematocrit by 9% (3% for each unit of PRBCs).

### QUESTION 3
It is prudent to begin blood products when the hemoglobin reaches 7 g/dL.

# Case Study 14

**INITIAL:**

A 40 y/o female is in her 3rd pregnancy and begins complaining of severe abdominal pain. The patient is 27 weeks gestation with 2 other normal term deliveries. The patient's skin is cool and pale. Just before your arrival, the patient discharges a large amount of fluid from her vagina. The fluid is mostly clear with a bloody tinge and streaks of dark green particulate substance. A vaginal exam reveals dilated 9cm, fully effaced, and a +2 station. Vitals: HR 110, BP 96/70, RR 22, pulse oximetry 98%. Pt wt.: 135 lbs.; Ht: 5'1''.

## BP: 96/70 | HR: 110 | RR: 23 | SpO2: 98 | EtCO2: 39

**ANY LIFE THREATS NEEDING ADDRESSED?**

| | | | | | |
|---|---|---|---|---|---|
| Na: | 140 | RBCs: | 5 | pH: | 7.38 |
| K: | 4.2 | WBCs: | 9 | pCO2: | 39 |
| Cl: | 101 | PLTs: | 179 | HCO3: | 23 |
| HCO$_3$: | 23 | HGB: | 16 | pO2: | 99 |
| Cr: | 9.0 | HCT: | 46 | BE: | 0 |
| BUN: | 1.0 | | | | |
| Glu: | 142 | | | | |

**OTHER LAB/IMAGE INFO:**

**MANAGEMENT PLAN:**

**UPDATE: Turn to page #380 for an update. Look for UPDATE #14. Use this information to continue with the case and this form.**

**ADDITIONAL MANAGEMENT:**

**FINAL DIAGNOSES/PATHO?**

**RSI REGIMINE:**

**VENT SETTINGS:**

**PERFUSION STATUS:**

**HEAD 2 TOE ASSESSMENT:**

**Scenario Question 1:**
At this gestational age, what complications should you be prepared to manage?

**Scenario Question 2:**
What is the chest compression rate and compression to ventilation ratio required in NRP?

**Scenario Question 3:**
What is the baby's initial (1 minute) APGAR score?

## CASE STUDY 14: RATIONALE

# Push It! Push It Real Good!

### PREDOMINANT PATHOPHYS
Imminent delivery,  NRP

### RSI REGIMEN
Sedation (ketamine, fentanyl); pain (fentanyl); paralysis (succinylcholine or rocuronium); continued sedation (fentanyl or ketamine); roc for continued paralysis.

### VENTILATOR SETTINGS
IBW: 47.8kg; SIMV or A/C; Target MV of 4-5 L/min as a starting point. PC (15-20 cmH2O) or volume control (TV 250-350 cc); RR 17- but if you use different RR and Vt, just make sure you are targeting the minute ventilation of about 4-5 L/min for this patient;  I:E 1:3; PEEP 3-5; FiO2 1.0.

### PERFUSION STATUS: STABLE

### CORRECTIVE ACTION NEEDED
This patient is in labor, and the fetus (who is trying to deliver) is incredibly premature. First- ensure the mother has ABCs maintained: high flow oxygen via NRB, ensure 2 large bore IVs, and be prepared to support mom's hemodynamics. The patient's amniotic sac and fluid rupturing indicate labor isn't far away.  The presence of meconium indicates the fetus is/ was in distress (hypoxic)- this should trigger you to be aggressive with oxygenation efforts for both mom and baby. Meconium also suggests meconium aspiration, so the baby's airway needs to be suctioned via meconium aspirator upon delivery. Be prepared to intubate, suction, ventilate, and administer surfactant upon delivery. Be prepared for NRP procedures. Fully effaced and 9cm dilated means that delivery is eminent.

### LABS
Serum: Hyperglycemic, otherwise normal. ABG: Normal.

### REQUIRED MANAGEMENT CHANGES BASED ON NEW INFORMATION
MOM: monitor for post– partum hemorrhage and shock. Treat shock with fluids, blood,  and potentially pressors. Treat post– partum hemorrhage with Pitocin.

INFANT: The infant is not breathing and blue, therefore, it's respirations should be immediately assisted. If the HR improves to > 60 bpm within 60 seconds, then ventilations only are to be continued. However, if HR remains below 60, then chest compressions will need to be started in addition to continuing ventilations.

### QUESTION 1
Fetuses of this gestational age will not be producing surfactant yet, and will require assisted ventilations, intubation, and most likely surfactant administration.

### QUESTION 2
120 in a minute using a 3:1 compression to ventilation ratio.

### QUESTION 3
APGAR (Appearance, pulse, grimace, activity, respiration rate) is graded as 0-10 with each of the five categories graded individually 0-2. At delivery, this patient was found to be: limp (activity 0), no respiratory effort (respiratory effort 0), peripherally cyanotic (appearance 1), no facial expressions (grimace 0), and a pulse rate of 42/ min (pulse 1). Minute 1 APGARs is therefore 2. An APGAR of 0-3 is termed severely depressed, 4-6 is moderately depressed, and  7-10 is excellent condition.

# Case Study 15

## BP: 106/74 | HR: 79 | RR: 16 (vent) | SpO2: 98 | EtCO2: 24

**ANY LIFE THREATS NEEDING ADDRESSED?**

| | | | | | |
|---|---|---|---|---|---|
| Na: | 137 | RBCs: | 4 | pH: | 7.42 |
| K: | 4.4 | WBCs: | 10.1 | pCO2: | 33 |
| Cl: | 99 | PLTs: | 201 | HCO3: | 24 |
| HCO$_3$: | 24 | HGB: | 13 | pO2: | 106 |
| Cr: | 7.9 | HCT: | 42 | BE: | 0 |
| BUN: | 0.8 | | | | |
| Glu: | 101 | | | | |

**OTHER LAB/IMAGE INFO:**

**MANAGEMENT PLAN:**

**UPDATE: Turn to page #381 for an update. Look for UPDATE #15. Use this information to continue with the case and this form.**

**ADDITIONAL MANAGEMENT:**

FINAL DIAGNOSES/PATHO?

**RSI REGIMINE:**

**VENT SETTINGS:**

**PERFUSION STATUS:**

**HEAD 2 TOE ASSESSMENT:**

**Scenario Question 1:** What are the morphological characteristics of early inflation?

**Scenario Question 2:** What are the morphological characteristics of late inflation?

**Scenario Question 3:** What are the morphological characteristics of early deflation?

**Scenario Question 4:** What are the morphological characteristics of late deflation?

# CASE STUDY 15: RATIONALE

# Pump Up the Jam

## PREDOMINANT PATHOPHYS
IABP timing

## RSI REGIMEN
Sedation (ketamine, fentanyl); pain (fentanyl); paralysis (succinylcholine or rocuronium); continued sedation (fentanyl or ketamine); roc for continued paralysis.

## VENTILATOR SETTINGS
IBW: 73kg; Target minute ventilation: 7-8 L/min since no acidosis is present); The patient vent settings indicate an expected minute ventilation of 7.5, however, the true minute ventilation is 9.4, therefore, look to see what's causing patient/ vent dyssynchrony: in this case, TV is set at 470, but Vte is only 450 (not too bad a difference). The RR is set at 16, and the f is 21 (this is the problem). Therefore, the true VE is Vte x f, which is 9.4 L/min.  The PEEP at 4 cmH2O and FiO2 of 1.0 is adequate (proven by a SpO2 of 98%). You could consider attempting to wean the vent if hemodynamics remains stable.

## PERFUSION STATUS: POTENTIALLY COMPROMISED

## CORRECTIVE ACTION NEEDED
This patient needs to have their IABP timing assessed and optimized, in addition, to ensuring that all treatments are appropriate. First, the patient's ventilator settings should be assessed (see above). Looking at the ABG, this matches- as the ABG reflects an acute respiratory alkalosis, therefore, sedate the patient to prevent over- breathing the ventilator. This will allow you to control the patient's respirations. Additionally, the FiO2 can be reduced because the O2 is 322 mmHg. Also, the IABP timing displays early inflation, therefore, adjust timing for inflation to be at the aortic notch. Consider RSI (sedative: ketamine or fentanyl; paralysis: Sux or Roc; continued sedation with ketamine or fentanyl; avoid any meds that would drop BP).

## LABS
Serum: Hyperglycemic, otherwise normal. ABG: Slightly hyperoxic; CO2 slightly low.

## REQUIRED MANAGEMENT CHANGES BASED ON NEW INFORMATION
This IABP reflects early deflation; therefore, the timing needs to move to a later deflation point, and then reassess the tracing. Early deflation means there is a is a loss of the increased coronary perfusion pressure. When the balloon expands, it forces blood above it backwards through the aorta, to the aortic root, and backwards still into the coronary arteries. When deflation is early, this coronary perfusion time is cut short. The benefit is minimized.

## QUESTION 1
Early Inflation: Balloon inflates way before the dicrotic notch. This violates IABP Rule #1. Result: this forces the aortic valve closed, ¯ stroke volume, and ↑ left ventricle workload.

## QUESTION 2
 Late inflation: the balloon inflates after the dicrotic notch and exposes the dicrotic notch for viewing. This also violates IABP Rule #1. Result: ¯ coronary perfusion pressure.

## QUESTION 3
Early Deflation: Swiftly down sloping diastolic pressure which causes a U– shaped diastolic curvature. Also, the augmented systolic BP is not lower, but the same as the patient's unassisted systolic BP. This violates IABP Rule #3.  Result: no ¯ in afterload = no real IABP benefit.

## QUESTION 4
 Late Deflation: there is a widened diastolic pressure. Also, the augmented end– diastolic pressure is not lower, but the same or higher than the patient's unassisted end– diastolic pressure. This violates IABP Rule #2. Result: ↑ left ventricle workload.

# Case Study 16

You are responding to a very small ER in rural America where a pregnant patient (G1, P0, A0) needs to be transferred to a higher level of care for PIH complications. She is 35 weeks gestation and is currently having abdominal pains. See the FHT monitor tracing in Appendix C, FHT #2. The patient weighs 220 lbs and has no other medical history. Pt height: 5'9''.

## BP: 162/104 | HR: 95 | RR: 14 | SpO2: 98 | EtCO2: 39

ANY LIFE THREATS
NEEDING ADDRESSED?

| | | | | | |
|---|---|---|---|---|---|
| Na: | 135 | RBCs: | 3.8 | pH: | 7.39 |
| K: | 3.6 | WBCs: | 10.1 | pCO2: | 40 |
| Cl: | 97 | PLTs: | 201 | HCO3: | 22 |
| $HCO_3$: | 22 | HGB: | 13 | pO2: | 93 |
| Cr: | 11 | HCT: | 42 | BE: | 0 |
| BUN: | 1.2 | | | | |
| Glu: | 144 | | | | |

OTHER LAB/IMAGE INFO:

MANAGEMENT PLAN:

UPDATE: Turn to page #379 for an update. Look for UPDATE #16. Use this information to continue with the case and this form.

ADDITIONAL MANAGEMENT:

FINAL DIAGNOSES/PATHO?

RSI REGIMINE:

VENT SETTINGS:

PERFUSION STATUS:

HEAD 2 TOE ASSESSMENT:

**Scenario Question 1:**
What is the treatment of choice for this patient should eclampsia develop and why?

**Scenario Question 2:**
What is the danger of administering the above medicine?

**Scenario Question 3:**
What other lab work should you be anticipating?

# CASE STUDY 16: RATIONALE

# Signed, Sealed Delivered

## PREDOMINANT PATHOPHYS
OB, FHT tracing, variability

## RSI REGIMEN
Sedation (versed, fentanyl); pain (fentanyl); paralysis (succinylcholine or rocuronium); continued sedation (fentanyl or versed); roc for continued paralysis. Avoid ketamine as it will worsen hypertension.

## VENTILATOR SETTINGS
IBW: 66kg; PC (15-20 cmH2O) or volume control (TV 400 cc); Target a minute ventilation of about 7 L/min; RR 17- but if you use different RR and Vt, just make sure you are targeting the minute ventilation of about 7 L/min for this patient; I:E 1:2; PEEP 3-5; FiO2 1.0.

## PERFUSION STATUS: STABLE

## CORRECTIVE ACTION NEEDED
This patient is stable, although he has the potential to develop an altered mental status and seizures. Provide supplemental oxygen to maintain a pulse oximetry > 95%. The FHT, in this case, is alarming: the late decelerations indicate a prolonged lack of placental oxygen and resulting in fetal hypoxia. In this FHT tracing, there is late decelerations, low-long term variability, and contractions every 2.5 minutes. Reposition the patient to remove the gravid uterus off the umbilical cord. If the water has broken, then rule out cord prolapse. Get a baseline on pregnancy– induced hypertension (PIH) labs: protein in the urine. Be prepared for preeclampsia and eclampsia.

## LABS
Serum: Hyperglycemic, otherwise normal. ABG: Normal.

## REQUIRED MANAGEMENT CHANGES BASED ON NEW INFORMATION
After repositioning the patient to displace the gravid uterus off the umbilical cord, the FHT have improved. In this new FHT tracing, we see early decelerations, improved variability, and contractions about 3 minutes apart. The improvement in variably comes with a return of good blood flow from the umbilical cord to the fetus, thus giving the fetus more oxygen. Still be cognizant of the mother– she is dangerously close to suffering eclampsia (high BP and high urine proteins).

## QUESTION 1
Magnesium sulfate; this is the treatment of choice for 3 different reasons. First, the mag will stop the seizure by reducing CNS nerves from being able to efficiently transmit signals; therefore, the seizures will stop. It acts as a tocolytic and will prevent labor should the seizure activity trigger labor. Mag will also reduce the BP/ MAP which is causing the seizures in the first place. [Mag gets you 3 bangs for your buck].

## QUESTION 2
The danger is magnesium toxicity. It can be diagnosed clinically by assessing deep tendon reflexes (DTR). The DTR assessment should be done before the administration of magnesium to get a baseline. Strike the thumb side of the forearm just above the wrist. Patients with high BP from PIH will have excitable reflexes (the nervous system is hyper-excited from the increased pressures and damaged distal tissues). Once mag toxicity is set in, respiratory rate will decrease, and there will be a noticeable difference in the DTRs from the pre– magnesium assessment. Counteract with calcium: 1-2 grams over 10 minutes.

## QUESTION 3
Urine protein—> if positive, then it can indicate pregnancy induced hypertension (PIH), which has progressed to preeclampsia.

# Case Study 17

A 62-year-old female with a history of diabetes and hypertension presents to the emergency department with two days of lethargy and malaise. She presents obese, experiencing shortness of breath, and with an intact right forearm fistula. Upon your arrival, the patient exhibits a GCS of 10 (E2, V4, M4). The patient has vomited twice prior to your arrival. Vital signs and lab work are provided. Pt weight: 310 lbs. Pt height: 6'0".

## BP: 155/94 | HR: 102 | RR: 29 | SpO2: 97 | EtCO2: 44

**ANY LIFE THREATS NEEDING ADDRESSED?**

| | | | | | |
|---|---|---|---|---|---|
| Na: | 142 | RBCs: | 5 | pH: | 7.33 |
| K: | 6.6 | WBCs: | 11.2 | pCO2: | 45 |
| Cl: | 99 | PLTs: | 222 | HCO3: | 20 |
| HCO$_3$: | 21 | HGB: | 15 | pO2: | 96 |
| Cr: | 26 | HCT: | 42 | BE: | -1 |
| BUN: | 4.3 | | | | |
| Glu: | 122 | | | | |

**OTHER LAB/IMAGE INFO:**

**MANAGEMENT PLAN:**

**UPDATE: Turn to page #380 for an update. Look for UPDATE #17. Use this information to continue with the case and this form.**

**ADDITIONAL MANAGEMENT:**

**FINAL DIAGNOSES/PATHO?**

**RSI REGIMINE:**

**VENT SETTINGS:**

**PERFUSION STATUS:**

**HEAD 2 TOE ASSESSMENT:**

**Scenario Question 1:**
The patient's repeat labs reflect a Na 141, K+ 5.3, Ca++ 97, HCO3 21, BUN 16, creatinine 2.3. The repeat 12 lead can be found in Appendix A, ECG #10.

**Scenario Question 2:**
At what serum level does potassium commonly become clinically pathological?

**Scenario Question 3:**
What ECG finding is consistent with clinically significant hyperkalemia?

# CASE STUDY 17: RATIONALE

# Fat Bottomed Girls

## PREDOMINANT PATHOPHYS
Hyperkalemia, altered mental status, metabolic acidosis

## RSI REGIMEN
Sedation (versed, fentanyl); pain (fentanyl); paralysis (rocuronium); AVOID SUX due to K+ being 6.6; continued sedation (fentanyl or versed); rocuronium for continued paralysis. Avoid ketamine as it will worsen hypertension.

## VENTILATOR SETTINGS
IBW: 73kg; Target minute ventilation: 8-9 L/min (upper end of normal or slightly beyond is prudent as patient is slightly acidotic); PC (15-20 cmH2O) or volume control (Vt approximately 450cc); RR 20- but if you use different RR and Vt, just make sure you are targeting the minute ventilation of about 7 L/min for this patient; I:E 1:2; PEEP 3-5; FiO2 1.0.

## PERFUSION STATUS: STABLE

## CORRECTIVE ACTION NEEDED
Due to the patient's history of dialysis (+ right arm fistula), in addition to the abnormally high potassium, this patient is experiencing hyperkalemia. Labs reflect a high blood glucose; therefore, hypoglycemia is ruled out. Primary treatment should be aimed at correcting hyperkalemia to include: calcium (protects the heart by stabilizing the myocardium), bicarb (attenuates acidosis), glucose and insulin (K sticks to the big glucose molecule, and insulin pushes the glucose- potassium molecules back into the cells). Additionally, ABCs must be maintained. This patient has vomited, and presents with AMS, which together presents a strong case to intubate this patient (protection of patient and airway).

## LABS
Serum: Hyperkalemic, high renal labs (from renal failure) hyperglycemic, otherwise normal. ABG: Acute metabolic acidosis.

## REQUIRED MANAGEMENT CHANGES BASED ON NEW INFORMATION
The patient is still hyperkalemic and requires repeat treatment and perhaps consider the second- and third-line medications for this patient, in addition to emergent dialysis.

## QUESTION 1
Other medications to treat hyperkalemia include: Albuterol (prevents K from leaving the cell), loop diuretics (helps to excrete K through urine), and kayexalate (pulls out potassium out of the bowels and excretes it in feces).

## QUESTION 2
Usually potassium > 5.0- 5.5 is deemed clinically significant. This will vary slightly from institution to institution.

## QUESTION 3
High amplitude T- waves. These are also discussed as tall, peaked T waves.

# Case Study 18

**INITIAL:**

You are called to a local ER within minutes of your base to a 32 y/o man who was found down while out walking around his neighborhood. EMS report via radio as you are taxiing to the hospital helipad that the patient has a GCS of 3, with difficulty bagging and wheezes, and is in PEA. Once you arrive and confirm PEA and wheezes with difficulty bagging. EMS crew and RN staff are performing good CPR and report they are in their 4th round of CPR (persistent PEA) where 3 epinephrine doses have been administered. Pt height: 6'5".

## BP: none | HR: none | RR: none | SpO2: none | EtCO2: none

**ANY LIFE THREATS NEEDING ADDRESSED?**

| | | | | | |
|---|---|---|---|---|---|
| Na: | XXX | RBCs: | XXX | pH: | XXX |
| K: | XXX | WBCs: | XXX | pCO2: | XXX |
| Cl: | XXX | PLTs: | XXX | HCO3: | XXX |
| HCO$_3$: | XXX | HGB: | XXX | pO2: | XXX |
| Cr: | XXX | HCT: | XXX | BE: | XXX |
| BUN: | XXX | | | | |
| Glu: | XXX | | | | |

**OTHER LAB/IMAGE INFO:**

**MANAGEMENT PLAN:**

**UPDATE: Turn to page #381 for an update. Look for UPDATE #18. Use this information to continue with the case and this form.**

**ADDITIONAL MANAGEMENT:**

**FINAL DIAGNOSES/PATHO?**

**RSI REGIMINE:**

**VENT SETTINGS:**

**PERFUSION STATUS:**

**HEAD 2 TOE ASSESSMENT:**

**Scenario Question 1:** You have a spontaneous return of circulation. If your vitals and vent observations were as follows, then what changes, if any, would you make? SIMV RR 16, TV 575, Vte 563, f 16, I:E 1:5, PEEP 7, FiO2 1.0, PIP 29, Pplat 25. Vitals: HR 102, BP 118/70; O2 91%, and EtCO2 48.

**Scenario Question 2:** You have a spontaneous return of circulation. If your vitals and vent observations were as follows, then what changes, if any, would you make? SIMV RR 19, TV 575, Vte 563, f 26, I:E 1:2, PEEP 5, FiO2 1.0, PIP 22, Pplat 19. Vitals: HR 102, BP 86/50; O2 88%, and EtCO2 71.

## CASE STUDY 18: RARTIONALE

# Take My Breath Away

### PREDOMINANT PATHOPHYS
Cardiac Arrest, Asthma, PEA

### RSI REGIMEN
Assume the patient wasn't in the arrest but was hemodynamically compromised: sedative: ketamine or fentanyl; paralysis: Sux or Roc; continued sedation with ketamine or fentanyl. Ketamine would be ideal for the asthma patient because it is a potent bronchodilator.

### VENTILATOR SETTINGS
IBW: 89kg; Assume acidosis from prolonged poor perfusion from cardiac arrest: SIMV or AC on volume ventilation (Vt ~550) or pressure ventilation (PC 15-20); Target a minute ventilation of ~ 10-11 L/min (good starting point for an acidotic patient); RR 20- but if you use different RR and Vt, just make sure you are targeting the minute ventilation of about 10-11 L/min for this patient; I:E 1:4-5 (asthma patients need longer E time); PEEP 3-5 cmH2O; FiO2 1.0.

### PERFUSION STATUS: COMPROMISED

### CORRECTIVE ACTION NEEDED
You immediately assess the patient and you've confirmed the PEA, wheezes, and difficulty bagging. The wheezing is most likely a clue indicating what's caused the PEA, so BVM ventilations is acceptable, and you need to maintain good compressions. Consider another epinephrine following the next rhythm check if PEA is still the problem. Next start considering what the problems are- wheezing is giving you the clue. Treat for status asthmaticus: consider albuterol, epi (already on board), methylprednisolone, magnesium, and forceful manual expulsion of the chest (put your hands on the patients chest, disconnect the BVM from the ETT if tubed, and push on the chest forcing all the air out).

### LABS
Serum: None available.

### REQUIRED MANAGEMENT CHANGES BASED ON NEW INFORMATION
Looking at the vital signs, the patient looks hemodynamically stable, but not for long if you don't start working to improve SpO2 and EtCO2. Increase PEEP to 6-8 cmH2O to improve pulse oximetry. RR and TV are too low therefore producing a lower minute ventilation (12 x 500 = 6L/min). Target a minute ventilation of 9 L/min to start to see to see how much that will reduce EtCO2. Remember, if our EtCO2 is not within normal range, then oxygen won't stick to the RBCs like normal, therefore, oxygen isn't taken to the cell or the oxygen can't get off the RBC. This results in acidosis and the patient is already acidotic, so do your part to clear out the acid so they can heal. Consider increasing the I:E to 1-4 or 1:5 since its asthma and air trapping. Continue to monitor closely .

### QUESTION 1
Increase PEEP to 8 to further push the pulse oximetry as close to 95% as possible. Just be ready for a drop in BP from the extra PEEP compressing the major vessels and reducing cardiac output. Vte x f = MV = 9 L/min. The EtCO2 is still only 48 mmHg. Don't give up here- keep pushing to get this as close to the normal range as possible.

### QUESTION 2
Your patient is over- breathing the vent (vent rate set at 19 and the patient frequency is 26): I:E should be a little longer since this is an asthma patient; PEEP needs to be elevated to increase oxygenation; support BP with fluids and pressors (perhaps norepinephrine or phenylephrine to not further increase HR); target a higher minute ventilation (10-11 L/min would be a good starting to point, then let EtCO2 guide further ventilation changes).

# Case Study 19

**INITIAL**:

You are responding to a scene flight where EMS is advising possible STEMI. Upon your arrival, you load the 51 y/o patient into the aircraft and obtain a baseline ECG (see Appendix A, ECG #8). The patient answers questions incorrectly and appears lethargic. The patient will squeeze your hand upon command and opens their eyes to loud verbal stimuli. The patient is short of breath and has no current medical history. Pt weight 195. Pt height: 5'11".

## BP: 92/55 | HR: 92 | RR: 14 (vent) | SpO2: 96 | EtCO2: 44

**ANY LIFE THREATS
NEEDING ADDRESSED?**

| | | | | | |
|---|---|---|---|---|---|
| Na: | 137 | RBCs: | 3.5 | pH: | 7.41 |
| K: | 3.9 | WBCs: | 9.2 | pCO2: | 44 |
| Cl: | 101 | PLTs: | 171 | HCO3: | 23 |
| HCO$_3$: | 23 | HGB: | 12 | pO2: | 126 |
| Cr: | 9.1 | HCT: | 43 | BE: | 0 |
| BUN: | 0.5 | | | | |
| Glu | 103 | | | | |

**OTHER LAB/IMAGE INFO:**

**MANAGEMENT PLAN:**

**UPDATE: Turn to page #379 for an update. Look for UPDATE #19. Use this information to continue with the case and this form.**

**ADDITIONAL MANAGEMENT:**

FINAL DIAGNOSES/PATHO?

**RSI REGIMINE:**

**VENT SETTINGS:**

**PERFUSION STATUS:**

**HEAD 2 TOE ASSESSMENT:**

**Scenario Question 1:**
What should you consider if you observe ST elevation in a majority of the leads?

**Scenario Question 2:**
Which coronary artery is most likely occluded for this anterolateral AMI to manifest?

**Scenario Question 3:**
n/a

# CASE STUDY 19: RATIONALE
# Don't Funk with My Heart

## PREDOMINANT PATHOPHYS
Anterior AMI

## RSI REGIMEN
Sedation (ketamine, fentanyl); pain (fentanyl); paralysis (succinylcholine or rocuronium); continued sedation (fentanyl or ketamine); roc for continued paralysis. Avoid benzodiazepines, as it will worsen hypotension.

## VENTILATOR SETTINGS
IBW: 75kg; SIMV or AC on volume ventilation (TV ~450 cc) or pressure ventilation (PC 15-20); Target a minute ventilation of ~7-8 (good starting point); RR 17- but if you use different RR and Vt, just make sure you are targeting the minute ventilation of about 7.5 L/min for this patient; I:E 1:2; PEEP 3-5 cmH2O; FiO2 1.0.

## PERFUSION STATUS: POTENTIALLY COMPROMISED.

## CORRECTIVE ACTION NEEDED
This patient is having an anterolateral AMI (ST elevation in V3-6 and ST depression in II, III, and aVF). This patient should have supplemental oxygen administered; RSI considered; 2 large IVs secured; and ASA, nitroglycerin (drip or spray), and potentially heparin should be administered. Fluid bolus to support BP but be careful in anterior AMI patients- they may have a backup of blood from the left ventricle into the pulmonary vasculature, they could quickly develop pulmonary edema.

## LABS:
Serum: Hyperglycemic, otherwise normal. ABG: Hyperoxia, otherwise normal. Cardiac enzymes would help confirm AMI, but it has essentially confirmed with (+) STEMI on the 12 lead ECG.

## REQUIRED MANAGEMENT CHANGES BASED ON NEW INFORMATION
The patient is waking up- potentially because you restored perfusion to the heart, so it began pumping better, which supplied your brain with oxygen, allowing the patient to start waking up. This patient should be sedated with versed or fentanyl, and paralysis with a non- depolarizing neuromuscular blocker is an option. Repeat the 12 lead en route.

## QUESTION 1
Pericarditis would be high on a differential if all (or most) of the leads showed ST elevation. Additional clues to look for to indicate pericarditis include PR depression, notching of the QRS complex, and ST elevation in Leads I and II concurrently.

## QUESTION 2
The left anterior descending artery (LAD), is responsible for this type of AMI.

# Case Study 20

**INITIAL:**

You have a patient that was involved in an ATV accident. The patient's face was smashed against the handlebars of the ATV, and he was not wearing a helmet. There is crepitus to the entire midface, including bilateral fractured zygomas. EMS has been clearing the airway with suction and by rolling the patient on their side but has had no success at establishing an airway. He has a very thick beard, is hypoxic, and hypotensive. Pt weight: 250 lbs. Pt height 6'4".

## BP: 88/62 | HR: 109 | RR: 25 | SpO2: 86 | EtCO2: 28

**ANY LIFE THREATS NEEDING ADDRESSED?**

| | | | |
|---|---|---|---|
| Na: XXX | RBCs: XXX | pH: XXX | |
| K: XXX | WBCs: XXX | pCO2: XXX | |
| Cl: XXX | PLTs: XXX | HCO3: XXX | |
| $CO_2$: XXX | HGB: XXX | pO2: XXX | |
| Cr: XXX | HCT: XXX | BE: XXX | |
| BUN: XXX | | | |
| Glu: XXX | | | |

**OTHER LAB/IMAGE INFO:**

**MANAGEMENT PLAN:**

**UPDATE: Turn to page #380 for an update. Look for UPDATE #20. Use this information to continue with the case and this form.**

**ADDITIONAL MANAGEMENT:**

**FINAL DIAGNOSES/PATHO?**

**RSI REGIMINE:**

**VENT SETTINGS:**

**PERFUSION STATUS:**

**HEAD 2 TOE ASSESSMENT:**

**Scenario Question 1:**
On back. Placed on back to not tip off the needed management.

## CASE STUDY 20: RATIONALE

# I Can't Feel My Face When I'm with You

## PREDOMINANT PATHOPHYS

### RSI REGIMEN

RSI regimen (even though in this scenario there is difficulty in ventilating- it is always important to consider HOW you would RSI every patient you encounter): sedation (ketamine, fentanyl); pain (fentanyl); paralysis (succinylcholine or rocuronium); continued sedation (fentanyl or ketamine); roc for continued paralysis. Exercise caution when administering medications that will lower BP as this patient is bordering on hemodynamically unstable.

### VENTILATOR SETTINGS

IBW: 87 kg; SIMV or A/C; PC (18-22 cmH2O) or volume control (TV 520-700cc); RR 13-17; targeting a minute ventilation of 8-9 L/min (hypoperfused patients typically indicates at least a little acidosis cellularly); I:E 1:2; PEEP 3-5; FiO2 1.0.

### PERFUSION STATUS: POTENTIALLY COMPROMISED

### CORRECTIVE ACTION NEEDED

This is one of the most difficult patients you could have: a hypoxic patient that has a multi-factor difficult airway. Obviously, your first goal is to attempt to open the airway, and with an unstable midface, it could pose to be incredibly difficult. On top of that, if you could open the airway, obtaining a good seal with a thick beard and multiple facial fractures would also be very difficult to achieve. In cases like these, it could be plausible to make an attempt at a rescue airway (King LT, LMA, etc), but your mind should already be considering surgical cricothyrotomy.

### LABS:

Serum: None available.

### REQUIRED MANAGEMENT CHANGES BASED ON NEW INFORMATION

Once you cannot intubate or ventilate, then it is important to be able to realize this and be ready to act. This patient requires a needle cric at a minimum and optimally requires a surgical cricothyrotomy. General practices call for a small size ETT (5 mm or so depending on the size of the patient), an incision, and then placement of the ETT. Savvy clinicians will use a bougie and place it in the airway as an introducer and slide the ETT over the bougie into the airway. It can be practiced with cow or pig trachs that are commercially available, or you can obtain some from your local butcher. Either way, be sure you are practiced for this for when this situation is presented to you. Next, ensure adequate ventilation and perfusion with the ventilator and adequate fluid resuscitation. Prevent any external bleeding from the trauma.

### QUESTION 1

**What are the anatomical landmarks for surgical cricothyrotomy?**

Begin by palpating the laryngeal prominence, which forms the superior edge of the thyroid cartilage. There is often a prominent "V-shaped" notch palpable. It is often more prominent in men. Next, identify and palpate the cricoid cartilage, which is a complete cartilaginous ring, shaped like a signet ring, with its widest part found posteriorly. The space between these structures is the cricothyroid membrane.

# CASE UPDATES:

**UPDATE 1**: After appropriate stabilization, the patient develops the following vital signs: HR increases from 102 to 118, BP drops from 102/70 to 72/46, and there is no longer a pulse oximetry reading. Radial pulses disappear.

**UPDATE 4**: You have RSI'd and intubated the patient. Your initial vent settings and monitored data is as follows: AC, RR 12, f 26, VE 12.7, TV 510, Vte 495, I:E 1:5, FiO2 1.0, PIP 18, PEEP 4, and Pplat 15. After receiving nitro drip and fentanyl, the patient's vitals are as follows: BP 90/58, HR 99, pulse oximetry 92%, and EtCO2 54.

**UPDATE 7**: You administer a fluid bolus of 1 L, get the patient set on your transport ventilator, administer fentanyl, and package the patient for transport. Vent settings: SIMV RR 18, PC, Vte 640, f 19, I:E 1:2, PEEP 5, FiO2 1.0, PIP 25. Hemodynamically profile: CVP 5/ PCWP 12/ CO 7/ SVR 500. Vitals: HR 100, BP 92/52; O2 89%, and EtCO2 62..

**UPDATE 10**: Just after you intubate the patient with sux and versed, he experiences a drop in pulse oximetry, EtCO2, and BP, and then develops ventricular fibrillation. With the information that is provided, what happened during intubation that would explain this situation? Secondly, what is the treatment for this condition (not v-fib, the condition that caused v-fib)?.

**UPDATE 13**: After appropriate stabilization, the patient develops the following vital signs: HR increases from 102 to 118, BP drops from 102/70 to 72/46, and there is no longer a pulse oximetry reading. Radial pulses disappear.

**UPDATE 16**: You reposition your patient and she states she is feeling more comfortable. Repeat vitals: BP 159/92, HR 100, pulse oximetry 99, RR 14. The updated FHT tracing is FHT #4 in Appendix C.

**UPDATE 19**: You RSI the patient and administer nitroglycerin IV by the pump. Within 10 minutes you notice the following: vent (RR 14, Vte 475, TV 510, PEEP 4, I:E of 1:2, f 23, minute ventilation 11.8) and vitals (BP 129/90, HR 122, pulse oximetry 100, RR 14 [on vent]. (+) curare cleft in the graphic EtCO2 waveform.

**UPDATE 2**: Your patient is now intubated and adequately sedated. The patient has the following vent settings: SIMV, RR 14, f 14, I:E 1:5, TV 500, Vte 480, MV 690, PEEP 3, PIP 18, Pplat 13, and FiO2 1.0. The updated vitals are as follows: HR 64, BP 102/80, O2 100%, and EtCO2 55.

**UPDATE 5**: Your patient is now intubated and on the ventilator. Assume the RSI meds were appropriate for the patient's hemodynamic status. Current vent settings/measurements: RR 14, f 21, VE 11.7, TV 425, Vte 445, I:E 1:5, FiO2 1.0, PIP 18, PEEP 4, and Pplat 15. Vitals: BP 104/60, HR106, pulse oximetry 93%, and EtCO2 32 with equal chest wall excursion..

**UPDATE 8**: As you are preparing the fluid resuscitation formula, the sending RN mentions the burn occurred 3 hours before and had been administered 300cc up to this point. Vital signs have essentially remained unchanged. The patient says the pain is 'not bad'.

**UPDATE 11**: You examine the CT (see Appendix D, CT #4 for this patient's head scan). The patient's seizure has now subsided. What other management obligations do you have?.

**UPDATE 14**: Your patient is now intubated and adequately sedated. The patient has the following vent settings: SIMV, RR 14, f 14, I:E 1:5, TV 500, Vte 480, MV 690, PEEP 3, PIP 18, Pplat 13, and FiO2 1.0. The updated vitals are as follows: HR 64, BP 102/80, O2 100%, and EtCO2 55.

**UPDATE 17**: The patient's repeat labs reflect a Na 141, K+ 5.3, Ca++ 97, HCO3 21, BUN 16, creatinine 2.3. The repeat 12 lead can be found in Appendix A, ECG #10.

**UPDATE 20**: After several attempts to create a seal, you are unable to ventilate the patient. NRB mask on high flow is yielding only 86% oxygen saturation. You attempt to intubate, and there are too much blood and trauma to the airway. What is your thought process in this situation.? How would you manage this terrifying situation?

**UPDATE 3**: The patient is now intubated and sedated. The patient's vital signs have remained stable throughout transport when suddenly you note the following findings: SpO2 drops to from 96% to 84% and the patient's extremities become mottled and cyanotic. You notice that you're so high in the air, you notice the cars look like ants.

**UPDATE 6**: En route, the mother rapidly progresses to imminent delivery. She begins crowning. After several contractions, the baby's head fails to progress forward. FHTs begin to drop (~110) and there are late decelerations occurring on the toco monitor. See FHT #2 in appendix C.

**UPDATE 9**: You improve compressions, intubate the patient, ventilate targeting a higher than normal minute ventilation, and are providing higher PEEP. Your patient has just recently regained a pulse and CPR has been halted. Here are your vitals and vent settings: SIMV RR 18, TV 250, Vte 190, f 26, I:E 1:2, PEEP 6, FiO2 1.0, PIP 34, Pplat 31. Vitals: HR 121, BP 88/50; O2 86%, and EtCO2 71..

**UPDATE 12**: The physician taking care of this patient inserts a Swanz– Gantz catheter prior to your arrival. You have the following patient data: HR 88, BP 82/60, RR 16 (on ventilator), pulse oximetry 86%, (+) troponin, Vte 425, MV 7, EtCO2 31, f 22, CVP 10, wedge pressure 14, CO 5, and SVR 1500. How will you manage this patient?

**UPDATE 15**: While you are removing the patient from the aircraft, the aircraft stretcher drops to the ground. You lift the patient back up and assess for any complications. You note the IABP as the following [see Appendix B: IABP waveform #3]. What needs to be done?.

**UPDATE 18**: Upon treatment for asthma, you get a spontaneous return of circulation. Your partner sets the patient up on the ventilator. The patient's vitals and vent setting & observations are as follows: SIMV RR 12, TV 500, Vte 475, f 13, I:E 1:2, PEEP 5, FiO2 1.0, PIP 27, Pplat 24. Vitals: HR 116, BP 122/62; O2 86%, and EtCO2 68.

# SECTION 3:
## DUMP SHEETS & MORE

# Dump Sheets, QuickLook Pages, Pharmacopeia, and Conditionopeia

## Instructions for the Quick Look Pages:

Alright! You have almost made it to the finish line. If you're looking at this section, then you have either studied the entire text or are crunched for time. Either way, you are quickly approaching your test date within days. It's time to start going over large chunks information very quickly. To successfully accomplish this, I have developed these "Quick Look" pages. These pages are designed so that the day of, or the week before, you have quick access to large amounts of information in a small space. This section makes it ideal to study quickly and prepare for the last-minute fortification of your knowledge on this material.

I have written down bite size pieces of information spanning each section of this text. If there is an abbreviation you seem unfamiliar with, then please see our web site (www.medspx.com) under the "Help" tab. This is where you will find an updated list of abbreviations with corresponding page numbers of abbreviations that are confusing. I wrote most of this section with verbiage and abbreviations that are commonly understood. It would be obtuse to consider this text flawless. However, my goal will be to continue improving it to achieve flawlessness. You will be able to add to this list of abbreviations, which a great help to me. So, let me know if there's anything confusing.

Otherwise, you should be ready to get started. I have enjoyed writing this text, and I love teaching. I remember studying those three manuals that I called my certification "study" Bibles, and one of the best things I did was to study large amounts of information very quickly. I was able to do this by studying these "Quick Look" pages. I wish you the best of luck and please, contact me if you ever have any questions, comments, concerns, or criticisms.

# NOW, GO PUNCH THE CLOCK AND KICK YOUR EXAM'S ASS!

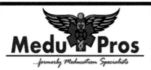
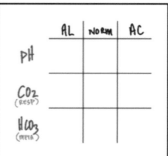

|  | AL | NORM | AC |
|---|---|---|---|
| pH |  |  |  |
| CO2 (RESP) |  |  |  |
| HCO3 (META) |  |  |  |

## HYPOXIA:
Moderate: 85-90%
Mild: 91-93%
SEVERE: ≤ 84%

**IBW**
**ADULT:** (2.3)(Ht > 5 ft) + 50 (if ♂) or 45.5 (if ♀)
**PEDS:** 8 + (Age in years/2)
**INFANT:** (9 + age in months)/2

### RSI-PREMEDS:
**Atropine:**
- Prevents bradycardia
- 0.01– 0.02 mg/kg IV (min. 0.1 mg ; max 0.5mg)

**Lidocaine:**
- Blunts ICP during intubation
- 1 mg/kg IV; max dose 3 mg/kg

### RSI-SEDATIVES:
**Ketamine:**
- Increases BP*; Bronchodilates
- 1-2 mg/kg IV

**Etomidate:**
- Avoid in sepsis- worsens adrenal insufficiency
- 0.3 mg/kg IV

**Midazolam:**
- Drops BP; has amnestic properties
- 2-5 mg IV, or 0.1 to 0.3 mg/kg

**Lorazepam:**
- Drops BP; lasts longer than versed
- 0.05 mg/kg IV

### RSI-ANALGESICS:
**Ketamine:**
- Increases BP*; Bronchodilates
- 1-2 mg/kg IV

**Fentanyl:**
- Avoid in sepsis- worsens adrenal insufficiency
- 0.3 mg/kg IV

**Morphine:**
- Drops BP; has amnestic properties
- 2-5 mg IV, or 0.1 to 0.3 mg/kg

### RSI-PARALYTICS:
**Rocuronium:**
- Non-depolarizing; lasts ~ 60 min
- 0.6-1 mg/kg

**Vecuronium:**
- Non-depolarizing; lasts ~ 45 min
- 0.08 to 0.1 mg/kg

**Succinylcholine:**
- Avoid in HyperK+, 24 hr s/p burn, crush injury, any patient who cannot move all 4 extremities
- 1-2 mg/kg

### RSI-REVERSALS:
**Dantrolene:**
- Reverses malignant hyperthermia (stops Ca+ release)
- 1 mg/kg IV (max10 mg/kg)

**Flumazenil:**
- Reverses benzodiazepines (can't fix Sz anymore)
- 1 mg/kg IV; max dose 3 mg/kg

### ETT SIZE CALCULATIONS
**ETT SIZE CALCS:**
Adults: 6.5-8.5 mm ETT size
Peds: (Age/4) + 4
Infants: 3.0-3.5 mm
Neo: Gestational Age/10

**ETT TUBE DEPTH:**
ALL: 3 x

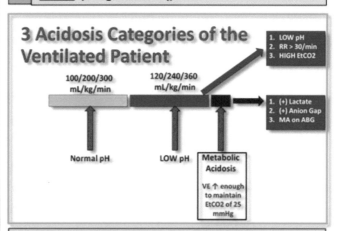

## 3 Acidosis Categories of the Ventilated Patient

100/200/300 mL/kg/min — Normal pH

120/240/360 mL/kg/min — LOW pH

Metabolic Acidosis
VE ↑ enough to maintain EtCO2 of 25 mmHg

1. LOW pH
2. RR > 30/min
3. HIGH EtCO2

1. (+) Lactate
2. (+) Anion Gap
3. MA on ABG

**SETTINGS:** [Vt = 6 mL/kg], [VE = see above], [I:E 1:2, unless peds or air-trapping], [PEEP 3-5], [FiO2 1.0]

**CONFIRM:**
RR vs. f → if f high, then sedate or increase sensitivity.
Vt vs. Vte → if Vte is low, check AutoPEEP, leak, then Dead Space
High PIP/Norm Pplat→ airway issue (correct for DOPE)
High PIP & Pplat→ Switch to PC at 15/5
**ADJUST:** [for SpO2: PEEP and FiO2], [For EtCO2: RR, Vt, or PC]

### COMMON RESPIRATORY PATHOS:
- SaO2 LOW w/ 100% SpO2= CO poisoning
- VQ match = CO equal to MV
- Dead space= 1cc per pound (Approx. 33% of Vt)
- COPD pts have polycythemia
- Isolated infiltrates = pneumonia
- Pneumocystis pneumonia = HIV/AIDS
- X-ray: ARDS: (-) costophrenic angles, (+) patchy; (+) ground glass
- Xray: Plum Edema: Kerley B

### CHEM RELATIONSHIPS
Δ ph 0.1 ↓ = Δ K+ 0.6 ↑
Δ ph 0.08 ↓ = Δ EtCO2 10 ↑
ΔEtCO2↓ 10 = ΔK+↑ 0.6

### ANION GAP CALC:
[Na + K] – [CL + HCO3]
If > 16, then Anion Gap Metabolic Acidosis present

### SPEED OF BUFFER SYSTEMS (FAST TO SLOW):
Bicarb buffer < resp < renal < phosphate

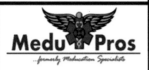

# MeduPros Dump Sheet

**HEMODYNAMIC PARAMETERS:**
- CVP= venous return; 2-6
- RVP= R Vent pressure; 25-30
- PCWP= L Vent pressure; 4-12
- CO= ejected blood; 4-8
- SVR= arterial squeeze; 800-1200

Overdampened

"Just Right"

Underdampened

**DAMPENING CAUSES:**
- OVER: kinked line, air in tube, pressure bag too full
- UNDER: hypothermia, catheter whip

**AMI PATTERNS:**
- Post. MI: RCA/LCx; ST ↓ V1-V3
- Inf.MI: RCA/Cx; ST ↑ II, III, aVF
- Ant. MI: LAD; ST ↑ V3-V4
- Ant/Lat MI: Cx/LAD; ST ↑ I, aVL,V4-6
- Ant/Sep MI: LAD; ST ↑ I, aVL, V1-V4
- Ant. MI: at risk for papillary rupture; presents with flash pulm edema and a holosystolic murmur @ heart apex 0-3 days after AMI
- Ant. MI: Significant ↓ in CO and BP
- **Sgarbossa** for ST ↑ w/ LBBB:
   - ST ↑ >1mm any lead w (+)QRS (5pts)
   - ST ↓ >1mm in V1-V3 (3 pts)
   - ST ↑ >5mm in lead w (-)QRS (2pts)

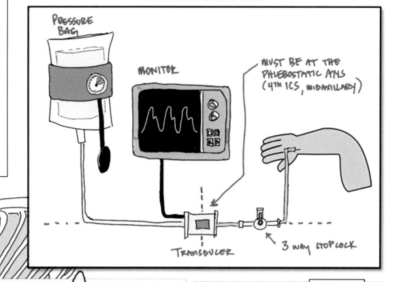

PRESSURE BAG

MONITOR

MUST BE AT THE PHLEBOSTATIC AXIS (4TH ICS, MIDAXILLARY)

TRANSDUCER

3 WAY STOPCOCK

PHLEBOSTATIC AXIS  4TH ICS

MID AXILLARY LINE

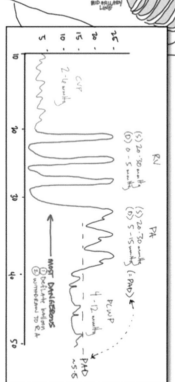

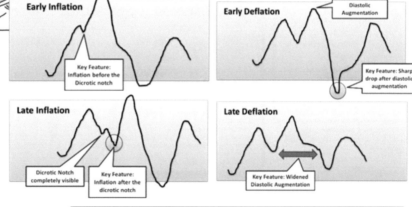

**Early Inflation**
Key Feature: Inflation before the Dicrotic notch

**Early Deflation**
Diastolic Augmentation
Key Feature: Sharp drop after diastolic augmentation

**Late Inflation**
Dicrotic Notch completely visible
Key Feature: Inflation after the dicrotic notch

**Late Deflation**
Key Feature: Widened Diastolic Augmentation

| | Hypovol | (R) Heart Failure | Cardiogenic | Obstructive | Distributive | Sepsis |
|---|---|---|---|---|---|---|
| CVP (2-6) | ↓ | ↑ | ↑ | ↑ | ↓ | ↓ |
| PCWP (8-12) | ↓ | ↓ | ↑ | ↑ | ↓ | ↓ |
| CI (2.5-5) CO (4-8) | ↓ | ↓ | ↓ | ↓ | ↓ | ↑ |
| SVR (800-1200) | ↑ | ↑ | ↑ | ↑ | ↓ | ↓ |
| HISTORY | Blood loss, fluid loss | Cor pulmonale | CHF Symptoms | Hx needed, Tension pneumo; pericardial tamponade | Sepsis, anaphylaxis, neurogenic ( ↓HR) | ↑ Temp; ↑CO/CI ; infection |

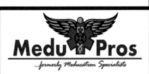

# MeduPros Dump Sheet

## HEART VALVES:

TOILET PAPER MY ASS:
Tricuspid → Pulmonic → Mitral → Aortic.

**AV Valves**: Tricuspid, Mitral

**Semilunar Valves**: Pulmonic, Aortic

## UTILITY OF CARDIAC OUTPUT:

- Atropine and beta 1 agonists will ↑ HR (thus ↑ CO); while beta blockers and calcium channel blockers will ↓ HR (thus ↓ CO).
- Isotonic fluids and vasopressors (w/ healthy hearts) will ↑ preload (thus ↑ CO); while hypotension and/ or hypovolemia will ↓ preload (thus ↓ CO).
- Improving preload and inotropes will ↑ contractility (thus ↑ CO); while reduced preload will ↓ contractility (thus ↓ CO).
- Any medication causing VASODILATION as a direct effect, (or a side effect) will ↓ afterload; however, any medication where VASOCONSTRICTION is a direct effect or a side effect will ↑ afterload.

## LVAD MANAGEMENT:

### A-BIRDS

**A**rrhythmias
**B**leeding
**I**nfections
**R**t. Ventric. Dysfunction
**D**evice Failure
**S**uckdown

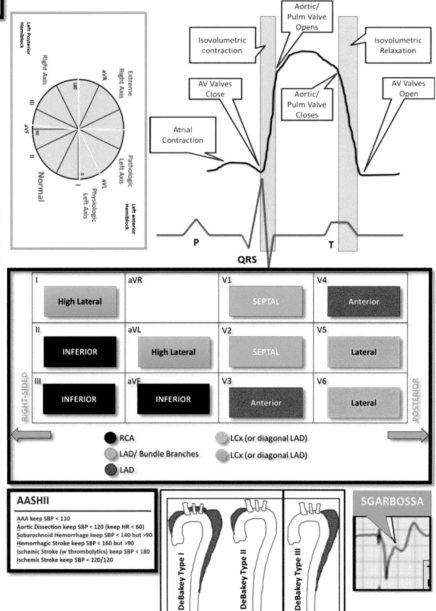

## AASHII

AAA keep SBP < 110
Aortic Dissection keep SBP < 120 (keep HR < 60)
Subarachnoid Hemorrhage keep SBP < 140 but >90
Hemorrhagic Stroke keep SBP < 160 but >90
Ischemic Stroke (w thrombolytics) keep SBP < 180
Ischemic Stroke keep SBP < 220/120

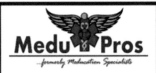

# MeduPros Dump Sheet

|  | Central Cord | Anterior Cord | Brown-Sequard |
|---|---|---|---|
| **Findings** | Sensory and motor deficits; Upper > Lower Exts | Complete loss of motor, pain, and temp below injury. | Ipsilateral motor loss & sensation; contralateral loss of pain and temp |
| **Mechanism** | Forced Hyperextension | Flexion or Vascular injury | Penetrating Trauma |

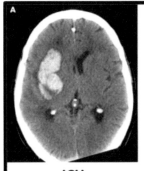

ICH

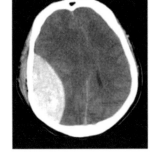

Eprdural

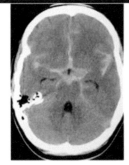

Subarachnoid

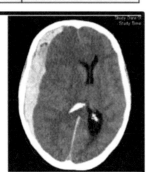

Subdural

### How to use CPP:

1. Calculate MAP
2. Plug in current ICP (measure if with a real patient)
3. Solve for CPP
   - If > 70: Do nothing
   - If < 70: Administer NS or LR boluses to raise MAP so that CPP is elevated to at least 70 mmHg.

| 1 | 2 | 3 | 4 |
|---|---|---|---|
| NOTHING | To Pain | To Verbal | Spontaneous |

| 1 | 2 | 3 | 4 | 5 |
|---|---|---|---|---|
| NOTHING | Garbled | Inappro. Words | Confused | A/O x 4 |

| 1 | 2 | 3 | 4 | 5 | 6 |
|---|---|---|---|---|---|
| NOTHING | Extension/Decere | Flexion/Decor | Withdraws | Localizes | Obeys |

## 9-12 = Moderate Head Injury

**Remember in TBI or CHI- Be aggressive to prevent HYPOXIA and HYPOTENSION. A single episode increases mortality by > 44%.**

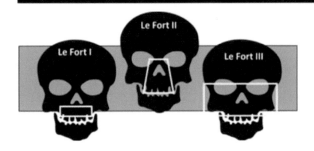

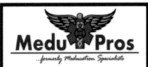
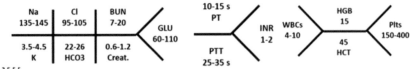

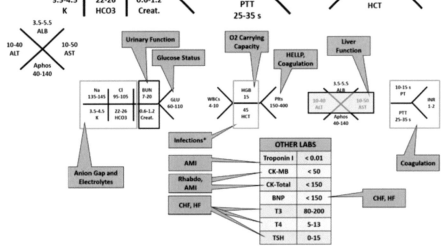

| OTHER LABS | |
|---|---|
| Troponin I | < 0.01 |
| CK-MB | < 50 |
| CK-Total | < 150 |
| BNP | < 150 |
| T3 | 80-200 |
| T4 | 5-13 |
| TSH | 0-15 |

---

## DELIVERY MANEUVERS

Mariceu's- used with breech Suprapubic pressure, hand in vagina, hook finger in mouth, gentle fetal head flexion to assist with delivery

McRoberts- knee to chest, raising pelvis to assist with shoulder dystocia

Woods' corkscrew maneuver- used only after McRoberts & suprapubic pressure; twisting of shoulders to facilitate the normal corkscrew motion of the fetus through the birth canal to correct shoulder dystocia

## EPI for Neonates: 0.1 mg/kg (using 0.1/mL)

### VEAL CHOP
- Variable = Cord Compression
- Early = Head Compression
- Acels = GOOD!
- Late Dcels = Placental Insufficiency

### PDA

**OPENS**: PGE1→KEEPS PDA OPEN; also causes apnea; 0.05-0.1 mEq/kg/min
**CLOSES**: (1) Indomethacin—> closes the PDA; 0.1-0.2 mg/kg; can repeat 0.1mg/kg up to 2 times. (2) Oxygen—> also CLOSES the PDA; which is why its acceptable to allow lower pulse oximetry in the kids with cyanotic lesions—> so oxygenated blood can be introduced into systemic circulation.

## Selected OB MGT:
- Palpating fetal parts through stomach after a trauma→ uterine rupture
- Boggy uterus → postpartum hemorrhage (requires fundal massage)
- Sinusoidal FHR pattern = very ominous & occurs with anemia and fetal distress → C-Section likely
- Terb (brethine) 0.25 SQ- relaxes uterus
- MgSO4- 4-6g over 10 min, relaxes smooth muscle. Therapeutic level: 4-8 mEq/L.
- Post-partum hemorrhage = 500cc blood loss or more
- Pitocin (oxytocin): contract uterus; 20-40u in 1000LR
- Fundal massage: contracts uterus
- PIH= protienemia, edema, HTN Tx: mag or benzos & muscle relaxer
- CaCl in mag toxicity: 1g over 2 min
- HELLP: hemolysis, ↑ liver labs, low platelets
- Isotonic fluids for resuscitation
- Consider hypothermia if ALL vital signs are low.
- Consider FLUID resuscitation with tachycardia.
- Consider SEIZURES with any infant 'bicycle pedaling' or eye twitching.
- Consider RESP DISTRESS with repeated sneezing or hiccupping.
- Premie's need surfactant. Usually < 26 weeks.

| Normal Vital Signs for Pediatrics | | | |
|---|---|---|---|
| Developmental Stage | RR | HR | BP |
| Infant | 25-50 | 70-160 | >70 |
| Toddler | 20-30 | 90-150 | >80 |
| Preschool | 20-25 | 80-140 | >80 |
| School Age | 15-20 | 70-120 | >80 |
| Adolescent | 12-16 | 60-100 | >90 |

### PALS:
- 1/3 depth of chest at 100-120 beats/min
- DEFIB: 2 J/kg, then 4 J/kg; Max 10 J/kg
- CARDIOVERSION: 0.5-1 J/kg
- Isotonic Fluid Bolus: 20cc/kg (neonates get 10 mL/kg)
- UO: 1-2 mL/kg/hr
- Dextrose: 2 cc/kg D25, 5 cc/kg for D10
- Epi: 0.1 mg/kg;
- Amiodarone: 5 mg/kg, may repeat twice
- Lidocaine: 1 mg/kg; maint 20-50 mcg/kg/min

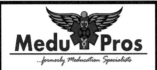

# MeduPros Dump Sheet

## TCAS (NA CHANNEL BLOCKERS)

- Cause Sz, ventricular arrhythmias
- ID TCAs: QRS > 100ms in Lead II, right axis deviation, sinus tach, pupil dilation, fever, dry mouth
- TCA Tx: serum alkalization: airway control, bicarb, fluids, benzos

## BENZOS

- S/S: ↓HR, BP & RR, (+) nystagmus
- Tx: activated charcoal & flumazenil
- CAUTION w/ flumazenil- it can make your patient prone to Sz.

## ANTIDOTES

- CO→ oxygen
- Cyanide→ amyl nitrate, Na thiosul.
- Organophos→ 2PAM, atropine
- Methemoglobin→ meth blue
- Anticholinergic→ physostigmine
- Coumadin→ Vitamin K, FFP
- Heparin→ protamine sulfate

## BETA BLOCKERS

- S/S: ↓HR & BP, ↑ asthma
- Tx: fluids, chrono and inotropes, glucagon, pacing
- -olol or –ol drugs

## CA CHANNEL BLOCKERS

- S/S: ↓HR & BP
- Tx: Suction gastric contents, 10 Ca gluconate, glucagon, insulin, atropine, vasopressors
- -il drugs

## DIGITALIS

- Dig. has a narrow therapeutic index
- S/S: yellow/green vision changes, V-tach, (+) ladle effect on ECG, PVCs
- Tx: : Suction gastric contents, treat any hyperK+ (insulin, glucose, Ca, bicarb)

## OPIATES

- S/S: ↓HR, BP, AMS & constricted pupils
- Tx: Narcan 0.4-2mg

## TYLENOL

- Ph1: 0-24h, v/v, malaise, subclinical until 12h
- Ph2: 18-72h, RUQ pain, serum ↑ transaminase, ↑ liver enzymes
- Ph3: 72-96h, abd pain, jaundice, liver damage, liver tender to palpation, DIC, Death
- Ph4: 4d-3 weeks, Complete resolution
- Tx: N-acetylcystine (mucomyst)

## SALICYLATE

- Ph1: 12h, hyperventilation, alkauria
- Ph2: 12-24h, continued respiratory alkalosis,
- Ph3: dehydration, hypoK, & meta. Acidosis
- S/S: n/v, hyperventilation, ↓ DTRs, hypoCa+, hallucinations

## Selected ENVIR. MGT:

- Hypothermia = hyperglycemia (insulin loses effectiveness), high pCO2/ EtCO2 (reduced RR from cold) = resp acidosis initially
- Profuse sweating & cramps = heat cramps
- Sweating & syncopal episodes = heat syncope
- Profuse sweating, 100.4-104 °F, & moist skin = Heat exhaustion
- No sweating, AMS, & > 104 °F = Heat Stroke

## IMPORTANT TEMPS:

Mild hypothermia: 90-95°F
Severe hypothermia: < 90°F
Shivering Stops: 91°F
Defib can resume: 86°F

---

Stop the cooling process @ 102°F (give antipyretics and passive cooling)

---

°F to °C:
(F°-32) x 0.5556 = °C

°C to °F:
(C x 1.8) + 32 = °F

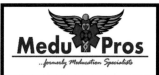

# MeduPros Dump Sheet

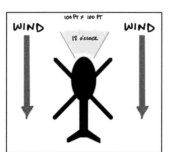

WIND — 100 PT × 100 PT — WIND
12 o'clock

## Emergency Info
- Emergency Freq: **121.5**
- Required Gs to activate ELT: **4**

## HYPOXIA TYPES:
- HYPOXIA- FBAO, ACE inhibitor reaction; throat closure in anaphylaxis
- HYPEMIC- anemia from blood loss, sickle cell anemia, CO poisoning
- STAGNENT- CHF/heart failure, obstructive shock
- HISTOTOXIC- CO Poisoning, cyanide

## HYPOXIA STAGES
- Indifferent <10k, 98-87%
- Compensatory 10-15k, 80-87%
- Disturbance 15-20k, 70-79%, S/S present
- Critical 20-25k, 60-69%, circulatory failure

Graph: [% O₂ Sats of Hemoglobin] vs [PO₂ (mmHg)]

LEFT
↓ Temp
↓ 2,3 DPG (from blood transfusion)
↓ H⁺ ions (Alkalbwsis)
↓ EtCO₂

Right
↑ temp
↑ Acid (H⁺ ions)
↑ EtCO₂

| Condition | Non- mountainous | | Mountainous | |
|---|---|---|---|---|
| | Local | Cross- country | Local | Cross- country |
| Day | 800' and 2 mi | 800' and 3 mi | 800' and 3 mi | 1000' and 3 mi |
| Night (NVG) | 800' and 3 mi | 1000' and 3 mi | 1000' and 3 mi | 1000' and 5 mi |
| Night (w/o NVG) | 1000' and 3 mi | 1000' and 5 mi | 1500' and 3 mi | 1500' and 5 mi |

## 760 torr = 14.7 psi = 101.3 kPa

## EPT vs TUC
- EPT Times:
- 22:10min, 25k:3-5min, 30k:1-2min, 40k: 15-30s; 45k: 9-15s
- (half these times for TUC times)

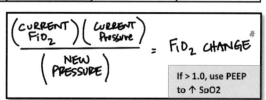

$$\frac{(\text{CURRENT FiO}_2)(\text{CURRENT PRESSURE})}{(\text{NEW PRESSURE})} = \text{FiO}_2 \text{ CHANGE}^*$$

If > 1.0, use PEEP to ↑ SpO2

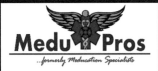

# MeduPros Dump Sheet

## NEWTON'S LAWS

- **1st:** Objects remain in Motion until acted on by outside force
- **2nd:** F=MA
- **3rd:** For q action, there is an equal and opposite reaction

## INJURY PATTERNS

- UP & OVER
- Head- CHI/Lacs
- Chest-Pneumo/Hemothorax
- Femur(driver): Fxs
- DOWN & UNDER
- Femur-Fxs/ hemorrhage
- Pelvis-Fxs/ hemorrhage
- ABD- liver/ hemorrhage
- ABD- spleen- bleed/ Kehr's
- REAR-ENDED
- C2-Fx
- Lumbar/Thoracic-Fxs
- Femur-Fxs
- Secondary impacts- mimics frontal
- SIDE IMPACT
- Likely to be very severe
- Entire anatomy on hit side affected
- Pelvic/femur/ext/head- Fxs/ blood
- ABD- liver/spleen- bleeding
- Chest- Pmx/Hmx, aortic injuries
- ROLLOVER
- Likely to be very severe
- Ejection-massive multitrauma
- Axial load- head/neck trauma
- Internal- Pmx/Hmx/liver/spleen/aorta
- MOTORCYCLE-UP/OVER
- Ejection-massive multitrauma
- Head trauma (less with helmet)
- Bilat femur fxs- bleeding
- MOTORCYCLE-LAY DOWN
- Much less likely to be severe
- Roadrash & Fxs to 'down' side
- FALLS
- Adults: tib/fib/femur/abds/Colles fx
- Peds: head injuries 2* big heads
- Critical Fall: 2.5-3x height

## UNIQUE TRAUMA PATHOS

- **BECKS TRIAD:**
  - Muff HR tones/JVD/↑pulse press.
- **FINDING: ↑ SQ AIR**
  - Assume bronchial injury
  - ETT right mainstem on purpose
- **TENSION PMX**
  - No BS, trah shift= late, SQ air, JVD
  - Tx- needle, 2nd ICS/ Cx tube 4-6th ICS
- **HEMOTHORAX**
  - No JVD, dull percuss, ~1500cc BL
  - Tx: fluid/blood/chest tube
- **FLAIL CHEST**
  - Paradox motion, 2 & 2
  - Allow self-splinting- no bulky dressing
  - (+) intubate to splint
- **CARDIAC TAMPONADE**
  - (+) Beck's Triad
  - Tx: pericardiocentesis- 60cc, long needle, xiphoid, 45* at left scapula
- **COMOTIO CORDIS**
  - Unexpected non-pen blunt force
  - Causes vent dysryth. At vulnerable state of repolarization
- **BURN W/LOSS CHEST COMPLIANCE**
  - A drop in Vt & increased PIP = escharotomy

## BURN PHASES

- **EMERGENT:** initial pathophysiologic phase of burn injury; Immediate problem is fluid loss, edema, reduced blood flow
- **ACUTE:** hemodynamically stable, has restored capillary permeability and has been showing signs of diuresis
- **REHABILITATIVE:** final phase of managing a burn injury. Most frequently, it overlaps the acute phase, and it continues after hospitalization; main goals during this phase are helping the patient to gain independence

## BURN DEPTH

- **SUPERFICIAL:** Only epidermis is affected; Red skin, pain at site
- **PARTIAL THICKNESS:** Epidermis & dermis are affected; Blisters, intense pain, white to red skin, moist mottled skin
- **FULL THICKNESS:** Epidermis, dermis, muscle, fat affected; Charring, dark brown or white, skin hard to the touch, little or no pain, pain at periphery of burn

## JACKSON'S THEORY OF BURNS

- **Zone of Coag:** center; membrane rupture; coagulation; proteins destroyed
- **Zone of Stasis:** injured cells w/ decreased blood flow; can become necrotic
- **Zone of Hyperemia:** outermost; likely will survive; best perfused

### THE PROCEDURE

**STEP 1: INITIAL FLUID RATE**
1. < 6 years old: 125 mL/hr of LR
2. 6-13 years of age: 250 mL/hr of LR
3. > 13 years old: 500 mL/hr of LR

**STEP 2: CALCULATE BSA**
1. Tabulate the total body surface area percentage (%TBSA)
2. Use Lund and Bauer or the Rule of Nines

**STEP 3: OBTAIN PATIENT WEIGHT**
1. Estimate the weight of the patient.
2. USE IDEAL BODY WEIGHT!

**STEP 4: CALCULATE TOTAL FLUID IN 24 HOURS**
1. 2 x KG x %TBSA for adults
2. 3 x KG x %TBSA for peds
3. 4 x KG x %TBSA for adults w/ myoglobinuria.

**STEP 5: DIVIDE BY 2**
1. The result is the volume needed in both the FIRST 8 hours as well as the volume needed in the NEXT 16 hours.

**STEP 6: DIVIDE BY 8- this gets the 'per hour' rate**
1. The result is the rate to needed to achieve the first 8 hours of fluid needed.
2. ADJUSTMENTS:
   a. This rate should be from the MOMENT of the burn. If there is a delay in fluid resuscitation, then do not divide by 8- divide by the remaining hours left in the first 8 hours.
   b. Example: if the patient was burned 2 hours ago, you'd divide the total volume needed in the first 8 hours by 6 hours, not 8 hours, because 2 hours have already passed.
   c. Also- any fluid administered prior to your fluid resuscitation rate should be accounted for- unless it was used to correct blood pressure.

**STEP 7: AMINISTER THE CALCULATED RATE**

| CURRENT FORMULAS |
| --- |
| *CONSENSUS FORMULA* |
| 2-4 mL/kg/%BSA burned |
| *MODIFIED BROOKE FORMULA* |
| 2 mL/kg/%BSA burned |
| *PARKLAND FORMULA* |
| 4 mL/kg/%BSA burned |

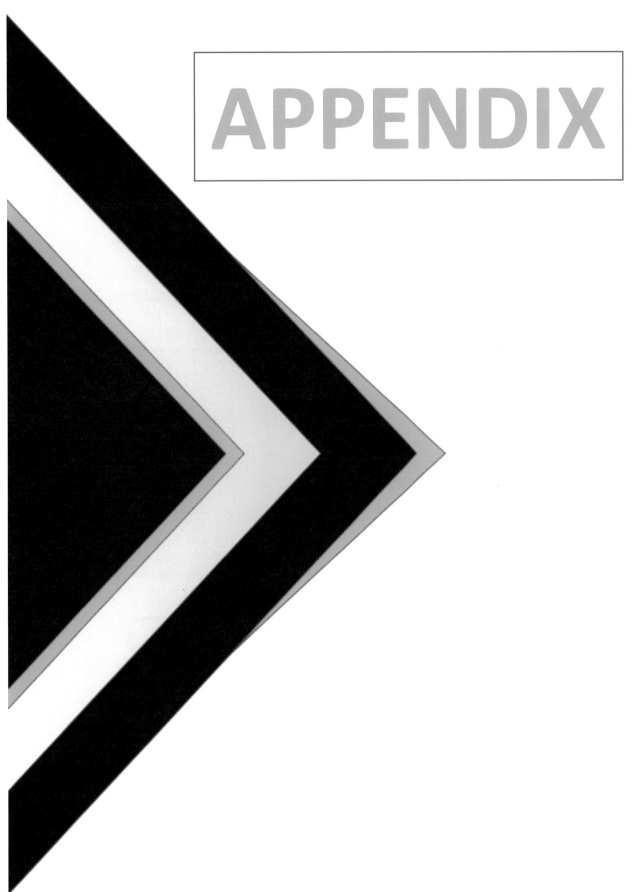

APPENDIX

# APPENDIX A: SELECTED 12 LEAD ECGs

## ECG #1

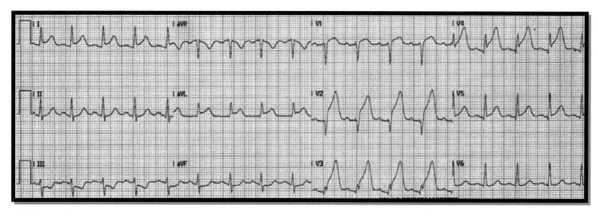

## ECG #2

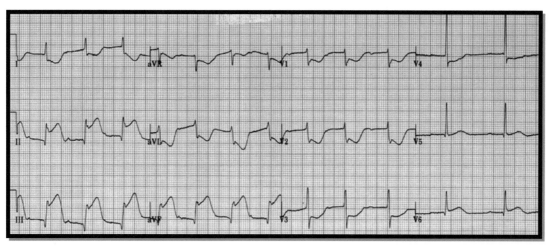

## ECG #3

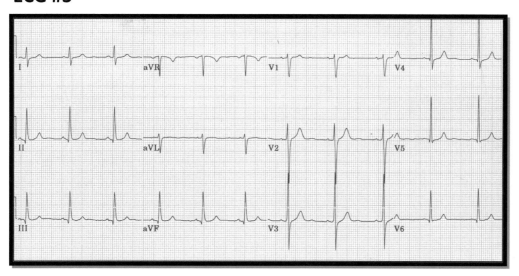

## ECG #4

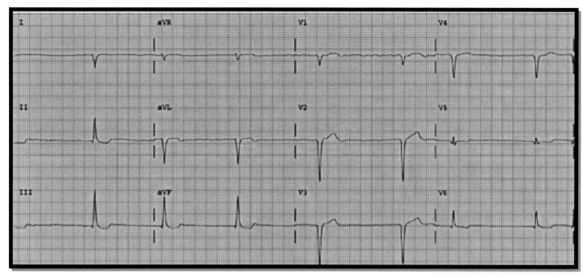

## ECG #5

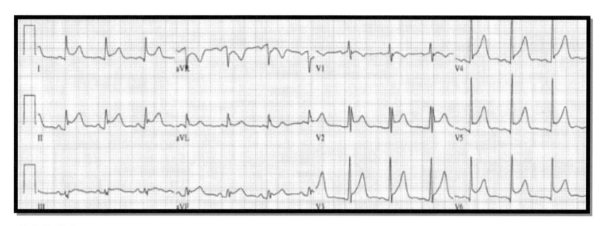

## ECG #6

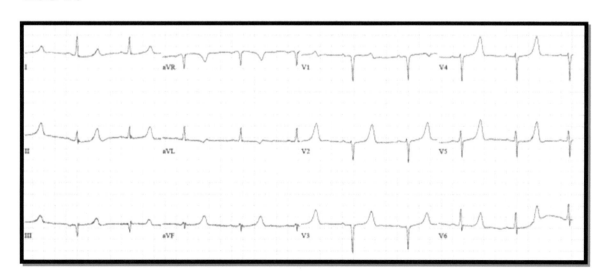

## ECG #7

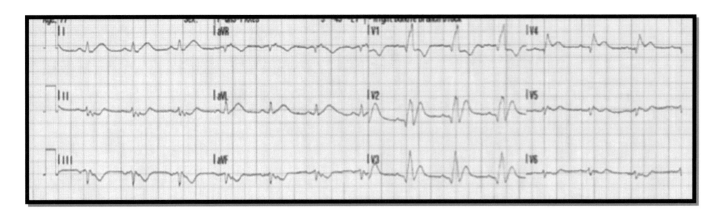

## ECG #8

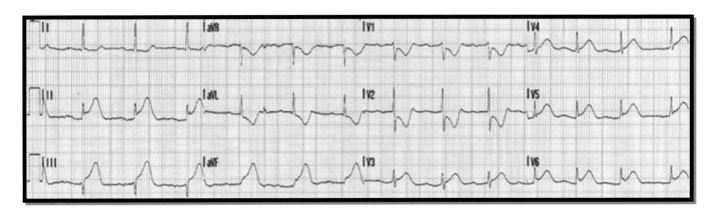

## ECG #9

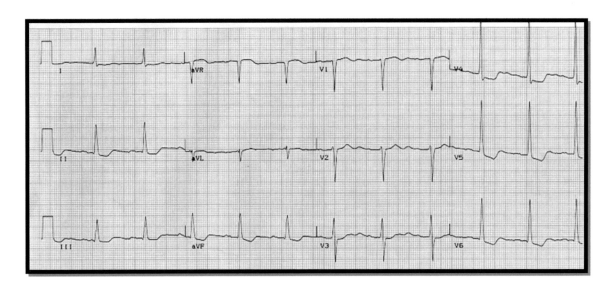

**ECG #9**

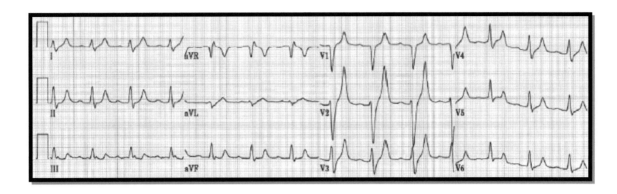

## APPENDIX B: SELECTED IABP WAVEFORMS

**IABP #1**

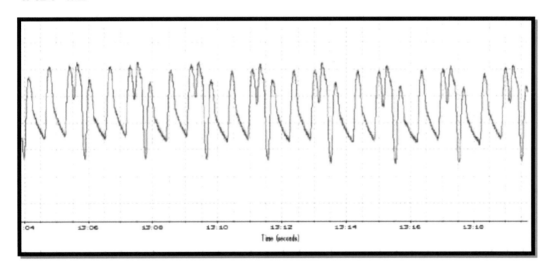

**IABP #2**

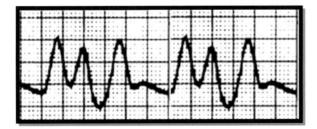

**IABP #3**

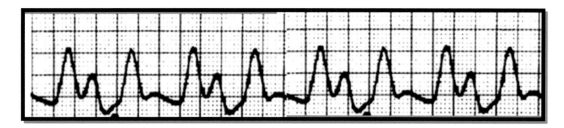

**IABP #4**

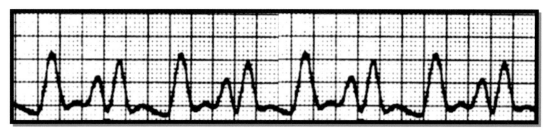

**IABP #5**

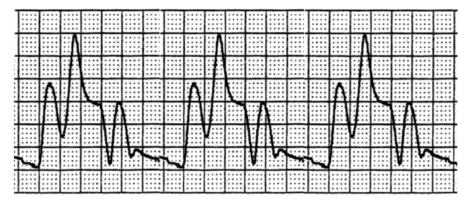

**IABP #6**

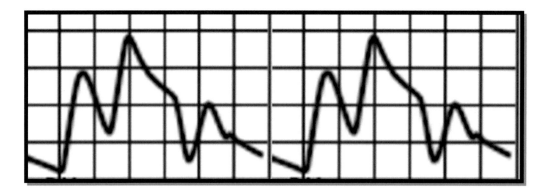

**IABP #7**

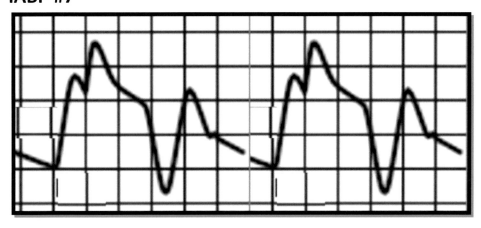

# APPENDIX C: SELECTED IABP WAVEFORMS

**FHT #1**

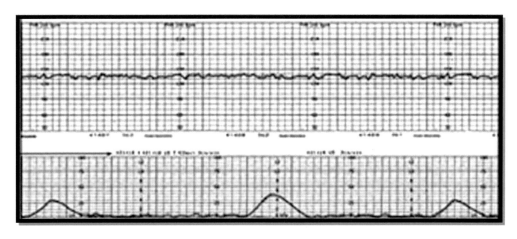

**FHT #2**

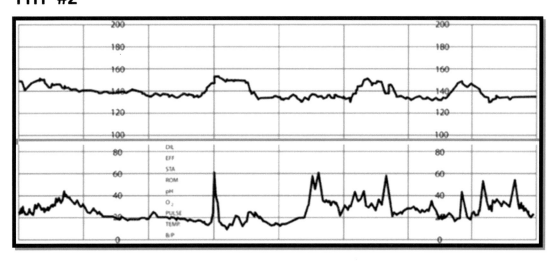

## FHT #3

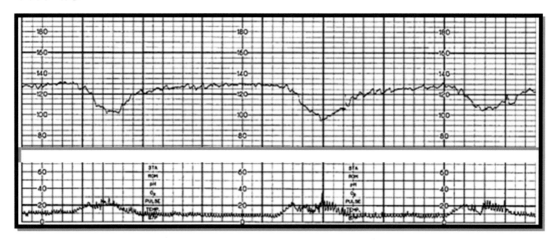

## FHT #4

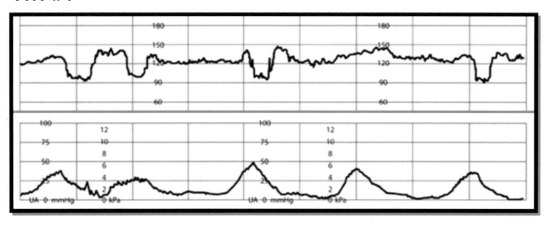

## FHT #5

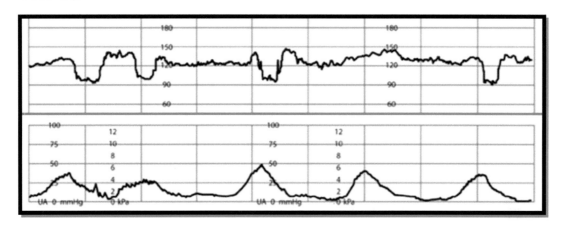

**FHT #6**

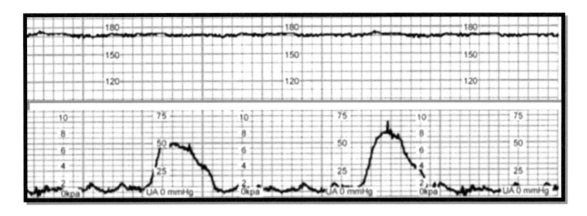

# APPENDIX D: HEAD CT SCANS

**CT #1**

**CT #2**

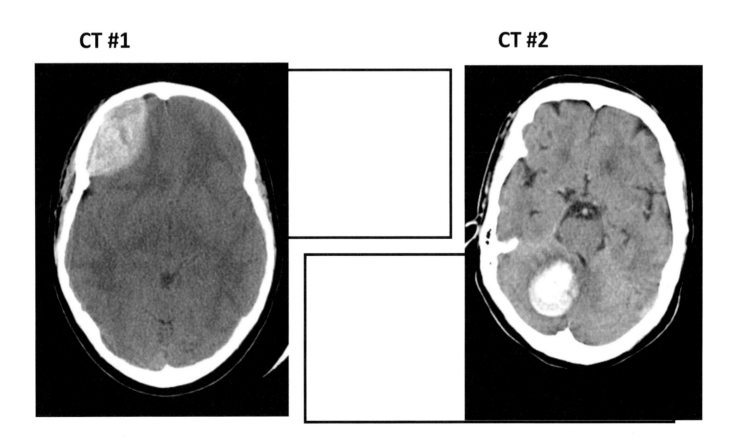

**CT #3**

**CT#4**

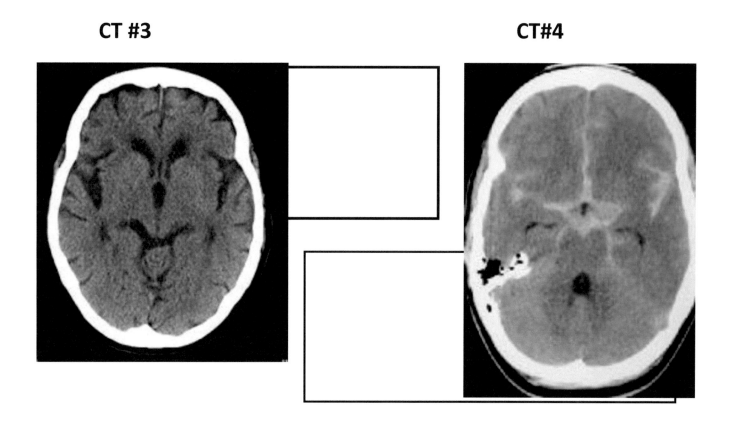

**CT #5**

**CT#6**

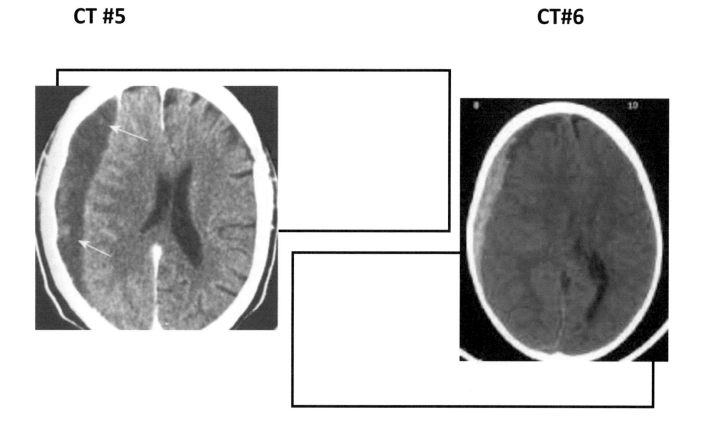

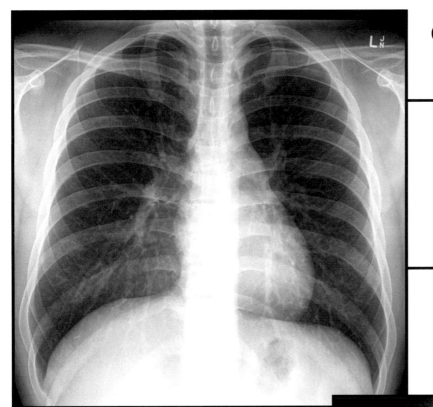

**CXR #1**

**CXR #2**

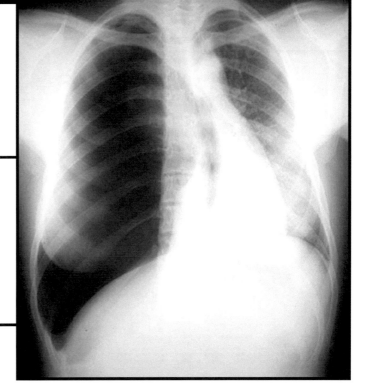

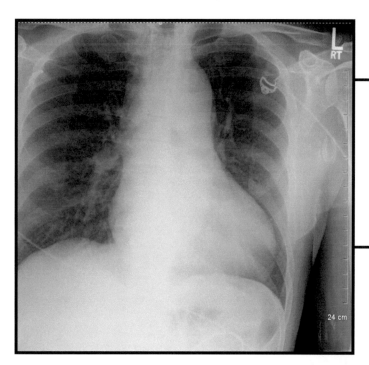

**CXR #3**

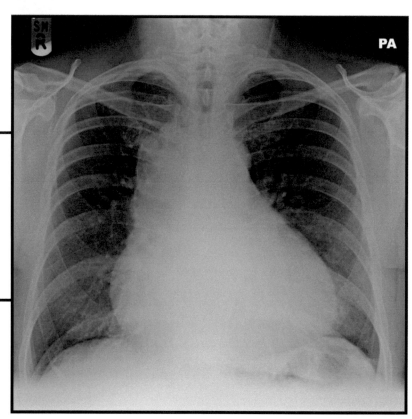

# KEY OF APPENDICES

**Appendix A– ECGs:**

1. Antrioseptal AMI

2. Inferior AMI

3. Normal

4. Digitalis Toxicity

5. Pericarditis

6. Hyperkalemia

7. (+) Sgarbossa Criteria

8. Inferior Wall AMI with

   lateral involvement

9. Digitalis Toxicity

10. Hyperkalemia

**Appendix B– IABPs:**

1. Normal IABP

2. Early Deflation

3. Early Deflation

4. Late Inflation

5. Late Deflation

6. Late Deflation

7. Early Inflation

**Appendix C– FHT Waveforms:**

Norm FHT no Decelera-tions/ Accelerations

2. with contraction

3. Late Decelerations and poor variability

4. Accelerations

5. Good variability and varia-ble decelerations

6. Fetal tachycardia with poor variability and no re-action during contractions

**Appendix D– Head CTs:**

1. Epidural hematoma

2. Intracranial hemorrhage

3. Normal

4. Subarachnoid hemorrhage

5. Subdural hematoma

6. Subdural hematoma

Made in United States
Troutdale, OR
01/02/2025

27524719R00247